EVERYTHING BELOW THE WAIST

Why Health Care Needs a Feminist Revolution

JENNIFER BLOCK

ST. MARTIN'S PRESS NEW YORK

First published in the United States by St. Martin's Press,
an imprint of St. Martin's Publishing Group

 Printed in the United States of America. For information,
address St. Martin's Publishing Group, 120 Broadway, New York, NY 10271

www.stmartins.com

Cover design by Francesca Messina
Book design by Steven Seighman

Library of Congress Cataloging-in-Publication Data

Names: Block, Jennifer, author.
Title: Everything below the waist : why health care needs a feminist revolution / Jennifer Block.
Description: New York : St. Martin's Press, [2019] | Includes bibliographical references and index.
Identifiers: LCCN 2019007959 | ISBN 9781250110053 (hardcover) | ISBN 9781250110060 (ebook)
Subjects: LCSH: Women's health services—United States. | Women—Health and hygiene—United States.
Classification: LCC RA654.85 B575 2019 | DDC 613/.04244—dc23
LC record available at https://lccn.loc.gov/2019007959

Our books may be purchased in bulk for promotional, educational, or business use. Please contact your local bookseller or the Macmillan Corporate and Premium Sales Department at 1-800-221-7945, extension 5442, or by email at MacmillanSpecialMarkets@macmillan.com.

First Edition: July 2019

10 9 8 7 6 5 4 3 2 1

Dedicated to my grandma Kay Block, who taught me to speak up

CONTENTS

ACKNOWLEDGMENTS

Writing this book meant countless days of feeling like it was an impossible undertaking. I have a network of loved ones that spans the globe, and these pages exist because people kept reminding me that they needed to be written. I can't name them all—many are strangers whose notes of praise for *Pushed* kept me going. Others are true friends, there with pep talks, honest feedback, a place to stay, a place to work, a meal, a drink, a book, emergency tech support, emergency childcare, research assistance. Some of those, in no particular order: Cris Parque, Annia Ciezadlo, Pagan Kennedy, Tracie McMillan, Karen Rose and Chris Stave, Jevon Nicholson, Phoebe Reilly, Mai Hoang, Manda Aufochs Gillespie, Ali and Don Kauss, Cynthia Caillagh, Lisa Selin Davis, Aaron Gilmartin, Roger Rothstein, Virginia Vitzthum, Bernardo Issel, Claire Kirk, Melissa Tapper Goldman, Barbara Katz Rothman, Maria Luisa Tucker, Andrew Boyd, Janis Brody, Joanna Wheeler, Rob Worthington, Jared Kelly, Carlitta Burrell, Tesa Mayorga, Wendy Geitz, E. J. Shu, Trish Hickey, Bill Bornstein, and Liz Canner.

In addition to my far-flung network, a slew of newly minted grandparents and aunties showed up in physical form when I was teetering in the work-life balance: Audrey, Roberta, Steff, Nonna, Ron, Steve, Shorna, Grandpa Lenny, and Uncle Adam. Ethan Murphy, thank you for being an incredible dad to our incredible kiddo. Brooklyn, thank you for being a village—with playgrounds and serendipitous playdates and friendly neighbors. To those parent-neighbor-friends in particular, I'm indebted to you for so many childcare "swaps" that ultimately weighed in my favor.

I'm so very lucky to have found my agent, Elizabeth Kaplan, early on in my career. Loyal and real, she firmly and patiently guided this blizzard of a book idea into something recognizable and found it a home at St. Martin's, where editors Karen Wolny and Elisabeth Dyssegaard brought it more rigor and clarity. Special thanks to Francesca Messina for the sharp cover design.

I want to express enormous gratitude to Ben Strader, Harriet Barlow, and the wide, wonderful family of Blue Mountain Center, which granted me space, community, and natural beauty to work out the thesis and structure; to the Whiting Foundation for its overwhelming generosity and vote of confidence in this work; to Sarah Blustain, Esther Kaplan, and the rest of the phenomenal crew at Type Investigations, which supported portions of reporting in chapters 4 and 6; and to Katie Orenstein and the OpEd Project for teaching and reteaching me how much our ideas matter.

This book wouldn't have been possible without my mother, Roberta Block, who is not only the sweetest person I know, but who enables me to take professional risks because I know she is there if I fall on hard times.

And most importantly, thanks to my son, Abe, who grew from babe-in-arms to dinosaur maven during the writing of this book, and who continuously reminds me that what we believe about our bodies and how they deserve to be treated is learned.

EVERYTHING BELOW THE WAIST

INTRODUCTION: THE PROBLEM WITH MEDICINE AS EMPOWERMENT

In Paso Robles, California, a woman returns to the clinic where she had an IUD inserted to have it removed, because, in her words, "I went from a happy-go-lucky 31-year-old to a depressed walking zombie in just 3 weeks." The clinician refuses—tells her she doesn't think it's a good idea, tells her to wait six months, says *what happens when you have an abortion?* After making her case and being denied multiple times, the patient, shaking with anger, turns the request into a demand. The clinician rolls her eyes, takes the device out, and wordlessly leaves the exam room.

In Somers Point, New Jersey, a woman having her second baby is nine (out of ten) centimeters dilated, on hands and knees with her midwife, feeling the urge to push, when the obstetrician on call enters the room, asks about the woman's previous delivery (vaginal), and tells her she'll need a C-section this time. When the woman asks questions, the doctor threatens to call "legal people" if she doesn't sign a consent form for surgery.

In Minneapolis, a 46-year-old woman at a renowned medical center has a robotic, "minimally invasive" hysterectomy. Two days later she tells the nurses of concerning symptoms: pain, elevated heart rate, increased respiration. Doctors note "anxiety" in her chart, administer Ativan through her IV without telling her, and discharge her with a prescription for the antianxiety medication. Two days later she wakes up in pain so unbearable she calls for an ambulance. It turns out her intestine had been damaged during the hysterectomy—she emerges from emergency surgery with a colostomy bag.[1]

You may already be familiar with a version of this story: Woman needs medical care. Woman is ignored. Woman has to fight.

The patient-doctor relationship is among the most sacred in the secular world. We surrender our modesty and trust our physicians—especially our OB/GYNs—with our most intimate needs and vulnerabilities. In return, at a minimum, we expect science, expertise, and respect. Elizabeth Blackwell, the first U.S. woman to get a medical degree, noted the gendered power imbalance inherent in the relationship and advocated for women's equal representation in the profession. "It is not only by what women will do themselves in medicine, but also by the influence which they will exert on the profession, that they will lead it to supply the needs of women as it can not otherwise," she lectured in 1859.[2]

Today, half of all medical students and some 60 percent of OB/GYNs are female, yet our dignity in the medical realm is no more secure.[3] Neither is our health. A 2013 Institute of Medicine report found that even as women's life expectancy has risen overall, U.S. women are "dying at younger ages" than our international peers, a trend that has been worsening for three decades.[4] And the quality of those years we are living is worse than men's, and worse than the previous generation's.[5] A 2013 study of some 2,000 mother-daughter pairs in the United States found that the daughters "entered adulthood at greater risk for the development of chronic illness than their mothers."[6] In 42 percent of U.S. counties, women's life expectancy is *decreasing*.[7]

Shocked? I was too. Hadn't we come a long way, baby, from the dark days when cervical cancer was the number one cause of cancer death in women, the days when breast cancer needed more "awareness"? Hadn't we conquered perpetual pregnancies? Aren't we all eating more fresh vegetables? And don't women have more power now, in medicine as well as in society at large?

To try to explain it, one can parse the generational and international differences: We live in a more toxic environmental "soup" now than in our parents' and grandparents' day, and the lack of guaranteed health care is a unique driver in the industrialized world. Another explanation, to be blunt, is racism. Black women are more likely to die of heart disease, breast cancer, and pregnancy, and when researchers drill down to determine why, the salient factor is the stress caused by the daily wear and tear of being a woman of color in twenty-first-century America. Health disparities hold true for men of color as well.

But why is our health slipping when women in the United States visit more doctors, have more surgeries, and fill more prescriptions than men?[8] Bias is a problem—women having heart attacks and strokes are more likely to be misdiagnosed by ER docs and sent home. "Women," concluded a 2017 article in *Glamour*, "are more likely to be misdiagnosed in pretty much any medical situation."[9] Hormones are a problem—not our own, necessarily, but the endocrine-disrupting chemicals that have infused everything from lotion to tap water. Research funding is also a problem—for example, autoimmune disorders affect a stupefying 10 to 20 percent of the population (depending on how many diseases you put under the umbrella) and some 75 percent of sufferers are women, yet these diseases claim a fraction of investigative efforts.

Another problem has emerged in recent years: *too much* treatment.

In November 2009, the U.S. Preventive Services Task Force (USPSTF), an independent group of physicians and researchers that makes recommendations on disease screening, ignited a firestorm when it recommended that women get *fewer* mammograms. The announcement came in the midst of a 15-year-long breast cancer awareness campaign. Pink ribbons were everywhere and the "early detection saves lives" mantra had been burned into the public consciousness. Despite this, the USPSTF announced that, based on epidemiological evidence, women would be better off if they held off screening until age 50 (rather than 40) and screened every two years rather than annually.

For many, it just didn't (and still doesn't) make sense: why would it be better for women to screen later and less often?

Sometimes, you wind up sitting next to just the right person at lunch. I was at a health conference around the time of the USPSTF's pink grenade, and that person was Ned Calonge, then the task force's director. Calonge gave me the cancer-screening spiel that he was frequently giving to audiences of clinicians at the time: there are five outcomes to a screening test, and four of them are not going to help you live longer or better. One, the test could be wrong—you don't actually have cancer—but you get unnecessary biopsies, surgery, or treatment, potentially causing harm. Two, the test could be right in detecting some abnormality, but what it detects is never going to progress into invasive cancer. Three, the test could also be wrong in the false-negative sense—you really *do* have an invasive cancer, but the test says you don't, so you ignore your symptoms. Four, if the test finds nothing and indeed you have nothing wrong, you are no better off than when you began. Only in the case that the test finds a bad cancer before you had noticeable symptoms are you potentially gleaning a benefit. Calonge's point? Think before you test.

In the case of mammograms, Calonge explained, the problem was that for every handful of lives saved, thousands of women were getting unnecessary, potentially harmful treatment. Years of annual screening, he said, had not delivered a *net* benefit.

In the connected realms of overtesting, overdiagnosis, and overtreatment, women are more vulnerable than men. We're recommended bone density scans and then prescribed drugs to treat "osteopenia," though the machines, diagnosis, and treatments were all manufactured by the pharmaceutical industry—and it turns out these drugs often *lead* to bone loss and fracture.[10] Routine thyroid cancer screening came into vogue in the 2000s, though now we know that some 80 percent of the resulting surgeries, in women specifically, were done unnecessarily.[11] Men and women are equally obese, yet women are more often recommended bariatric surgery. We're more likely to be prescribed antidepressants and antipsychotics and recommended electroconvulsive therapy.[12] We're also more likely to be prescribed opioids, and 40 percent more likely to become dependent on them.[13] We are prescribed more drugs and are recommended more surgery in general.

In particular, we endure a lot of surgery on our sex organs. For the past several years, roughly one-third of U.S. women giving birth have done so via cesarean section—major surgery that carries serious short-term and long-term risks to baby and mother, particularly for future pregnancies. While some of these operations are necessary, many are not. There is a statistical threshold at which the harms outweigh the benefits, and public health authorities agree that at our rate of 32 percent cesareans, we're well above that threshold. This trend raises questions not only of appropriateness but of consent. There are hospitals in places like northern New Jersey and Miami, Florida, where there are more C-sections than vaginal births, and hundreds of hospitals have de facto bans against vaginal birth if women have had a previous cesarean or are carrying a baby in the breech position, leaving them no choice but surgery.

The cesarean rate is now a public health crisis—a likely contributor to the rising number of maternal deaths. And most maternity care is still largely an outdated, one-size-fits-all assembly line: clinicians frequently induce and speed up contractions, immobilize women on their backs, restrict food and water, and tell them when and how to push—if they aren't pushed into the operating room first. "If overtreatment is defined as instances in which an individual may have fared as well or better with less or perhaps no intervention, then modern obstetric care has landed in a deep quagmire," maternal health leaders warned in a 2014 report.[14]

At least this scenario has been getting more attention recently. A wave of headlines have asked why practice standards vary widely across states, counties, even individual hospitals; why so many mothers are dying in childbirth; and why countries with better outcomes employ more midwives than doctors.

In this book, I ask similar questions about everything from fertility treatment to contraception to pelvic surgery to the way miscarriages are handled. In many cases, we're being denied the most appropriate treatment. As one physician put it to me, "covering up the symptoms, bypassing the normal functions, or removing the organs is generally the treatment protocol." The second most common major surgery after the C-section is hysterectomy—it is estimated that one-third of women in the United States will lose their uterus before age 60.[15]

If you're a woman, reading this book may lead you to question everything about your "well-woman" care. Consider a typical workweek for an OB/GYN practice: most patients are coming in for an annual exam, including a pelvic exam, Pap test, breast exam, and perhaps a mammogram. Prescription pads are full of orders for hormonal contraceptives for the premenopausal and hormone therapy for the postmenopausal. Interspersed with routine preventative care are treatments for abnormal Pap results and fibroids. Over at the hospital, common GYN surgeries are hysterectomy and transvaginal mesh for pelvic prolapse and incontinence, and more and more women are choosing to have prophylactic breast and ovary removal based on genetic testing.

How much of these bread-and-butter practices have been subject to the rigors of scientific scrutiny? Some more than others, this book will show, but what's surprising is that much of what we think of as bedrock, preventative women's health care has resulted in the same kind of overtreatment that's been burdening health care more broadly—overscreening leading to overdiagnosis leading to overtreatment leading to more harm than benefit.

You may have heard that it takes an average of 17 years for scientific evidence to change medical practice. A 2013 CDC survey of primary care doctors and OB/GYNs found that around 75 percent continue to offer yearly Pap tests, even though USPSTF recommended in 2003 that they be done every three years.[16] This is because most cervical abnormalities and HPV infections clear up on their own and do not progress to cancer, while the freezing/burning/biopsy procedures that follow from abnormal results can cause scar tissue, sexual pain, and pregnancy complications like preterm birth.

The routine manual pelvic exam (often conducted by doctors in concert with the Pap) has been found over and over again to deliver only discomfort, anxiety, and a 98 percent false-positive rate.[17] In 2014, the American College of Physicians reviewed seven decades of studies and recommended that physicians stop doing them without cause.[18] The American College of Obstetricians and Gynecologists responded that it "firmly believes in the clinical value" of annual pelvic exams, even if they are "not evidence-based."[19] One (female) obstetric leader told the *Washington Post* that it "is a time of intimacy between the patient and care provider," when patients might disclose problems they would otherwise keep mum about.[20]

Long-held beliefs are difficult for us patients to give up, as well. The truth is, women seem to want and expect an annual exam—surveys show we find it reassuring. Even if we know mammograms are a poor test, we figure it's better than nothing, and advocacy groups like Susan G. Komen openly contested the USPSTF recommendation for years. Women often lament that hormonal birth control spins their moods out of control, but we accept these consequences as necessary rites of passage—or more disturbingly, because we feel we have no choice. Do we sometimes confuse medical technology with empowerment?

There are no sacred cows in this book. Part of my hope is to offer a corrective to what I've noticed is a tendency in the mainstream media and among those with feminist sensibilities in particular to trust medical opinion over evidence, to embrace the latest reproductive technology without a careful weighing of the costs, and to dismiss sources that don't comport with the dominant narrative. I've seen this happen time and again with reporting, for example, on epidurals, egg freezing, the latest libido drug, IUDs, the HPV vaccine, infant formula, and the grandmother of all medical liberators, the Pill. I've also noticed a reflex to discount any elevation of the "natural," be it childbirth, birth control, or approaches to treating illness. Some feminist scholars have denounced the "new maternalism" of women seeking home births and "attachment" parenting—they've even taken aim at the vast evidence on the benefits of breastfeeding.[21]

I should say here that in discussing "women's" health I'm referring mainly to those born with female sex organs, however they identify. People who have hormonally or surgically transitioned are an exception to many of the concerns of this book, as they may welcome the full use of medical technology in the service of maintaining their gender identity, and I respect that choice. The unique health risks of reassignment surgeries and transition hormones are beyond the scope of this book, though people who have transitioned or are in the process of doing so may still find value in knowing the health impacts of many treatments and procedures discussed here.

In these chapters I take the reader into the fertility lab to examine, at the cellular level, what it means to freeze the biological clock. I ask why we still remove more wombs in America than any other major organ, of either sex, and what that means for women's quality of life—especially our sex lives. I report on discoveries and technologies largely unknown or dismissed, from the wonders of fertile cervical fluid to the vastness of the clitoris to the causes of and remedies for our most intractable pelvic pain. To understand typical GYN care, I retrace its history as a profession that has spread itself thinner and thinner and gets far less hands-on training in the operating room than any other surgical specialty.

And I go back to the 1970s women's movement to understand how, in this supposed age of empowerment, our bodies are still so vulnerable to medical control and double standards.

That movement did advocate for the medical establishment to drop the "doctor-knows-best" attitude. It educated women about their bodies and urged them to take more control in the doctor's office—or walk out if need be. It fought for more prudent research and less wholesale experimentation on women. And it sent women in droves into previously all-male medical schools. By some measures, things improved. But even as the #metoo movement has forced a reckoning of how women's power is systematically undermined by sexism and violence, we haven't examined what role the medical system plays.

There is an entire subgenre of reportage and memoir about our failing American health care system, in which pharma has outsize influence on research, costs are out of control, and good physicians are bullied by administrators with what are called perverse incentives. Contextualizing the $3.5 trillion we spend on health care has become a parlor game (Equal to Germany's entire economy! One and a half times the *global* auto industry![22]). Feminists have been agitating for decades about how research still mainly happens on male bodies—even male rats are used more than female rats.[23] But the problems in women's health are not just political or economic. They are ideological and cultural. The failure to listen to a patient's request to remove an IUD, or to accept her refusal of surgery, or to recognize her symptoms as life-threatening rather than psychological is a problem that can't just be blamed on capitalism or medical orthodoxy.

In the last 25 years, feminists around the world have developed a language of human rights that includes not only the right to contraception and abortion, but the right to fertility and sexuality—to sexual health and agency and pleasure and the right to *create* a family and to raise that family with dignity. This framework of "reproductive justice" recognizes that people have uneven access to these rights and advocates to remedy those broader injustices. Reproductive justice puts people at its center rather than a product or procedure.

If we look at typical U.S. health care within this reproductive justice framing, a troubling picture emerges, one that challenges the empowered-consumer, post-sexual-revolution narrative. Yet mainstream feminism hasn't been out front on this issue. As we'll explore, instead of practicing solid patient advocacy, groups like Planned Parenthood and the National Organization for Women (NOW) are often in the awkward position of defending and sometimes even helping to market poor, redundant, and even harmful products and practices because they fit under the banner of gender equality. And the medical industry has deftly waved that banner over everything from estrogen to "pink Viagra" to infant formula.

Sometimes the person you're meeting for lunch hands you a perfect metaphor. Last spring, that person was Carol Downer, cofounder of the Federation of Feminist Women's Health Care Centers, and what she handed me was a brown paper bag; inside, there was a Lucite speculum. Downer, at the time 86, is one of the most influential 1970s feminists you've probably never heard of. And this practice—handing another woman a gynecological tool over coffee, as if it were a pastry—was one that she helped spread throughout the country in the early 1970s. Her epiphany was that if women could access their own anatomy, they wouldn't have to rely on the patriarchal medical system. Downer and others led "self-help" clinics in which they hopped up on tables with a mirror, flashlight, and speculum to show other women how to view their own cervices, and even how to perform a "menstrual extraction," which also happens to function as an early abortion.

At the time, feminists were somewhat divided over biology. On one side was the idea that women were not only oppressed by men but also by their own bodies, which suffer "barbaric" childbirth and a host of other indignities that limit equal participation. If biology was destiny, that destiny was a prison. Modern medicine, on the other hand, offered liberation: our bodies are different from men's, but science could make them equal.

This idea had precedent. One interesting footnote to the suffrage movement is that women rallied for "twilight sleep" anesthesia to deliver them from the physiological oppression of childbirth, which they tied to political oppression. Margaret Sanger envisioned a "magic pill" decades before the oral contraceptive. In *The Second Sex*, Simone de Beauvoir sharply cast female biology as a destiny of "servitude," and second-wave leaders like Betty Friedan drew on her ideas in urging women to reach "beyond biology."[24]

There was logic here: if women were being reduced to their biological functions, one response was to transcend them, negate them. "Women are defined, valued, judged, in one way only: as women—that is, with sex organs that must be used," wrote Andrea Dworkin. "Women's work is done below the waist; intelligence is higher. Women are lower; men are higher. It is a simple, dull scheme; but women's sex organs in and of themselves are apparently appalling enough to justify the scheme, make it evidently true."[25]

Downer and her camp had the opposite reaction: embrace biological difference, demand acceptance, seize control. Self-helpers believed that fluency and control over one's own biology was fundamental to the pursuit of civil rights. "An extraordinary social movement has developed around the idea that women should control their own bodies," wrote the journalist Claudia Dreifus in 1977. "What unites these women is . . . their belief that self-knowledge of anatomy and bodily functions can be liberating . . . None of us can be healthy in a system that creates sickness out of normal life functions and that profits from illness."[26]

Conflict with the mainstream women's movement was almost immediate. When Downer attended her first NOW conference in 1971 in Marina del Rey, California, with other like-minded activists, bags of specula in hand, "they weren't even going to give us a table," she told me. The activists ultimately got the table but were forbidden from getting too graphic. So they did workshops quietly in two rooms, 20 women at a time. "Over the course of the conference, every woman came in. And they left with a plastic speculum in a little paper bag," Downer said. "So by the end, all the women were walking around with paper bags."

This radical arm of the women's movement won many gains. It led to the publication of *Our Bodies, Ourselves*, still considered the mainstream feminist health bible. It led to direct actions against high-dose birth control pills, diethylstilbestrol, the Dalkon Shield, the exclusion of women from clinical research, and the isolation of women in maternity wards.

In Chicago, the self-trained underground group Jane Collective performed thousands of at-home abortions without incident before *Roe*.

But once abortion became legal, self-help came to be seen by many as a growing pain. It was navel-gazing, essentialist, retro. It glorified difference when the point was to prove how women deserved the *same* treatment as men. Movement energy went toward concerns outside the body. In essence: women should *become* doctors, not play doctor.

"The minute you started grounding something in the body, a body inherently different from the male body, there's this fear that we're all going to be barefoot and pregnant in the kitchen again," explains scholar Wendy Kline.

Feminist health activists regret this turning point, for it had wider implications, even in terms of what was researched. There was fear "that if we knew about sex differences they'd be used to discriminate against women," says Sue Carter, who is a professor of biology at Indiana University and director of the Kinsey Institute and has been in the field for 50 years. The women's health community pushed back hard on this in the '90s, and some things changed—the National Institutes of Health (NIH), for one, created an Office of Research on Women's Health (though it is barely funded). "But the basic science, the basic understanding of women's health, fell in the cracks. It didn't get the sort of head-on interest that it should have right from the start. So here we are in 2019, and we don't really have a fundamental understanding of sex differences, much less women's health."

Today, overtreatment and mistreatment flourish in the absence of a strong watchdog apparatus, revealing a medical system that has not fully overcome its patriarchal, paternalistic origins. But is something even deeper going on? If women and our providers have at all internalized the view that our biology is the source of social inequality, and there is evidence that we have, how might that be affecting women's participation in this system? Does regarding our bodies as oppressive render us more vulnerable to the overuse of medical technology? Are we relying on medicine as a workaround for social change?

This is a book about feminism's unfinished revolution in women's health. To be sure, some are leading the way. A growing contingent of women and providers are advocating for more "body literacy" and a more functional approach in medicine, focused on the root causes of disease. There is grassroots political momentum for paid parental leave and tax-free tampons, and popular outrage when Facebook or Instagram censors images of birth or breastfeeding. Routine abuses of power in maternity wards now have a name that's showing up in peer-reviewed medical journals: *obstetric violence.* And a new underground of community abortion providers is enabling women to take matters back into their own hands.

The ideal of "reproductive justice" is being adopted, at least in name, by more mainstream groups. "Reproductive justice is a truly universalist framework, because it's based on human rights," says Loretta Ross, one of the creators of the framework. "There is no variation in what rights you are entitled to, what varies is your ability to access those rights."

Still, there are forces pushing back, and one of them is how patients and providers both conflate medicine with liberation. This book makes a case for health care that's more respectful of female physiology and for a more health-conscious feminism—one that reframes empowerment to include not only "control" of our bodies but also our right to support, protect, and enjoy them.

1: THE CHURCH OF THE MAGIC BULLET

THE FIRST SYMPOSIUM of the Uterine Cervix was organized by a young, male scientist on January 25, 1958, at the University of Malmo, in Sweden. Erik Odeblad had graduated medical school and held a PhD in physics—he had written his dissertation on cervical "crypts," the microscopic pockets within the neck of the uterus that produce cervical fluid. As a med student, Odeblad had become thoroughly entranced by the stuff while involved in a study of vaginal microbes. He had peered at the cervices of 153 women, often several times, collecting 520 fluid samples in all. He quickly lost interest in the microbes but was transfixed by the varied cervical secretions: clear and viscous at times, opaque and lotion-like at others, and sometimes barely present.

The accepted medical wisdom of the time was that these changes were just varying dilutions of the same "mucus" (we'll come back to this word choice) and not significant, but Odeblad and other scientists suspected they had a close relationship with ovulation.[1] They were right. Many years later, Odeblad would prove that cervical fluid enables sperm to reach an egg. But before he could do that, he needed a way to analyze the secretions.

Like any good scientist, he searched the literature for what was already known. Other scientists publishing in the 1940s had noted the cyclical variations, but had not been able to explain their purpose. It is likely that midwives going back to antiquity noted cervical fluid, and as male physicians began peering under women's skirts, they too began to notice it and to speculate in newly established medical journals. In 1855, the physician W. T. Smith pointed out that conception is most likely to occur at that time of the menstrual cycle when the mucus content of the cervix is "in its most fluid condition." J. Marion Sims, who surgically experimented on enslaved women without anesthesia, observed in 1868 that sperm swam best in the mucus that he described as "clear and translucent, and about the consistency of the white of egg."[2] But these were just hypotheses based on observation, not lab science.

Odeblad wanted to know the how and why—what function did these fluids serve, and how did they relate to reproduction? One thing that fascinated him, but which he did not mention in his first published paper, was that the bacteria he had been studying were only present in the cervical mucus collected *prior* to ovulation. This was, in other words, "an indication that post-ovulatory mucus was able to exercise an antimicrobiological effect," he would later write.[3]

This observation hinted at high-level functioning and at molecular variation among the fluids produced by the cervix. But a typical lab with microscopes wouldn't be of much help in proving or disproving his hypothesis. He needed to know what elements were present in these fluids—how much hydrogen and oxygen, for instance—and he needed to see them in action. Another paper caught his eye, on a new method for measuring viscosity: nuclear magnetic resonance (NMR), which would later evolve into magnetic resonance imaging (MRI) technology. Odeblad was probably also well aware of the 1952 Nobel ceremonies in Stockholm, where Felix Bloch and Edward Purcell were awarded the prize in physics for discovering NMR.[4]

If Odeblad could study the different cervical fluid samples with NMR, then he could figure out their material composition and structure, which would help unlock the properties of each—and prove that they indeed had discrete functions. So in 1953 Odeblad traveled to California as a Rockefeller Foundation fellow at UC Berkeley to study the technology. The Rockefeller Foundation had been investing in science for some years, bringing scientists from around the globe to Berkeley. Also notably, the year 1953 was when the foundation began cautiously investing in "family planning," under longtime pressure from John D. Rockefeller III, who had personally helped launch the Population Council.[5]

The fellowship turned out to be a bust. One of Odeblad's main goals had been to get access to the NMR machine across the bay at Stanford, where Bloch was tenured. But when Odeblad met with the esteemed professor and asked if he might use the spectrometer on human samples, Bloch held his technology close. "He made it clear that NMR was a tool for physicists, not for research into physiology, medicine, or biology," wrote a scientist who talked to Odeblad about the encounter.[6]

Back in Sweden, Odeblad found another potential collaborator, this one more of a sharer. Gunnar Lindström, who had just received his PhD from the Nobel Institute of Stockholm, essentially let Odeblad hack his NMR machine. By December 1954, the two had applied NMR to study liver, muscle, fat, tendon, cartilage, and other bodily tissues, and they submitted a paper detailing their studies. With its publication in 1955, they accomplished a "first" in medical science—they were the first to use NMR to study the human body—though this probably wasn't clear to either at the time.[7]

Lindström quickly bored of academia and went to work for SAAB, the auto company; Odeblad took his new skill and went back to studying cervical mucus, his primary goal all along, and the one to which he would devote the rest of his career. He would become the first professor of medical biophysics at his university, a brand-new field he himself had pioneered. In order to continue his work, he built his own NMR machine in the OB/GYN department of the hospital where he worked. We should probably add inventor to his list of accomplishments—he constructed three over the course of his career.

By 1957, Odeblad had accumulated enough breakthrough knowledge on cervical fluid that he convinced his colleagues to host the symposium in Malmo. They invited OB/GYNs from across Scandinavia. There was "increasing interest in the uterine cervix" that prompted the meeting, where Odeblad unveiled "The Physics of the Cervical Mucus."[8] He reported on its density, the optical transparency, its color, and its index of refraction. He discussed its viscosity and fibrosity, its rate of flow and "flow elasticity," all of which, he noted, "are of considerable importance to the molecular physics of the cervical mucus." He performed "more complicated physical studies such as diffusion measurements and proton magnetic resonance phenomena of cervical mucus."[9]

At the time, cervical fluid had never been given such monumental respect or granular attention. It was merely "discharge," a waste product at best, a sign of infection at worst. In the years since Odeblad's first paper, another scientist made the observation that the size and shape of the cervix changes at mid-cycle to allow for a greater volume of fluid. Here was this dynamic organ—the mouth of the womb, to be clear—gesturing, signaling, and Odeblad was trying to decode her language.

Odeblad would publish some 60 papers over the next several decades, thereby confirming many of his then radical hunches: number one, that the cervix secretes distinct types of "mucins" that serve distinct functions; number two, that they are produced in individual microscopic glands within the cervix, which had already been named (dismally) "crypts"; number three, that each secretion is stimulated by sex hormones released by the ovaries; and number four, that each type of cervical fluid has an important function in reproduction, most notably, the watery, viscous, egg white–like substance that is made around the time of ovulation, which he and others would later refer to as a "hydrogel" because of its extremely high water content.

One of Odeblad's most stunning discoveries was that this hydrogel is both portal and selector of sperm. At another symposium in 1976, he presented a taxonomy of the fluids. The stretchy egg-white secretion is actually two types of fluid combined, types L and S. The S type, he observed, has a long "string"-like molecular structure, while the structure of L is more oval. Those strings provide streams for the sperm, with a swift current that draws them into the cervical canal. L mucus is structured "like pebbles in a brook, and the watery S mucus running between them," he wrote in 1983.[10] He suspected, rightly, that "one of the physiological functions of L mucus is probably to capture morphologically abnormal sperm." Meanwhile, what he called G mucus both precedes and follows ovulation, is thick and acidic, kills sperm on contact, and blocks the cervical os, which "aids in retaining the sperm which have colonized the cervix after swimming up from the vagina."

In other words, thanks to Odeblad's inquiries, we gained concrete scientific evidence that fertile cervical fluid is actually what enables sperm to meet egg. Cervical fluid, not semen alone, should equally qualify as "baby batter." It's not clear that sperm can even get close to the egg without it.

What Odeblad discovered amazed him and could have amazed the world had it been aware of his discovery. People already suspected that women are fertile for only a handful of days each month; Odeblad made it clear that those days are marked by a reliable, observable physical sign—that is, the presence of fertile cervical fluid. This also meant that for the rest of the month, when there is neither egg nor medium, it is impossible to become pregnant. For more than three-quarters of a cycle, women might as well be on a 100 percent effective contraceptive.

This was nothing short of a breakthrough in human knowledge of fertility, which for a long time had been hazy on the details. Though we had figured out that vaginal intercourse with male ejaculation led to pregnancy, the dominant thinking for centuries was that men deposited little humans in women. In order to prevent or end pregnancy, midwives and healers recommended all sorts of pessaries, poisons, and treatments in the vagina: they attempted to block the semen from reaching the womb; douche, steam, or smoke it out; or shake the "seed" loose once inside. Failing that, various herbs were used to "restore the menses." One study counted upward of 400 remedies, both contraceptive and abortive, dating from ancient times.[11] Withdrawal was mentioned in both the Torah and the Hadith (and is much more effective than we usually give it credit for—more on that later).

In various places at various times, women (and couples) were successful at limiting the number of children they had, so we know that some methods worked.

Still, we only had a fuzzy idea about the window of fertility. Early physicians recommended women stick to a "safe period," but that period was only a slightly educated guess, based on animal research, and in humans it turned out to coincide more with the fertile period. Then in 1929, two gynecologists—Kyusaku Ogino, in Japan, and Hermann Knaus, in Austria—each following his own independent line of inquiry, both studied ovulation and found that it occurs 12 to 16 days before the next menstrual period, which is accurate.

Two years later, Ogino and Knaus joined forces to propose an algorithm so that women could apply this science to determine their own safe period. The next year, a Catholic gynecologist in Chicago based his book *The Rhythm of Sterility and Fertility in Women* on these calculations. It sold over 200,000 copies in the next ten years, and the rhythm method was born. "These findings of modern science disclose a rational, natural, and ethical means to space births and to regulate intelligently the number of children," wrote physician-author Leo Latz. In 1951, Pope Pius XII endorsed the method. And by 1965, a majority of Catholics were practicing it.[12]

Of course, the rhythm method notoriously failed to prevent many large Catholic families because it is a prognostication. The calculation works backward from the perceived onset of the *next* menstrual cycle, based on the last several menstrual cycles. While ovulation is somewhat predictable, the body throws curveballs. It is sensitive to sleep disturbances and sickness, stress and light. And the algorithm really only works for a very regular 28-day cycle, with ovulation around day 14 (which most women don't have), and still not always. It is not and was never a reliable method of birth control, because it had nothing to do with a woman's individual "rhythm." Furthermore, during this period, physicians and formula companies were discouraging women from breastfeeding, which made them more prone to multiple pregnancies in close succession (because exclusive breastfeeding can halt ovulation for as long as two years).

It might not be an exaggeration to say that Odeblad's work had the potential to change the course of history. Along with other research that had documented the relationship between body temperature and ovulation, the work revealed observable, measurable, physical signals the female body gives when it is fertile: egg white–like cervical fluid leading up to ovulation, and a slight rise in temperature following ovulation until menstruation. These two signs, if closely observed, are two main components of "fertility awareness-based methods" of contraception (also known as fertility awareness method or natural family planning) in which women track their cycles (a task now aided by dozens of apps) and either abstain or use a barrier method for intercourse during their "fertile window." In skilled hands it is upward of 95 percent effective.

But Odeblad's work and the work of other scientists drawn to crack the code of female ovulation did not find their way to the mainstream. *Our Bodies, Ourselves* was several years away. And "cervical mucus" still struggles for ink in even the most progressive publications.

Furthermore, the Western zeitgeist in the 1950s was less interested in the intricacies of human biology than in mastery of it—*better living through chemistry*. The world wasn't quite ready for contraception based on body literacy. It was ready for the Pill.

"MODERN LIFE IS BASED ON CONTROL AND SCIENCE"[13]

By 1950, Margaret Sanger had coined the term *birth control* and planted it firmly in the public conversation. She had established a network of clinics around the country and shifted public attitudes about sex and reproduction. But the movement still had little to offer in terms of practical tools. Diaphragms and cervical caps were difficult to obtain and often poorly fitted. The condom required amenable men. Most of the research and development that was happening was on impractical, unsexy spermicidal foams and jellies.

Sanger was 70 years old and had recently survived a heart attack. She was feeling her own mortality and was somewhat desperate to see her vision of sexual freedom through. This is the most likely explanation for her appeal to the renegade scientist Gregory Pincus. Pincus had successfully created in vitro rabbit embryos and, as a result, had been rendered a monster in the press, been banished from Harvard, and gone rogue with his own start-up lab in working-class Shrewsbury, Massachusetts.[14]

Sanger's vision, which she proposed to Pincus, was very clear: she wanted a contraceptive that was inexpensive, easy to use, discreet, and 100 percent effective. Something scientific, something that wouldn't hinder sexual spontaneity, or mitigate pleasure, or harm a woman's future fertility. And she was very specific that it be a pill, something a woman could "swallow with her morning orange juice."[15] She had in fact been dreaming of this "magic pill" for most of her adult life.

Pincus was one of the most knowledgeable scientists in mammalian reproduction and had little to lose in taking up the cause. He also didn't need anybody's approval. And he had an idea of how such a pill would work: more than a decade earlier, researchers at the University of Pennsylvania had shown they could prevent ovulation in rabbits with the hormone progesterone. With a pittance of a donation from Planned Parenthood, he began replicating this research on rabbits and then rats. By 1953, while Odeblad was trying to get his hands on an NMR machine in California, Pincus had begun testing different compounds of progestin—synthetic progesterone—on women, several of whom he sourced from a Worcester insane asylum. Three years later, the Pill as we know it would be approved by the FDA for menstrual disorders, and by 1960 it would be sanctioned as a contraceptive.

What's interesting, and rarely noted, is that Pincus and his collaborators, Min-Chueh Chang, a reproductive biologist, and John Rock, a Catholic physician in Boston who tested the compounds on his own patients, and the physicians who later carried out their experiments in Puerto Rico, all grounded their work in the same science in which the progenitors of fertility awareness-based methods grounded theirs: they tested women's temperatures as a proxy for ovulation—if the temperature didn't rise, they knew the woman didn't release an egg.[16] They observed women's cervical mucus and found that under the influence of progestin there was no period of stretchy fertile hydrogel but rather a constant thick mucus, very "hostile" to sperm (what Odeblad called "G mucus"). They also observed that the women stopped having periods, thus their uterine linings were too thin for implantation of a fertilized egg.[17]

Pincus and Rock and the other investigators found that progestin acted on the pituitary gland, preventing it from releasing the hormones that signal the ovaries to ripen and release eggs. But it also had these other effects, so they were not clear by which mechanism it worked to prevent pregnancy. They also had very little awareness of how it was impacting other bodily systems. But even in the mid-1950s, they had reason to wonder.

Beginning in the late nineteenth century, with the rise of physiology, scientists became very interested in the body's glands—pituitary, thyroid, pancreas, adrenal, ovaries—and their excretions, that is, hormones, which scientists realized directed much of the body's systems. Hormones are often called "messengers," but this term really doesn't give them enough credit. They cause tissue to grow or recede; they determine the building or breakdown of muscle, bone, and fat; they convert glucose; they affect blood pressure, pH, and electrolytes; they determine sleep or wakefulness, hunger or satiation, euphoria or relaxation, fight or flight. In a word, hormones greatly influence how we *feel*, and whether we are well. Researchers at this time tried to isolate each excretion and decode its function, then replicate it in the lab. The discovery of insulin, for example, was a game changer because it made diabetes a manageable disease. This was the beginning of endocrinology.[18]

By the 1920s, gynecologists believed that the ovaries were very important for women's health and well-being, not only for their reproductive cycles but for their physical and mental health, as well as their femininity. They also believed many diseases and conditions to be the *result* of diseased ovaries (just as they'd blamed the uterus prior) and removed them often. As an alternative to *ovariotomy*, which keen physicians noticed was a "cure" worse than the disease, researchers were interested in isolating and extracting ovarian hormones, so if a woman was ill or infertile they could supplement. Scientists who sought to extract "the female principle," as estrogen was called, housed their labs near slaughterhouses so they could recover cow glands (the larger the animal, the more they could extract); then they realized estrogen could be found in animals' urine, and thus began "hormone therapy." (Premarin is still made from the pee of pregnant horses.)[19]

Pincus and Chang were not yet working with estrogen—they would eventually add it to the mix after some accidentally contaminated a batch of progestin and seemed to result in fewer side effects. They had been focused on progesterone because physiologists had determined that its rise in pregnancy prevented ovulation. From this fact, we get the oft-repeated explanation that the Pill works by "tricking" the body into thinking it is pregnant.

But this is misleading. A woman in early pregnancy is bathing in progesterone, and her ovaries are churning out estrogen—pregnant women will ultimately generate 100 times the amount of estradiol that the ovaries would produce each month in the buildup to ovulation. As anyone who's experienced pregnancy will tell you, it can be extremely taxing. But in addition to months of luscious hair and that full body "glow," the hormones of pregnancy (not just estradiol but two other forms of estrogen we never talk about, estrone and estriol) are protective. For every baby a woman births and breastfeeds, her breast cancer risk drops.[20] Her risk of endometrial cancer drops as well.[21] Her brain maps new neural pathways.[22] Looking at a woman's long-term health, pregnancy can be a net gain.

The Pill's one major upside is that it reduces a woman's lifetime risk of ovarian cancer (which is already very low). But synthesized versions of estrogen and progesterone do not have the same protective effects as those produced by the human body.[23] Ethinyl estradiol and progestin are similar enough to fit into the same receptors as estrogen and progesterone, respectively, which are located on cells throughout the body, and those receptors then signal to the pituitary that they're occupied. This causes the ovaries to stop producing either of these hormones. And physiologically, this is a net loss, argues Jerilynn Prior, an endocrinologist and founder of the Centre for Menstrual Cycle and Ovulation Research at the University of British Columbia. Prior writes about the "preventative powers" of ovulation, specifically to prevent osteoporosis, breast cancer, and heart disease.

On a graph, a healthy ovarian cycle looks like lapping waves of estrogen, progesterone, and two pituitary hormones: follicle-stimulating hormone, or FSH, and luteinizing hormone, or LH. All are bottomed out on day one of a menstrual cycle (which explains why many women *feel* bottomed out), and then FSH begins to rise, which stimulates estrogen. Estrogen peaks just before ovulation (along with a peak amount of cervical fluid), which is roughly in the middle of the graph, and then begins to taper off along with FSH as progesterone and LH ascend, until progesterone declines, which releases the menstrual flow, and the cycle begins anew. On the Pill or any hormonal contraception, however, this graph looks very different. For one, there are no waves of estradiol and progesterone—the pituitary stops making LH and FSH; instead, there is a static dose of ethinyl estradiol and progestin.

Critics talk about this in ways that can seem contradictory. Lara Briden, an Australian naturopathic doctor and author of *Period Repair Manual*, points out that one's hormonal profile while on the Pill looks more like menopause than pregnancy. On the one hand, this makes sense: if pregnancy is a hormonal garden enjoying an extended summer, the Pill invokes a steady dormant winter. A woman's own sex hormones are flatlined. But on the other hand, the amount of synthetic estrogen a woman is receiving while on low-dose hormonal birth control is four times as high as the amount of estrogen that she would normally have, which counters the notion that the Pill is "low dose."[24] Her own estradiol may be near menopausal levels, but the amount of estrogen is not.[25]

Drug manufacturer Searle originally appealed to the FDA for approval of the Pill to treat menstrual irregularities—it was a way to sidestep the politics of birth control, but the application was not based on any evidence.[26] And yet that cover story has been fulfilled, as one of the Pill's primary roles in medicine is to "regulate" the cycle. According to the Guttmacher Institute, more than half of women are taking hormonal contraception for reasons other than contraception, including to treat cramps, irregular cycles, and acne.[27]

We can call the clockwork bleeding women get while on the Pill a period, as many do, but we should probably call it something else. It is an engineered bleed, not the result of a cycle that's come into regulation. Because there is no cycle. The "period" wouldn't happen at all were it not for the placebo pills included in birth control packs. This was part of the Pill's design, because at the time of its development, women were thought to be reassured by a monthly flow. And John Rock thought the Catholic Church would be persuaded to sanction the Pill if it were simply mimicking the "natural" cycle (it was not persuaded). But 28 days could just as easily be 44 or 103—the brand Seasonale has a 91-day cycle; Amethyst dispenses with the placebos altogether. Those who make a distinction call it a "withdrawal bleed," because it is the result of withdrawal from the hormones.

Why does this matter? Aren't too many periods actually *un*natural and *un*healthy, because if women were really following nature's plan, we'd be pregnant or breastfeeding most of our adult lives? Isn't it true that now, without hormonal intervention, we bleed *too much*?

This argument for "menstrual suppression" has had its own impressive shelf life, but rarely mentioned are the conflicts of interests of its promoters: Brazilian physician and scientist Elsimar Coutinho, who is most famous for his research that led to Depo-Provera, and American scientist Sheldon Segal, who developed Norplant. (Both products, not coincidentally, suppress bleeding.) In 1999, they coauthored a book whose title asked *Is Menstruation Obsolete?*[28]

The book, which was a media sensation, argued that the "incessant ovulation" of modernity has no physiological purpose and only causes women pain, suffering, inconvenience, and anemia. Coutinho has said his "greatest contribution to humanity was to realize that menstruation was unnecessary, a disposable phenomena. Women can reproduce without bleeding because menstruation is not a condition to pregnancy. Menstruation is unnecessary, ovulation is necessary."[29] Malcolm Gladwell was so taken by this epiphany that he wrote in a famous *New Yorker* piece that "there is no medical reason" to menstruate. "The real promise of the Pill was not that it could preserve the menstrual rhythms of the twentieth century but that it could disrupt them."[30]

Among the problems with this theory is that the hormones of the ovulatory cycle have multiple functions. They affect more than reproduction. The physiological ratio of estradiol and progesterone maintains bone mass, clears arteries of plaque, and regulates insulin. The endocrine system affects our neural pathways, fat distribution, and gut microbiome. Chandler Marrs, who holds a PhD in neuropsychology and founded the web site Hormones Matter, points out that the mitochondria in our cells, the very building blocks of our bodies, need estrogen to function properly. And then there's the little matter of our sexual function.

Here is a statement that has somehow become radical in the last 20 years: ovulation is healthy. And if women are on the Pill or even just under too much stress, they're not ovulating regularly, not getting the monthly dose of sex hormones that's beneficial to so many of the body's systems. "I'm increasingly convinced that these silent ovulatory disturbances and the stress that causes them are related to women's earlier risk of heart attack," says Prior. Furthermore, she says, the balance of progesterone to estrogen in the body's own cycle offers cancer protection that the Pill regimen does not. "So I think if we don't start understanding about ovulation, we're putting women at risk for early osteoporosis, early heart attack, and also increased risk for breast cancer."

If a person is on the Pill (or patch, ring, injection, or implant), the ovaries go offline. Though she can still produce these hormones in smaller quantities elsewhere in the body, the Pill won't make up for what the ovaries are not providing. Ethinyl estradiol and progestin are like keys that fit into locks (receptors) but only open some of the doors, and sometimes they open the wrong doors. They have different effects than endogenous hormones (produced by the body), sometimes even the opposite effects.

Case in point: the body's own progesterone enables implantation of an embryo, while levonorgestrel, used in many pills, IUDs, and the morning-after pill, thwarts it. Progesterone is a natural anticoagulant, while the newer "fourth-generation" progestins increase the risk of blood clots.[31]

A typical "informed consent" conversation between a person and their doctor includes mention of the clot risk, a question about smoking, and perhaps a conversation about body mass index. Blood clots and strokes are rare, but known, accepted, established risks. But the hormones have effects on other bodily systems that get little to no attention. They may not be as life threatening as a stroke, but some we could still fairly call "risks." Others we might call drawbacks. All of them qualify as major bummers for something that is still presented to young women as preventative medicine, if not a rite of passage.

WARNING: SEXUAL LIBERATOR MAY CAUSE SEXUAL (AND OTHER) DYSFUNCTION

As a PhD candidate at McGill University, in Montreal, Cynthia Graham was curious about the Pill's effectiveness in treating PMS, for which it was, and still is, widely prescribed. To her surprise, she found no placebo-controlled trials in the literature, which meant there was little evidence supporting this use. "So a bit ambitiously I did a placebo-controlled trial, using a widely used low-dose hormonal contraceptive, and we looked at mood and looked at hormone levels as well," says Graham, now a professor of sexual and reproductive health at the University of Southampton and a research fellow with the Kinsey Institute. "What came out of that study unexpectedly was that a subgroup of women in the pill group were experiencing decreased sexual desire."[32] (Her results also showed the Pill had no clear impact on negative mood.) Graham has spent a good portion of her career researching this connection, and there is now "consistent evidence," she says, that the Pill lowers libido in some women. She won't make an official estimate, but mentions one study that reported 25 percent and another that reported 12 percent. "There's no doubt it's a minority," she says.

If you've ever wondered why we still don't have a male Pill, the answer is sexual side effects—research has shown that manipulating male sex hormones can dampen libido, cause erection trouble, and diminish orgasm. Similar side effects may manifest in women, too, yet most of us are never warned. "Most research done in the early days tended to see sexually related side effects as 'trivial,'" says Graham. "There's a kind of reluctance not only to investigate it but to report it when found." For research in men, however, sexual response was in fact the primary concern—one of the largest studies of a male Pill, she tells me, surveyed subjects on *20* different sexual criteria. "There's never been a study like that on the Pill."

Any decrease in libido is an ironic bummer for a product credited with spurring the sexual revolution. There's still no consensus about why exactly it happens. The suspected reason is that the Pill lowers testosterone, the "hormone of desire," in two ways: first, it puts the ovaries on hiatus, and the ovaries are a woman's main source of testosterone. The other reason has to do with sex hormone–binding globulin, or SHBG. When someone is on the Pill, their liver increases production of SHBG to clear excess estrogen from the blood. But SHBG also binds to testosterone. "So you're in double jeopardy, your ovaries are no longer making it, and SHBG is binding to testosterone made by the adrenals. There's nothing physiologically available," Irwin Goldstein, a urologist, told me at a sexual medicine conference. The effect on testosterone explains why the Pill is so great at clearing up acne (OK, one more upside), but it is also the price we pay, he said, because testosterone plays a role in female arousal, lubrication, and general well-being.

Goldstein made his career promoting Viagra and working for parity in sexual dysfunction drugs for women—he's taken in hundreds of thousands of dollars in consulting fees, so he's hardly anti-pharma.[33] Yet he wants a black-box warning placed on the Pill. When I asked Jerilynn Prior what is the most important thing women need to know about the Pill's impacts, she pointed to the same libido effect: "The evidence is pretty clear that there's a decreased interest in sex on the Pill," she said.

To be clear, this doesn't mean every woman will lose her mojo. The freedom of not worrying about getting pregnant can be a powerful aphrodisiac, and everyone's response is different. Still, the potential for the side effect is there, and it's not the only one.

Another big downer: depression. "These days, when I meet a patient who complains of flat mood, low libido, weight gain, irritability, and anxiety, one of my first questions is, 'Are you on the Pill?'" says Kelly Brogan, author of *A Mind of Your Own* and a functional psychiatrist. A vocal minority of Pill users have been complaining for decades that the Pill "makes them crazy," and in 2016, an enormous study out of Denmark lent powerful credence to previous studies and anecdotal reports: it looked at more than one million women and found that hormonal contraception was associated with more diagnoses and treatment of depression. The patch and ring seemed to have a more profound effect than the Pill. One of the most striking findings was that the risk of depression was 80 percent higher for teenagers.[34]

What is the mechanism that would cause mood disturbances? In addition to raising levels of SHBG, the Pill increases thyroid-binding globulin, which means "you are essentially driving a hypothryroid state, and that hypothyroid state is well documented to include an experience of flat mood, cognitive fuzziness, changes in sleep, changes in appetite, changes in libido, and depression," says Brogan.

"So, remarkably little is known about the physiology of hormonal contraception," says Steven Kushner, a UCLA- and Columbia-trained psychiatrist now based at a research center in the Netherlands focused on the biology of mental illness. In 2017, he and a group of researchers conducted a series of studies to try to suss out the link between hormonal contraception and mood. They took three groups of women—on the Pill, on the Mirena IUD, and normally cycling—put them through a stress test, and took hair and blood samples. They were particularly interested in the IUD, which has been marketed as having only "localized" effects on the uterus and is considered safe for those who didn't tolerate "systemic" hormonal methods. "We showed definitively that the hormones released by Mirena have systemic effects, and those effects exist in the brain. Basically, there's a sensitization of the stress response system," Kushner explains. That is, the same way a diabetic becomes resistant to insulin, a person can become resistant to cortisol, which is associated with depression and anxiety. Kushner's work demonstrates that synthetic hormones have effects on the brain, but it still doesn't nail down the mechanism.[35]

Julie Holland, also a psychiatrist and author of *Moody Bitches*, has a theory that disrupting the estrogen balance may disrupt the seratonin-dopamine balance. "Estrogen and seratonin are yoked in the brain. When one is up the other is up, when one is down the other is down," says Holland. The brain is chock-full of estrogen receptors, but high seratonin doesn't mean that everything is peaches and cream. "There is this thing that happens when people are on high dose SSRIs that they don't feel anything, they feel numbed out," she says of drugs like Prozac, "because seratonin and dopamine are on opposite sides of a seesaw, so the higher you push on seratonin, the lower the dopamine. And dopamine is what gives you drive and pleasure and reward." She calls estrogen the "hormone of accommodation." After cortisol, it operates like a stress hormone, "it calms you down, makes you resilient," which is great when you need to take on a lot without getting overwhelmed. "But it can also make you super complacent and accommodating and whatever-you-want-honey. Without the balance of drive and reward, you may not get where you want to get to in your life," says Holland.

That said, remember that the estrogen in the Pill doesn't behave in all the same ways as the body's own estradiol, and for women who experience not only depression but anxiety, it would seem that the synthetic hormone is not as accommodating. Meanwhile natural progesterone can have a sedating effect (which may be one of the reasons why newly pregnant women need so many naps), "and synthetic progesterone may be a bigger problem," Holland points out. "Women who have progestin-only devices, like the implant and Depo, really tend to get depressed, fat, and sleepy." The mechanisms aren't totally clear. "It's not just a question of what are these synthetic hormones doing to you, because what is also affecting you is that your natural cycle has been turned off," says Holland.

Brogan points out that in addition to causing an endocrine imbalance by design, the Pill is associated with inflammation and also inhibits absorption of nutrients like magnesium, selenium, vitamin B6, and folic acid. (Folic acid is the "preconception" vitamin that public health campaigns urge young women to take. The pill Beyaz was Bayer's attempt to remedy the depletion effect by adding folic acid to an oral contraceptive.) "Micronutrient depletion, at least in the vitamin B realm, has been correlated with risks for depression," says Brogan.

At the end of the day, how hormonal contraceptives impact mood isn't easy to tease out, and may have different pathways depending on the person's genetics and epigenetics. To add to the complexity, synthetic hormones produce different metabolites than endogenous hormones, Marrs points out, and we don't even know what they all are or what they do. "The relationships between sex hormones and brain and mood go beyond our understanding," says Brogan. "I mean, I think we are entering into the great abyss of the unknown in systems biology." Kushner reiterates this: "We really should know more about the effects of hormonal contraceptives on the body overall, not only on the reproductive system itself, which is the target, but with the increasing appreciation that there are effects on other physiologic systems, and we really need to understand that in exquisite detail." And we don't.

Like Brogan, Holland steers her patients away from hormonal contraception if she can. She's seen the Pill lead women to antidepressants, which she calls the "low-libido double whammy." In her book, she urges patients who must be on antidepressants to "please consider a nonhormonal form of birth control . . . (Or you can stay on this combination of medicines and become a nun. Your call.)"

"The thing I'm really worried about is that my private practice and those of all my colleagues are filled with women in their 30s and 40s—women who are single and want to be married and have kids, and I'm afraid that because they're on antidepressants and the Pill, they're not capable of mating the way we've been mating for thousands of years," Holland says, "which is, we're mid-cycle, we're horny, and we know who has a good smell and who will give us a healthy baby."

This may sound too "woo-woo" for some readers, but Holland is referring to longstanding evidence that the Pill affects how we process pheromones—most famous is the "T-shirt study," in which women on the Pill performed worse than their cycling sisters in sniffing men's sweaty T-shirts and reporting attraction to those deemed by researchers to be the best genetic match for them.[36]

Less woo-woo is how the Pill affects metabolism. "Oral contraceptive agents can induce substantial metabolic changes that resemble those seen in persons at increased risk for premature coronary heart disease," begins one study.[37] This can mean higher cholesterol, triglycerides, and insulin resistance, and it can also mean flab.[38] When the body can't convert glucose to energy, it converts it to fat.

A 2009 study took two groups of women to the gym for ten weeks in a row and gave them trainers who put them through chest presses, leg extensions, arm curls, and crunches. One group was taking oral contraceptives, the other was not. The group on the Pill gained 60 percent less lean muscle and had higher levels of cortisol, the stress hormone, too much of which can lead to glucose intolerance and insulin resistance.[39] A recent study found that women who'd taken the Pill were more prone to getting gestational diabetes in pregnancy.[40] Another found that Pill use predisposed women to type 2 diabetes in menopause.[41]

The relationship between metabolism and the ovaries works in the inverse as well—insulin resistance inhibits ovulation. If eggs are ripening but not releasing, they form little "cysts" on the ovaries, hence the diagnosis of polycystic ovarian syndrome (PCOS, discussed further in the next chapter), which often also means an overabundance of androgens, which cause hair growth, acne, and weight gain. More and more, PCOS is being understood as a metabolic problem that manifests as a reproductive problem, not the other way around. The common treatment PCOS? The Pill.

There are concerns about hormonal contraception and bone health, particularly for young women. Progesterone increases the osteoblast cells that make new bone, while estrogen maintains that bone, explains Prior. They work hand in glove. But the progestins in hormonal contraceptives don't behave like progesterone in this regard. Prior cites three large studies that have shown increased fracture risks (of 10 to 20 percent) in menopausal women who previously took hormonal contraceptives.[42] Meanwhile, other studies show lower bone density in Pill users compared to non-users.[43] And depot medroxyprogesterone acetate (DMPA), the active agent in Depo-Provera, is so strongly associated with bone loss that the FDA requires a "boxed warning" on the product label that reads: "Women who use Depo-Provera Contraceptive Injection may lose significant bone mineral density."[44]

Ovulation strengthens bone. So bone density is also a concern for women who aren't necessarily on the Pill but whose hormones may be out of whack for whatever reason. "We've shown with the strongest kind of evidence that if women have regular cycles but aren't ovulating most of the time, or if they're not having a long enough luteal phase [which follows ovulation], they'll be losing almost 1 percent of bone mass each year," says Prior. "That silent bone loss means that we end up at menopause already at risk for fracture."

Another downside of the Pill is that it causes inflammation, which over time may weaken the immune system.[45] This may put Pill users at greater risk for autoimmune diseases like lupus, cancer, and even HIV.[46] In 2017, another enormous study out of Denmark surprised researchers by suggesting that even the "lower-dose" pills, assumed to be safer, confer a heightened risk of breast cancer.[47] This "upends widely held assumptions about modern contraceptives for younger generations of women," reported the *New York Times*. In a letter to the editor, a group of physicians and researchers out of the University of California, San Francisco, countered that "given the existing literature showing that hormonal contraception reduces both cancer-related and all-cause mortality, raising false alarms about the safety of contraceptives is a disservice to women. Scares about the safety of contraceptives predictably decrease contraceptive use and increase unwanted pregnancies."[48]

Daniel Grossman and coauthors at the UCSF-based research group Advancing New Standards in Reproductive Health take issue with the Danish study because, he told me, it could simply be measuring the doctor-visit effect—women who are on the Pill have more opportunity for diagnosis and treatment of other things. But couldn't this also be said of studies showing a relationship between Pill use and lower "all-cause mortality"? I asked him. "It may be that they get more care and get detected earlier, that has not been clearly determined," he said. "It's very clear that there's a significant reduction in the risk of ovarian cancer, and there's definitely a decreased risk of uterine cancer," and possibly less gastrointestinal cancer associated with oral contraceptive use. Not that he'd recommend the Pill for cancer protection (though he does bring up the theory that perhaps "ovulation isn't a good thing"), but the point is that "the data of the safety of the Pill is very, very strong." That of course depends on what's meant by "safety." Prior points out, "There's a lot of hype about the Pill decreasing the risk for ovarian cancer, but there is little hype for it increasing the risk of stroke."

The National Cancer Institute—which runs cancer.gov—warns that "long-term use of oral contraceptives (5 or more years) is associated with an increased risk of cervical cancer." That risk is three-fold for five to nine years of Pill use and four-fold for ten years or more. "Hormones in oral contraceptives may change the susceptibility of cervical cells to HPV infection, affect their ability to clear the infection, or make it easier for HPV infection to cause changes that progress to cervical cancer," the Institute explains in its fact sheet.[49] Equally concerning, a large study of couples in which one partner was HIV positive and the other negative found that hormonal contraception doubled the odds that the negative partner would become infected.[50] In addition to changing the cervix, another likely mechanism is that the Pill thins the vaginal lining, making it more prone to scratches and cuts that create pathways for the virus.

Odeblad was concerned about the Pill's effect on the cervix and began to study it, though these studies were published in Catholic natural family planning publications, not mainstream, peer-reviewed journals.[51] He summed up his findings like this: "a pregnancy rejuvenates the cervix by 2-3 years, but for each year the Pill is taken, the cervix ages by an extra year."[52] Several physicians I've talked to have also noticed changes as well, even in the vulva. "It looks whiter and thinner, it won't look moist and lubricated," Andrew Goldstein, an OB/GYN in New York, told me. "Usually [the] vulva is a glistening, beautiful color." Adaline P. Satterthwaite, an American doctor who tested the Pill in Puerto Rico, noted a common side effect was inflammation. "Whatever you call it," she remarked, "the cervix looks angry."[53]

More than half of teenagers have used the Pill—it's available as a chewable tablet—or implant or IUD, even though a majority are not yet having sex.[54] Prior is especially concerned about the side effects on immature bodies. "Teenagers are still gaining peak bone mass, which is sort of a bone reserve for rest of their lives, and they're still developing normal menstrual and ovulatory cycles. In other words, they're in a time of maturation," says Prior. The optimal situation for bone mass is having a period that starts not too late and menopause that's not too early—it takes a few years for the cycle to normalize, and normal ovulation maintains bone reserves. "Now what if you come along with this huge force and suppress the whole shebang? The evidence is it's not good. It's not good for bones and it's not good for reproduction," she says.

That statement goes against the dominant view that hormonal methods have no negative impact on fertility, but the long-term research that would truly answer that question has never been done. There are, however, studies that point to the need for it, like one that looked at some 900 women aged 19 to 40. The ovaries of those who were taking hormonal contraception were half the size compared to non-users, and they had significantly lower measures of "ovarian reserves" compared to non-users, a predictor of their ability to conceive.[55] Another study looked at more than 100 women who were undergoing embryo transfer at a fertility clinic and found a correlation between the thickness of their endometrial lining and how long they'd been on the Pill. The women with thin linings were more likely to have been on the Pill for ten years, while the group with the normal lining had a mean six years on the Pill. The authors noted that they could find only one previous study examining long-term Pill use and fertility, which found no correlation, and suggest their findings show a previously "unidentified side effect," one that "may be of importance when counseling women considering long-term contraception."[56]

Marrs, Prior, Kushner, and Holland all echo the same concerns. The Pill works by disrupting a key endocrine system, the hypothalamic-pituitary-adrenal axis. That's not a side effect, it's the intention. "When you shut down the body's own mechanism and replace it, the gist is all sorts of things go wrong," says Marrs. Not the same things to the same degree in every woman—that depends on genetics and epigenetics. But it explains why a drug intended to affect the reproductive organs winds up affecting all sorts of other systems.

Still, sweeping defenses like the *Times* letter are common. "What's clear is that the Pill did usher in a gender revolution, and moved women's equality forward at an astounding pace," wrote Jill Filipovic in the *Guardian*. "Scaring women away from highly effective forms of birth control with inaccurate claims isn't radical or brave." In Slate, Jessica Grose argued that "the birth control scare story" is its own magazine genre.[57] Even the 2005 edition of *Our Bodies, Ourselves* (on which I served as an editor) reports, "The birth control pill is considered the most intensely researched medication in history" and cautions readers to reject "alarming stories from friends, trusted adults, or the media." Prior says, "There's a sort of feeling like to criticize the Pill is to criticize motherhood and apple pie. It's just not allowed."

CLEVEREST OF ALL INVENTIONS

The wide-ranging effects of the Pill beg the question: what did we know and when did we know it?

In 1970, Wisconsin liberal senator Gaylord Nelson called for congressional hearings into the Pill's safety, after he was handed a copy of Barbara Seaman's book *The Doctors' Case Against the Pill.* The most famous thing about the closed-door "Nelson Pill hearings" is that a group of feminist activists stormed them, loudly protesting the lack of firsthand testimony from women—all the presenters were male physicians, some consultants to pharma. The women shouted things like "Why isn't there a male pill?" "Why have 10 million women been used as guinea pigs?" "We will no longer tolerate intimidation by white-coated gods antiseptically directing our lives!" They were dramatically carried out by guards; Seaman later wrote that the action "became the Boston Tea Party of women's health."[58] The women who met there went on to found the National Women's Health Network. The other upshot was that an informational package insert would be included in every Pill pack—and all drugs from that point forward.

But that insert was heavily redacted, only mentioning the risk of blood clots, which was significant. With the help of Senator Bernie Sanders's office, Chandler Marrs obtained thousands of pages of transcripts from the hearings and, with research assistants, delved in. The risk of blood clotting and lodging in the lungs (pulmonary embolism) or blocking an artery to the brain (stroke) seems to be the stickiest in our collective memory, but those "white-coated gods" had actually testified about much more: metabolic disturbances and cases of Pill users developing diabetes; its impact on cancer in animal studies; delayed fertility and increased rates of miscarriage, stillbirth, and birth defects; the effects on the immune system; and even how it made women more susceptible to sexually transmitted infections. There was also lengthy testimony about the Pill's impact on mental health, with one doctor testifying that "three patients have stated they were desperately afraid that they were going to kill themselves," but after they stopped using the Pill, "the depression and suicidal fears disappeared."[59] It turns out that at least one woman committed suicide in the original trials, though, according to Marrs's research, "her case, along with 18 other deaths, were omitted in the reports filed to the FDA."[60]

Of course, the Pill that was tested on about 800 women in Puerto Rico (Pincus thought it "a place where women wouldn't ask as many questions"[61]) and won FDA approval had about four times the estrogen and ten times the progestin of the "second-generation" pills, which went on the market in the 1980s.[62] That evolution decreased the number of blood clots and allowed women a certain level of comfort that the Pill was "low dose." Still, even today, a good 60 percent of women who try hormonal contraceptives quit within the first six months because of side effects, and another 30 percent will try up to five different brands for the same reason.[63] As Marrs and other researchers have pointed out, dozens upon dozens of brands on the market suggest an abundance of choice, "but from a pharmacological standpoint, not much has changed in hormonal contraceptive technology over the last half-century."

By the late 1960s, researchers in England found that the Pill put women at six to seven times the risk of a blood clot as normal. While the second-generation, lower-dose pills brought the risk down, the 1980s also saw less study of this relationship, even though the risk had hardly been eliminated. Then came the so-called third generation of pills, which were even lower in dosage, the theory being they would lower the risk even further. Instead, they did the opposite. A World Health Organization study published in 1995 found that they had *doubled* the risk of the previous generation's Pill, with many more studies confirming this finding.[64]

Now we also have a "fourth-generation" progestin called drospirenone, found in brands like Yaz and Yasmin, made by Bayer. These were so popular that they topped the contraceptive charts in 2009, with combined sales of $1.78 billion, yet studies have shown that drospirenone puts women at the highest risk of blood clots since Enovid came on the market. Bayer reportedly spent more than $2 billion settling lawsuits in the following years, all the while denying any flaws in the product.

NuvaRing and the implants Nexplanon and Implanon, which all contain the third-generation progestins, are also higher-risk than the Pill of the 1980s. More than 230 deaths associated with NuvaRing have been reported to the FDA, and 77 deaths associated with the implants. The FDA has received nearly 100,000 official "adverse event reports" related to the hormonal IUDs Mirena, Skyla, Liletta, and Kyleena, including 132 deaths.[65] Depo-Provera is so risky the FDA wouldn't approve it for 20 years, and many believe that it never should have. In other words, we may now have all these choices about how we take "the Pill," but the technology is just as clunky as it was 40 years ago.[66]

Holland hears this frustration from patients all the time. "As soon as they mention the words 'birth control' they're given a prescription for the Pill. There is zero time spent talking about diaphragms and caps, those days are gone. Maybe if my patients push a bit, they'll get Mirena, and less often they'll get the nonhormonal IUD. It used to be in the '80s and '90s, they'd tell you all your options," she says. "What I want to know is, who killed the cervical cap?"

Among feminist health veterans, cervical cap nostalgia is strong. What happened was basically that the medical industry abandoned barrier devices after the Dalkon Shield, an IUD that caused pelvic inflammatory disease and led to several deaths (and thousands of lawsuits), was pulled from the market in the 1970s. This was also the impetus for the FDA to begin regulating devices. With industry spooked, feminist health centers took over to fill the market void, obtaining "investigational device exemptions," that is, permission from the FDA to run trials. One small trial found that among 100 women fit with the cap, most considered it a superior method.[67] But the FDA shut down another study (and product) after it showed the cap caused minor abrasions on the cervix. Women were again reliant on doctors for cervical caps, and for the most part, physicians had no interest in prescribing them.

Virginia Reath, a women's health physician assistant in New York who began as a radical feminist health activist in the early 1970s, explains that enthusiasm for the cervical cap—basically a smaller diaphragm—existed within the larger feminist health movement because it allowed women to take back control of their bodies, a corollary to the "self-exam" with the speculum. And she locates physicians' abandonment of female-controlled barrier methods as part of a medical backlash.

The self-exam was "so transgressive," she says. "You were taking a medical thing that no one was supposed to know about anyway, and you were saying it was like a game—'Hey, you want to see your cervix?'" (In the late '80s, the performance artist Annie Sprinkle took the show on the road with her "Public Cervix Announcement.") Reath, for her part, was an art student at Bard in 1971 when she learned how to do it from Lolly Hirsch and her daughter Jeanne, activists who learned from Carol Downer and went on to found *The Monthly Extract: An Irregular Periodical.* Reath brought it back to her consciousness-raising group. "We'd have our flashlights and mirrors, we'd look at it, crack up, and have some wine. I was the one who drove it, because I was fascinated, I was hooked." She led workshops for years. "There was this huge movement of know your body," she says. The women's health movement was prompting women to demand a share of the power in their doctors' offices, to bring their partner or an advocate with them, and to ask questions. Physicians recoiled, "because you were in their business," says Reath. "I think in a way that clinicians fought back by not wanting to fit the cervical cap, by pushing the Pill."

By the late 1980s the "cervical cap renaissance" was over, and by 2002 fewer than 1 percent of women had ever used it.[68] In 2016 it reemerged as the silicone FemCap, though it is not exactly taking the market by storm. So nobody killed it, but the mainstream medical field never championed it either, even after women changed the specialty's demographics. The focus became contraceptive effectiveness—and reducing the number of abortions. Reath points out that "diaphragms with backup abortions are safer than the more effective contraceptives, the Pill or the IUD." Not every woman is comfortable with that, and there are certainly other downsides to the cap, like having to fumble with insertion and spermicide. But at the same time not every woman wants to trade safety for effectiveness.

For the feminist health-minded, the Pill was a mixed bag. For the mainstream, it was revolutionary and remains so. "It's magic, a trick of science that managed in one fell swoop to wipe away centuries of female oppression," wrote Vanessa Grigoriadis in *New York* magazine on the Pill's fiftieth anniversary.[69] "The advent of the pill, probably more than any other event, has enabled women the world over to prevent or delay pregnancy and, in doing so, to complete our educations, choose our careers, and create more egalitarian relationships," wrote the authors of the 2005 edition of *Our Bodies, Ourselves.* "Every morning of the month / You push a little tablet through the foil / Cleverest of all inventions / Better than a condom or a coil," sings feminist rocker Tracey Thorn.

When the Pill was approved, abortion was illegal and dangerous. Contraception was only legal if you were married and your doctor would prescribe it. It wasn't even easy to get information about basic female biology. Perhaps back then the Pill deserved its pedestal. But today? Many women don't even take it for sexual liberation. They take it for pimples. As historian Elaine Tyler May put it: "Without the political and cultural upheavals of the last fifty years, particularly those brought about by the feminist movement, the pill would have been just one more contraceptive—more effective and convenient than those that came before, but not revolutionary."[70]

If anything is nudging the Pill off its pedestal, it's the IUD—more effective than the little tablet, it can outlast a president's term in office. Indeed, one lasting legacy of the Pill has been the shift in focus to long-acting reversible contraceptives, shorthand LARCs. These include hormonal IUDs and implants—products that decrease the potential for user error—and now the American College of Obstetricians and Gynecologists and even the American Academy of Pediatrics recommend them as "first-line" methods, even for adolescents. In the United States, the primary users of LARCs and the long-lasting but less reversible Depo-Provera are low-income women of color.

Another legacy is the international community's push to spread this concept to resource-poor women with Depo in particular, now in a self-injectible form called Sayana Press, both made by Pfizer. This complicates the idea of "international aid" when DMPA is associated with so many negative health effects, and there's evidence suggesting it makes woman more prone to contracting HIV.[71] It also contradicts the world's evolution on "sexual rights." DMPA is "the same type of hormone—not the same dosage—but the same type of hormone exactly that's used to treat male sex offenders, to dampen their sexual interest," says Cynthia Graham. "Yet it's really being pushed a lot now, particularly for young women."

Margaret Sanger wanted magic, but what we have is reality. Messy, complicated reality. Because, of course, "the Pill" is not just a pill. It's control, independence, power, equality, sexual freedom. It's progress. In 2019 in the United States of America, women are still fighting for all of it. So it's not surprising that those who've asked tough questions about the Pill's contemporary merit have been met with fierce resistance. Laura Eldridge, author of the 2010 contraceptive guide *In Our Control,* was lambasted in the feminist blogosphere for discussing the Pill's risks. A direct disciple of Barbara Seaman, Eldridge dared to point out that "the lack of serious examination of the Pill has created an environment where women live with life-disrupting side effects for decades, unaware that a large consumer health movement has been asking questions about the dangers of hormonal contraception for the past four to five decades . . . Blindly worshiping at the church of the 'magic bullet' is never the best thing for female consumers."[72]

"Eldridge's life's work is trying to scare women about the birth control pill," wrote Amanda Marcotte on her prominent blog shortly after *In Our Control* was published. "She's not doing this from an anti-feminist perspective, but from a feminist one that fetishizes the notion of 'natural,' a common problem on the left." Marcotte went on to be a regular Slate contributor, and in 2015 branded Ricki Lake "the newest hero of the antichoice movement" for announcing plans to make a documentary about the Pill, which codirector Abby Epstein said would challenge "the taboo around questioning the mainstream acceptance of hormonal contraceptives."[73]

The forthcoming documentary is based on the 2013 book *Sweetening the Pill: Or How We Got Hooked on Hormonal Birth Control,* by Holly Grigg-Spall, a film critic turned feminist pariah. Grigg-Spall was on the

Pill for about two years when she began suspecting it of causing her sudden depression, brain fog, and panic attacks. She went off it for a couple months and felt "lighter. A rush of positive emotions let me feel happiness, excitement and enthusiasm. I became stable in both my thoughts and feelings . . . Yet, like a victim of Stockholm Syndrome, I returned to taking it."[74] She began blogging about the symptoms as they returned, in 2008, and the cultural pressure she felt to stay on the Pill, and she received comments and emails from women noting the same. In the book, she conveys her own and other women's negative experiences and poses a broader question: for whom is the Pill liberating—women? Or men, who are relieved of the burden of contraception? Or capitalist society, which profits? As her subtitle indicates, she suggests we've become hooked on the idea more than the reality, at the expense of our health.

I've met Grigg-Spall and she does not want to ban the Pill, nor is she anti-abortion. She does, however, challenge the Pill's elevated status in mainstream feminism, what she describes as "the paternalistic tone of much contemporary feminist discussion of contraception in the US that treats women as though they were hysterics unable to handle the responsibility and complexity involved in truly informed consent . . . Any criticism is considered irresponsible, playing into the hands of those on the Right who want to see [hormonal contraceptives] banned."[75]

Needless to say, her book did not open a dialogue. Instead, reviews of *Sweetening the Pill* were scathing. Some amounted to "a willful character assassination," in Grigg-Spall's words. In Slate, Lindsay Beyerstein wrote, "Sexists have been trying to reduce women to incubators since time immemorial, but recently some self-proclaimed feminists have jumped on the bandwagon, arguing that true liberation means being left alone to experience feminine bodily functions like ovulation, childbirth, and breast-feeding in all their natural glory," adding, "a feminism based on the fetishization of bodily functions is no feminism at all."[76] Jennifer Gunter, an OB/GYN with more than 85,000 Twitter followers, called it "that atrocious pill book" and suspected "a pro-life agenda."[77]

One woman started a Care2 petition, asking the publisher, Zero Books, to stop publication. "Birth control is an effective method that *women should have the right to choose.* And that claim about birth control being dangerous? Total bogus," it stated, citing "multiple, extensive trials." The petition nearly met its goal of 7,000 signatures.[78]

The book had its shortcomings, but Grigg-Spall's big point was that we should be having a more honest conversation about the Pill. I'd add that we should also be having an honest conversation about why it's been so difficult to have this conversation. Where is the skeptical, critical eye of the feminist health movement, the one that got us that package insert in the first place?

One reason the Pill is such a sacred cow is of course politics. "Many, many organizations that work on reproductive health issues are so under attack from the right that they are reluctant to acknowledge any problems with a product," says Amy Allina, a women's health advocate in Washington, DC, who spent many years as the program director at the National Women's Health Network. The Network, for example, "deviated from the line," warning consumers about drospirenone-containing pills, finding itself on opposite sides of the aisle from Planned Parenthood (more on this in chapter 6). As Laura Wershler, a longtime activist who served on the board of Planned Parenthood in Canada, put it in an interview with Grigg-Spall in *Bitch*: "Ultimately our inability to present the downside of hormonal contraception and champion the growing research on the benefits of healthy, continuous ovulation comes from a belief that our pro-choice stance will be questioned."[79]

Ricki Lake also got flak in 2015 for announcing her forthcoming film: according to Lake, she was "abruptly" let go from the celebrity advisory board of the National Campaign to Prevent Teen and Unplanned Pregnancy, the group behind Bedsider.org, on which she had served for some 20 years. Lake summed up how a former leader of the organization called her up and explained the decision: "You ladies don't understand. I'm on the Hill fighting for reproductive rights, the conservatives are attacking us. You're going to make it harder for me. The population [whom] we really need to take these products are high-risk, they're already suspicious, they don't want to take these products." Merck, Johnson & Johnson, Wyeth, and Pfizer were all contributors to the campaign, which has since been rebranded as Power to Decide.

Meanwhile, on the medical side, the leadership wants "gold standard" evidence before it will address negative side effects: a double-blind randomized controlled trial, to prove each and every one. Jenny Higgins, an associate professor of gender and women's studies at the University of Wisconsin and a leading contraceptive researcher, told me that she came up against this in coauthoring a chapter of *Contraceptive Technology,* the bible of the field, with a physician colleague and wanting to include a line about there being "very good quality studies" that show the hit to libido. "Every time I tried to put a sentence like that into our chapter, my coauthor wasn't comfortable with it." The chapter walked the "conservative line," Higgins said, of "we need more data."

Similarly, clinicians typically tsk-tsk DIY methods, though around one-third of women at some point rely on withdrawal, and the dirty little secret is that it's a smidgen less effective than the male condom.[80] Higgins has authored several papers on the subject. Fertility awareness-based methods—when women "chart" their temperatures and cervical fluid to pinpoint their fertile days and act accordingly—are similarly "far more effective than people in the public health community or medical community give [them] credit for," Higgins says. Or, generally, the media. In a 2013 *Guardian* piece author Hadley Freeman skewered a friend who gave up approved methods for fertility tracking and withdrawal, a combo Freeman equated with using "no method at all" and "voodoo."[81] Among clinicians, the focus is on effectiveness, as so perceived. And the most "effective" methods tend to be the technologies with the least amount of involvement from the woman herself: those which are inserted, implanted, or injected by professionals. "We are trained to want to prevent unwanted pregnancy and prevent disease; we're not taught to sexually liberate our patients," says Higgins.

CYCLE EVANGELISM

"We're not taking people's bodies seriously enough," Emily Varnam says as we head north on Interstate 75 toward Flint, Michigan, for the free "Fifth Vital Sign" class she is coleading with Kelsey Knight. The two millennials raised $6,000 in a Kickstarter campaign (including a large donation from the mother of a young woman who died of a blood clot while on NuvaRing), bought a used Honda, and left New York City in January 2016. They spent several months on the road, traversing the country giving talks. In Flint, they'll talk to the female residents and staff of a group home for homeless teenagers. We arrive at a modest house on a perfect spring afternoon. Varnam and Knight carry in a purple plastic bin with a laptop, clay model uteruses, a fertility thermometer, a Planned Parenthood contraceptive kit, several books (including Grigg-Spall's), and hand-drawn vagina-uterus-fallopian-tube T-shirts that say "Tell Me I'm Beautiful."

At the time, Flint was a national story because of the lead in the city's water system, and the women saw a direct connection between the disempowerment of Flint's citizens and their mission. Varnam, a birth doula, and Knight, a labor and delivery nurse, had the idea for the trip because "we were coming to the conclusion that the foundation from which we were asking women to advocate for themselves in pregnancy and childbirth had already been broken. They already distrusted their body," says Varnam. She was also called to it by her friend circle. "They're all coming to me saying, 'I don't know what to do about my birth control, I'm having really bad side effects. Can you help me?'" So she started calling herself a "birth control doula," helping her friends "transition off hormonal birth control and find what works for them."

On their web site is a picture of the two women side by side in jeans, pointing to their groin with the same two fingers you'd use to take a pulse. Their gesture is meant to communicate that the menstrual cycle is as much of a vital sign as the heartbeat or temperature, that it is a proxy for a woman's health overall, an idea that is spreading. Even the American College of Obstetricians and Gynecologists has called for its members to consider the menstrual cycle "as an additional vital sign."[82]

In their presentation, Varnam and Knight explain the cycle with excitement and reverence, especially the cervical fluid part. "Cervical fluid extends the fertile window," Varnam says in her British lilt, showing a PowerPoint slide with a dozen pictures of cervices at various points, oozing blood or milky fluid or just shiny and pink.[83] "Every one of us would be such a miracle if we didn't have cervical fluid to keep the sperm alive!" We already all are miracles, of course, but the egg is only viable for 24 hours, she points out. Drawing directly from Odeblad's work, the women report that the "egg whites" are pH matched to the sperm and also contain "snacks" in the form of sugars, so the sperm can keep swimming for days before the egg is released. "We don't talk enough about cervical fluid," says Varnam. "But we talk about sperm all the time! We think cervical fluid deserves respect and awe."

After a slide showing how the cervix becomes softer and pulls up higher around ovulation (another, more subtle, sign of fertility), they name the practice of tracking all this knowledge, the fertility awareness method (FAM). "Fertility awareness can be just about you—a journey with yourself," says Varnam. "It can also be birth control."

Knight talks about "perfect" use versus "typical" use success rates—the way methods are categorized by researchers. Sometimes this is also expressed as "method" failure versus "user" failure. For example, if you know how to put on a condom, check the expiration date, and don't try to reuse one, you're a "perfect" user. If the condom breaks the failure will be purely mechanical (the rate is 2 percent). Perfect use effectiveness of FAM is estimated at 99.5 percent.

There are at least a dozen fertility awareness-based methods, as they are called by researchers, and each uses one or more criteria (e.g., charting, cervical fluid, temperature) and its own rules to determine the fertile window; users may add a barrier method during that time. This makes it challenging to estimate effectiveness. A recent systematic review of more than 50 studies found "typical use" rates as low as 2 pregnancies per 100 women during a year and as high as 33 pregnancies per 100 users in a year. With "perfect use," the rate of pregnancy was often under 5 percent. The authors of one of the larger studies remarked that it "is comparable to the method effectiveness of modern contraceptive methods like oral contraceptives."[84] Natural Cycles, a fertility tracking app approved as a contraceptive medical device by the FDA in 2018, claims its data show a "typical use" failure rate of about 7 pregnancies per year per 100 users.[85]

Varnam returns to the idea of tracking the cycle as a health tool, a form of "listening to the body." She gives the example of one woman who discovered she had a thyroid problem because her temperature remained low all month, and another who learned she was miscarrying because she saw her steady high pregnant temperature take a dive, and another who detected early cervical cancer before a Pap smear because she was spotting outside her period.

Listening to women is a central tenet of feminism. And to Knight, Varnam, Grigg-Spall, and others, fertility awareness is so inherently feminist. As a form of birth control, it's cost-free, side-effect free, and more equitable because it requires communication between partners—shared decision-making, if you will. "When I first started teaching fertility awareness, 95 percent of students wanted this for birth control," Toni Weschler, author of the FAM bible, *Taking Charge of Your Fertility*, told me. "There was such a demand, such a hunger for something that didn't wreak havoc on the female body, that didn't cause women to deal with side effects and ramifications of other drugs. And women were fed up with having sole responsibility for birth control. When they realize they're the ones who are rarely fertile, and that men are fertile every day, it changes the whole equation."

In Flint, much of this information is new to the room of teens and staffers, who open up about their own experiences and uncertainties. One teen reports that she's been on Depo since age 15. "I bleed for the entire third month and then it stops when I get the next shot. I'm getting tired of it." A 40-something woman asks about orgasms—she's not sure she's ever had one. Another woman talks about her PCOS, infertility treatments, and emergency C-section, "My stuff doesn't work," she says, to which Varnam shoots back, "Nobody has figured out how to help you make it work."

Back in the Honda on our way to Detroit, we debrief. The class is comprehensive and diplomatic, covering all contraceptive methods matter-of-factly. "I don't want to take away access, I want to communicate risk," says Varnam. "When I look back, I was on birth control for four years before I even had sex. I'm angry about that."

"I feel like there's this expectation that girls be on birth control," says Knight, but this is problematic because these methods don't protect against sexually transmitted infections, and they put women in a weaker position to negotiate condom use—something Varnam has experienced personally.

"Men will say something like, 'But you're on birth control,'" she says.

"And the female condom is a joke!" adds Knight. "Is there any way to make the condom better? I want the Thinx of nonhormonal birth control."

While many feminist health practitioners promote fertility awareness and have tried to expand its reach, the method didn't originate with second-wave feminism. It is very much scientific, yet it was not born out of Odeblad's lab work either. The group most interested in using the signs of fertility to prevent pregnancy was the Catholic Church. And that story begins in 1953 in Melbourne, Australia.

John and Evelyn Billings, he a neurologist, she a pediatrician, were Catholics and parents of a large and growing family (they would ultimately have nine children). John was "drawn reluctantly" to spend one night a week as a medical consultant to the local archdiocese, advising women who were trying to space their pregnancies. At first he committed to just three months, but was quickly called to find something better than the rhythm method or the Pill (which the pope had not yet decreed immoral), so he spent his other evenings searching the medical literature. "The more I read the more I found myself becoming convinced that it was the activity of the cervix during the cycle that was the most constant and positive indication of fertility and the time of ovulation, and that there we might find a solution," he wrote.[86] With the support of the archdiocese, the couple began enlisting women to "chart" their temperatures and cervical fluid changes.

The Billingses would later team up with chemist James Boyer Brown, who developed the first method of measuring estrogen levels in urine and other technologies that enabled modern fertility medicine. Brown had turned down "many attractive offers from the USA," including one from Pincus, to continue his work in the OB/GYN department at Melbourne University.[87] There, according to WOOMB International, the Billings method organization, he conducted more than 750,000 "hormonal assays" on the women who were charting, confirming the relationship between the ovulatory cycle and cervical fluid. With this large body of evidence, Evelyn Billings began formally teaching the natural family planning method, and John authored a book in 1964, titled *The Ovulation Method: Natural Family Planning*, which went through several printings and was translated into Chinese, Spanish, and Italian.

In 1977, Erik Odeblad crossed paths with the Billingses while giving a lecture to veterinarians in Sydney. It's not until this moment that the Swedish scientist learned his work had a very practical application:

women can tell whether they are near ovulation depending on which type of mucus they have, which means they can calculate when they are fertile. He also learned that the Billingses' group had been teaching this as a method of birth control for several years, and he subsequently created a training program at his university.

The Billings method took off throughout the Catholic world. Meanwhile, the science trickled down to obstetrician-gynecologists like John Rock, the Boston doctor who would go on to test the Pill; Rock used it to help patients with infertility. These physicians instructed their patients to track their cycles, take their temperatures, check for cervical mucus, and time sex with ovulation.

In 1976, Margaret Nofziger, a denizen of the Farm commune in Tennessee (also the locus of the resurgence of midwifery and home birth), published *A Cooperative Method of Natural Birth Control,* one of the first secular books in North America to instruct women in fertility awareness. In a later iteration, published in 1992, Nofziger added a preface with a mea culpa for not acknowledging the Church's contribution. "I am sorry to admit that I knew nothing of the Catholic research and involvement with basal temperature, etc. I had the mistaken but widespread impression that the Catholic Church only sanctioned 'rhythm.'" Nofziger attributed her knowledge to the medical infertility workups she went through herself: doctors had instructed her to take her temperature and look for fertile mucus. "I thought I was very clever to turn this information around for purposes of birth control," she wrote.[88]

Nofziger wrote that the Catholic Church "had a highly scientific, well developed body of information" that was so solid it formed the basis of the World Health Organization's 1967 report *Biology of Fertility Control by Periodic Abstinence.* "Fortunately, I had arrived at the same conclusions," she wrote. "We were, after all, dealing with the same physiology."

Nofziger's book led the way but stayed fringe. *Taking Charge,* on the other hand, is an international bestseller and is now in its twentieth anniversary edition. Weschler continues to get fan mail from around the world. But most of the praise is from women who read it in order to get pregnant, not for contraception.

FAM never took off as contraception the way the restrictive and moralistic "natural family planning" (NFP) did. While FAM encourages women to use barrier methods during their fertile period, NFP proscribes everything but abstinence. And NFP instruction comes with a dose of heteronormative, anti-abortion rhetoric. NFP classes are often limited to married, heterosexual couples.

The Billingses' research also led to the protocols behind "restorative reproductive medicine," which uses women's charts as a diagnostic source and personalizes hormone treatment to try to restore the cycle (more on this in chapter 2). Billings claims 50,000 teachers in China alone (for some perspective, we have fewer than 35,000 obstetricians in the United States) and a presence in 100 countries. An American competitor, the Couple to Couple League, has more than 1,000 instructors in the United States. Also under the NFP umbrella is the Creighton Model, developed by Catholic physician Thomas Hilgers, who also pioneered a restorative reproductive medicine called Natural Procreative (NaPro) Technology. A couple can learn Creighton at one of 300 Fertility*Care*™ Centers of America. In the late '80s, Weschler told me, feminist American FAM instructors created the Fertility Awareness Network and held a "conference" each year. There were eight members.

One of those members was Geraldine Matus, who trained with Creighton ("I was kicked out," she told me) and founded Justisse in 1988 as "the first systematized secular method of fertility awareness." But she encountered feminist resistance to body literacy when she would give lectures to local college students and brought up the downsides of the Pill. "I was considered a Catholic demon who was trying to destroy feminism, I literally had things thrown at me," she said.[89] "But something in me knew there was an absolute truth to how this would empower women. I know how it empowered me."

"*Our Bodies, Ourselves* was a major step forward, but even this amazing source paid scant attention to FAM's initial development and validation, even though it had begun to gain a sizable number of adherents in Europe as early as the 1960s," wrote Weschler.[90] In 1999, New Mexico–based feminist writer Katie Singer documented her search for a FAM class. "In many areas, Catholic organizations seem to provide the method's only teachers," she wrote.[91] This has changed in recent years, as organizations like Justisse, in Toronto, and Grace of the Moon, in Washington, offer online training for fertility awareness educators, and the Association of

Fertility Awareness Professionals is now standardizing instruction. Matus told me she's seen 50 percent more enrollment each year in recent years, likely because of the Internet and social media. The knowledge inspires a fervor to share it. "I wanted to stop women on the street. 'Do you know what your body does between periods?'" Weschler told me.

The learning curve poses a barrier to entry—any fertility awareness-based method requires someone who's motivated and can afford to either take classes or read a book—but it may also be a perceived one: clinicians may unconsciously draw on their own biases and assume a person lacks the discipline or intelligence to use the method. A midwife who works part time at a Planned Parenthood told me "'it feels good" to send clients home with the Pill or an IUD. Sending them home with a course pamphlet may feel like not doing enough.

The method also requires sexual agency. And clinicians are often faced with clients who lack it. Amy Willen, a nurse-midwife who works in a nonprofit clinic on Chicago's West Side, tells me many of the women she sees have little power to negotiate when sex happens. "Obviously there are better things than hormonal birth control. There's healthy relationships, there's tracking your cycle," she says. "I can't undo centuries of oppression in 15 minutes, but I can give her something that will help her not come back pregnant in six weeks." Willen agrees that in this context, hormonal contraception is a method of harm reduction, not exactly empowerment.

On the other hand, knowledge can lead to power. "These methods by definition aren't going to be effective [if women can't negotiate intercourse], but that doesn't mean you shouldn't tell them about it," says Rachel Peragallo Urrutia, an OB/GYN and lead author of the systematic review of fertility awareness-based methods mentioned above. "We can have all kinds of ideas about what's good for the public health and spacing and population control, but it's really not appropriate for us to put that on our patients."

Lisa Hendrickson-Jack has interviewed more than 100 experts on her Fertility Friday podcast and is also a FAM educator based in Toronto. There's a general concept that everybody should know, "which is that a woman is not fertile all the time. That there is only a specific window in her menstrual cycle when she is capable of getting pregnant, and if she learns to identify when that is, then she can use it to prevent pregnancy," she tells me. "Most women don't have the most basic knowledge about their menstrual cycle, and every woman who learns it says that they wish they would have learned this in junior high. They wish someone would have taught them."

In one of the more memorable podcasts, Hendrickson-Jack interviewed Laura Wershler, and they discussed ideological resistance to the method. Wershler had strong words for that camp: "If you're a doctor who serves women, if you're a nurse who works in a sexual health clinic, if you're a health care provider or counselor in any way and you're not acknowledging FAM . . . then you're not doing your job, you're not a pro-choice sexual and reproductive health advocate," she said.

It seems strange, and worth examining, why FAM struggles for feminist cred. "I think part of the reason FAM is not available everywhere and not in every textbook is because of where it came from," meaning the Church, says Hendrickson-Jack. The people who've dismissed it on these grounds also "don't believe it works, they don't understand the science behind fertility awareness."

Geraldine Matus, who also has a doctorate in psychology, believes there's something more fundamental at work, that even feminists have internalized a patriarchal framing of medical technology, in which we look to it for power over nature. And so we embrace the Pill and dismiss the "natural," even if that means interfering with our health. "In our intention to get our bodies out of the patriarchy, we've actually put upon ourselves the same injuries. Because we're trying to control our bodies rather than living in harmony with nature," she says.

"You have to recognize what the Pill meant for people and what it has done for the world," says Hendrickson-Jack. "I'm not anti-Pill from a philosophical standpoint. I don't think that women shouldn't have access to birth control," she adds. "What I do advocate for is full and complete understanding, full disclosure and informed consent," and a more nuanced approach to health. "If you go to the doctor's office with menstrual pain, you get the Pill. If you go with a problematic cycle, you get the Pill. Nobody's asking, why do you have pain? Why do you have acne? What are the underlying factors? Women are not being served fully by this ideology," she says.

FAM's limited acceptance could also just be a question of branding. Men get the discrete words "semen" or "seminal fluid" for their distinctly mucosal ejaculate (and also the perfectly fine word "ejaculate"), but women get "mucus"—ever so slightly preferable to the medical/militaristic horror of "discharge," which Weschler calls "the D-word."

The stretchy, translucent, slippery-slick wonder substance that will carry and protect sperm is not pourable or drip-droppy, like fluid. It's tougher than that. But it is definitely not snot. I'm thinking we need to steal a word from the beauty aisle. Cervical gloss? Serum? The French "gelée"? There is "hydrogel," which sounds almost space age. Or we could co-opt a term from reproductive technology (so often it's the other way around): How about "cervical medium"?

Because a medium is exactly what the fluid is, providing sperm a portal to their destination. And it is smart, in the way that technology is smart. It gums up underperforming sperm, transports the crème de la crème, and feeds and cares for those tiny flapping germ cells. It is a gatekeeper. And when the medium is not present, the cervix makes a smart lotion that exfoliates and keeps the vaginal walls supple, that is also like a veil whose acidic pH stops sperm in their tracks. This we could call a contraceptive moisturizer.

(Cervical "crypts" are another problem. When I hear that word I think death. Medieval churches. Horror films. "Pockets" sounds too casual. Maybe these are little purses, or hideaways, or clutches. They are protective of potential life, not sealants of decay. Alas, Odeblad was a scientist, not a copywriter.)

The radical thing about FAM is that it allows people to achieve the same contraceptive outcome through less *control* of our bodies and more of a relationship—with oneself, with one's partner(s)—that requires curiosity, respect, and agency. Women can learn to distinguish the lotion from the gelée. We've all taken our temperature. And now, dozens of apps make it simple to chart, prompting you daily to record whether your fluid is "dry," "egg white," "creamy," or "atypical" (data that will be shared with the app's developer, of course). Though the technology of the Pill may have upstaged fertility awareness for 50 years, technology may bring it back by the light of the smartphone.

2: FERTILITY INSURANCE

A HANDFUL OF SPERM are swimming across the screen in no particular direction. A sharp pen-like device enters the screen from the right. I'm standing a few steps behind Adrienne Reing, an embryologist at the Institute for Reproductive Medicine and Science at St. Barnabas Medical Center, in Livingston, New Jersey, watching the modern miracle of in vitro fertilization. Reing has her right hand on a joystick and her left hand on a dial. She eyes her target, one out of maybe five swimmers, though I'm not yet sure how she sets them apart, and takes a jab.

"She just disabled it," John Garrisi, the lab director, explains. She breaks it? I ask, somewhat startled. "It does break the tail, but it's OK, because the tail is unnecessary, and because we're going to perform the function of the tail." The tool she's using is actually a needle the width of a human hair, with an even finer tip.

Reing sucks the fin-less swimmer into the needle's chamber with the dial. She repeats this on four more screens, each with just a few sperm spread out, choosing, striking, and collecting four more sperm into the same needle. "She's lining them up in the tool," Garrisi says.

She then rotates the "drop" under the microscope, bringing her next target into view: the egg, so large it just fits on the screen. "What we're doing right now is working against the clock," says Garrisi. "Those eggs are very sensitive to pH, to temperature, and there in not the best environment right now, they belong in the incubator. So she's working to get them back as soon as possible."

The eggs are so sensitive to their environment, I'm told, that my very presence may be having an effect. Earlier that day, I suited up in a blue paper "bunny suit" and hair net in the locker room with Serena Chen, a reproductive endocrinologist and director of reproductive medicine at St. Barnabas, who set up the lab visit. I asked if this is what the partners wear. "You know, we do not let them in," said Chen. "They get a picture [of the embryo being transferred that day], and they're told to positively visualize in the waiting room. The less people we have in the lab, the better it is for the embryos." A medical resident is with us as well, but only because of my visit. "We hardly ever give tours," I'm told. I try to send good energy to the eggs. "Energy matters," said Chen.

This particular egg has a nice shape, all agree. Spherical, with a billowy cloud around it. I want to keep watching but Garrisi draws my attention to the island in the middle of the smallish lab—it is not much bigger than a modern kitchen, with many beige fridge-like appliances decorated with multicolored labels. He wants to explain the egg's role in physiological conception, so I can appreciate the embryologist's role in the dish. Wearing a black surgeon's cap and teal scrubs, he has the aura of a judo master—soft-spoken, looks you in the eye, confident, and kind. He grabs a paper and pen and draws a circle with a ring around it. The cloud surrounding the egg is the zona pellucida, he explains, and in a physiological conception, it serves as the gatekeeper through which just one sperm will ultimately pass, a complex molecular event. The zona pellucida is sticky. Each sperm head has a special sauce of enzymes that are released upon encounter with it, and the sperm with the best sauce and swimming action will essentially "digest its way through the zona pellucida."

The sperm that makes it through will then touch the egg membrane itself, which causes an electrical reaction. "Calcium ions go out, the electrical pulse spreads in either direction," says Garrisi. The egg will respond by opening what's called the perivitelline space, a kind of foyer between the egg's front door and the egg itself. Once this happens, the egg hardens its outer gate, he says, essentially closing the door to any more suitors. If more than one sperm happen to breach the zona pellucida at once, the runners up will be locked in the foyer. In 2014, researchers at Northwestern University observed that millions of zinc atoms are released at this point, "in a display that looks just like tiny fireworks and lasts about two hours after fertilisation," as one report put it.[1]

So reproduction really requires electricity and movement.

In physiological conception, only around 100 sperm out of tens, perhaps hundreds, of millions complete the journey through the cervix, up into the uterus, down into the fallopian tube, to meet the egg soon after it's released from the ovary. Think about this—100 out of 100 million is just .0001 percent. That means various mechanisms are in play so that it's not a pile-on.

The biology of conception has launched a thousand metaphors of sperm racing to the finish line, competing for first place, vying for the prize, the trophy, and others. And if not sports comparisons, it's military metaphors (sperm become missiles, warheads). But the biological reality is that the female body is actively guiding and selecting at every stage of the journey. The substance at least as interesting as semen is the fertile cervical "mucus" Erik Odeblad studied, which the cervix produces in the days leading up to ovulation. It plays an essential role in conception: it washes the sperm of its seminal carrier fluid (which the egg wants none of), traps sperm that are misshapen or slow, carries the ideal candidates up its molecular strands, and can even preserve choice candidates in the cervix's "crypts," keeping them alive with sugars and carbohydrates. Some 70 percent of the sperm don't make it past this point. Their population is further reduced at the velvet-rope entrance to the fallopian tube, which bounces even more.

"Basically, the fastest sperm don't fertilize the egg because they are immature," Scott Gilbert, a professor of biology at Swarthmore College and author of many papers and chapters on the subject, explains. Rather, the sperm spend hours or days being matured by cells inside the fallopian tube: it's called "capacitation." The cells initiate chemical reactions that change the sperm's membrane, "allowing the sperm to sense the presence of the egg (and to travel toward it) and to fuse with the egg cell once it finds it. So there is cooperation between the sperm cells and the mother of the baby!" To his credit, Gilbert coauthored a paper critical of sexist metaphors in 1989, pointing out that scientists knew of the female's role starting in the 1950s.[2]

The egg, once released, signals its arrival, possibly with progesterone carried from the ovary on its cumulus cells, which "hyperactivates" the sperm, allowing them to detach, finally turning them into the Olympic swimmers of their mythology. Perhaps then and only then is it really a race to the finish line. Still, the sperm must navigate the cloud of cumulus cells to even reach the zona pellucida.

Assisted reproductive technology mimics or obviates many of these mechanisms. Millions of sperm (hopefully) are collected, "washed" with a synthetic mucus-like compound, and filtered. In IVF, the sperm that make the cut—ideally more than one thousand—are "matured" in a special medium, mimicking capacitation. Then they are deposited directly onto their single-cell maid in waiting (somewhat of a pile-on).

"To see it, it's interesting because they're all stuck, they've all got beating tails, and they're spinning the egg," says Garrisi. He likens the sperms' action on the egg to "a bunch of dogs playing with a beach ball."

In intrauterine insemination, or IUI, which requires a sperm tally in the millions, pre-washed sperm are brought past the cervix (and cervical fluid) directly into the uterus. Still, the remainder of the choosing and capacitating is done by the egg and its allies, as it would be after intercourse.

What I'm about to watch on screen will skip all of that, because Reing is about to inject a single sperm directly past the egg's protective zona, right into the center of the egg itself. That is what Garrisi meant when he said, "We're going to perform the function of the tail," though that's not even the half of it. In intracytoplasmic sperm injection, or ICSI (ick-see), the embryologist does the selecting and initiates the movement. She opens the electrified door by mechanical means.

Reing positions the egg, which has been "denuded" of its cumulus, with a pipette on the left holding it in place while she lines up the sperm-loaded needle on the right. Slow and steady, the needle is poking the egg, a triangular fold revealing the pressure—Garrisi pokes his own scrubs with a pen to help me visualize what I'm seeing in two dimensions. "We need to break the membrane in order to deposit the sperm inside. When you just poke it like that, it actually doesn't break, it just gives," he says.

The sperm is a visible dot in the needle, and as the needle is poking, the sperm looks as if it's retreating, trying to swim away from its fate, though that's not actually what's happening (because it can no longer swim). "She's pulling back the suction in order to break the zona pellucida," explains Garrisi. "That tool, even though it's sharp, will not break the membrane. Sucking it past the sharp needle is what breaks it." Something too subtle for me to notice tells the embryologist that the membrane is broken, and propulsion sends the sperm right into the egg's middle. Reing then retracts the needle, the next sperm waiting near the tip. She rotates the drop, bringing another round egg into focus, and repeats the process in under a minute.

"So what happens now is the egg becomes activated by the process of the stick," says Garrisi. "Normally the electrical impulse will initiate egg activation, but it turns out that the physical stick will do the same thing. So now the egg knows it's been fertilized." If all goes well, Garrisi explains, the sperm's nucleus will soon transform into a pronucleus. Then the two pronuclei will fuse and the fertilized single-cell egg will divide into two, then four, then eight, and by day five it will be a roughly 60-cell blastocyst.

SAFER SEX?

For millions of parents worldwide each year, this laboratory or one like it is the bedroom in which their child was conceived. For women, assisted reproductive technologies offer an extension on the biological clock—a technological workaround, especially for those who've devoted their 20s and 30s to building a career.

ICSI—with fresh eggs, with frozen eggs, with donor eggs—is the most high-tech workaround possible, and it is the method used for about three-quarters of all cycles in the United States.[3] For about 10 percent of cycles, the "micromanipulation" of the cells does not end there. More and more clinics are offering preimplantation genetic screening and diagnosis (PGS and PGD) in which an embryologist biopsies a days-old blastocyst—removes one of those 60 or so cells and inspects it for all 46 chromosomes; they can even look for markers for a handful of horrible, fatal diseases, like cystic fibrosis, Tay-Sachs, and Huntington's.

Garrisi leads us to a smaller adjacent room with four human-size stainless steel thermoses: freezers full of eggs and embryos. He opens one, and like a theatrical cauldron, fog spills over. After biopsy, he freezes the cleared embryos. If a clinic is offering biopsy without this technology, they're doing a disservice to the patient, he says. "This allows us to transfer one embryo at a time." Which allows them to prevent twins, which ups the overall success rate. The way Chen explains it to her patients is that "two transferred at the same time is a 75 percent pregnancy rate, and two embryos in two separate transfers has an overall 90 percent chance of pregnancy."

PGD testing began as a way for couples with grave genetic inheritances to ensure they didn't pass on a disease (or go through an abortion following prenatal testing). But more and more, it's just another step in the reproductive technology process after you've already come so far.

"I feel like a lot of patients who we have right now who are high-risk, they say why would I ever transfer an untested embryo after everything I've been through?" Chen says. A few weeks after we meet, she'll participate on a panel at the famed 92nd Street Y in New York City called "The End of Sex," along with Stanford bioethicist Henry Greely, author of the book by the same name, and they'll seriously consider the possibility that in the not-too-distant future, even fertile heterosexual couples will prefer needle-pipette conception over skin-to-skin. "People will say, well, it's much safer and much more cost effective to get pregnant this way than any other way," she says.

Her point is that, theoretically, the screening technology will reduce the risk of miscarriage and birth defects. Greely argues the technology is already here. "If we can do that, why would you take those risks? Then sex becomes a little bit of a reproductive Russian roulette," says Chen.

This of course presumes so many things, for one, that miscarriage is worse an ordeal than IVF, neither of which I have ever heard any woman call a picnic. In order for the embryologists to have eggs to work with, those eggs need to be "harvested" from a human, who must take ovary-stimulating hormone injections for weeks prior, travel to the clinic for multiple transvaginal ultrasounds to check on progress, and then return to have a needle threaded through her vagina into her ovary (under anesthesia) to extract eggs from each follicle. Then another visit for the embryo insertion, more hormones, and waiting in the hopes of a pregnancy (and not another cycle). The other big problem with the "Why risk sex?" argument is that it presumes that we know all the risks of these procedures and micromanipulations, which we don't.

IVF has been in wide use for 30 years; ICSI for 15. Studies on the long-term outcomes of all "are scarce."[4] Biopsy is still experimental, according to the American Society for Reproductive Medicine. While some studies have detected no problems in toddlers who were biopsied as embryos, others have detected neurodevelopmental abnormalities in areas such as fine and large motor function and muscle tone.[5] And of course there is no long-term evidence yet—these children aren't old enough to reproduce. In 2012, Michelle LaBonte, then a biologist at Wellesley College, now at Harvard, surveyed the web sites of more than 250 fertility clinics offering the test. Nearly 80 percent did not mention risks at all, and two-thirds of those that did still said the procedure was safe regardless.[6] In a piece she wrote for the *Journal of Medical Ethics*, she raises the possibility that PGD is being oversold, the same way amniocentesis was assumed safe until studies showed that it increases the risk of miscarriage.

We make this mistake not infrequently with new medical technology, especially in OB/GYN. For a long time cesarean sections were thought to be safer for the baby, but then it turned out that bypassing vaginal birth raises the risk for asthma, obesity, and a host of other conditions nobody ever could have imagined until there was long-term data to show a connection. We think we can do it better than nature, and then nature says, I told you so.

Studies show that babies conceived with assisted reproductive technology (ART), either IVF or ICSI, have roughly double the rate of birth defects, even among singletons who are not premature.[7] Twins categorically have worse outcomes, and while there has been a definite movement over the past decade among fertility clinics toward "single embryo transfer," twins still account for one-quarter of technologically assisted pregnancies in the United States.[8]

"There is a gap in our knowledge about the long-term outcomes of ART," says Judith Stern, a professor of obstetrics and gynecology at Dartmouth Geisel School of Medicine. "We've been doing this for well over 30 years at this point, and about 15 years ago we started realizing that there really were adverse outcomes, at least in the short term for babies." Those include low birth weight, increased risk of prematurity, and possibly birth defects. That said, she and a team of researchers in Boston are finding that it's difficult to separate the effects of ART from the effects of infertility—in other words, the poor outcomes in babies may have more to do with the biological fitness of the parents than the technology per se. "But we really don't know anything about the long-term effects, not only on the kids but on the women who undergo treatment," she says. There are lingering questions about links to cancer, diabetes, and cardiovascular disease.

All these concerns apply to egg donors as well, and to women now sold on the promise of egg freezing, who are essentially donating eggs to their future selves. Donors have even less research to go on, because the only studies of long-term risks like breast and ovarian cancer are in women undergoing IVF, and those studies are inconclusive. Infertility itself is associated with a higher risk of cancer, whereas egg donors tend to be healthy. As some researchers and advocates argue, "The clear and ethical solution to extrapolating from infertile women is to actually carry out long-term studies of egg donors."[9]

Neither Chen nor Garrisi show much concern about risks. "Nothing I do is anywhere near as risky as the process of pregnancy and delivery," Chen likes to say. Yet she does tell me about "the dish effect," which points to some added risk for IVF/ICSI babies. The most obvious sign of a dish effect is the rate at which dish embryos cleave into identical twins: it is four times the rate of natural twinning (2 percent versus 0.5 percent). "Those are very high-risk and have a higher rate of birth defects," Chen tells me. "The fact that we make more of them with IVF, it has to be the dish effect."

I ask Garrisi what the risk is to the human embryo, removing one-sixtieth of its minuscule form. "Virtually zero," he says. "Yeah, but that's for him, that's not for everybody," Chen interjects. If it were that easy, every fertility clinic around the country would be offering it, but it takes tremendous skill, coordination, and hours of clinician time. "Patients come to me all the time and say my doctor said PGD would not be good for me, and I'm like, 'Well yeah, because you're at a program where the lab is not comfortable doing PGD,' they don't have the skill or experience to feel comfortable and make the benefits outweigh the risks. Because there *are* risks—you're doing microsurgery on the embryo. If it's someone with decades of experience doing it"—she nods at Garrisi—"he can say zero, but it's really not zero." She cites a large Dutch study in which "they killed six percent of their embryos."

ICSI originally developed as a way for men with too few sperm to genetically father a child, what's called "male factor" in the biz. The technology can help a man who's diagnosed as azoospermic, having a semen sperm count of zero—as long as a surgeon can extract a single sperm from within his testes, fertilization could happen. But ICSI may also have driven its own ascendance.

This is because the "egg denuding" process became irresistible for embryologists simply preparing an IVF. For the eggs to be easily penetrated in ICSI, an embryologist must remove the outer cumulus cells. To do this they suck an egg into a needle and propel it out in various medium solutions—rinse and repeat, rinse and repeat—until the zona pellucida is the only barrier remaining.

It seemed logical that by stripping the egg, they could better tell whether it was mature, ready for union. So embryologists began denuding eggs en masse. What they didn't realize (and many may not still, because nothing is standardized in fertility medicine) is that the act of stripping makes fertilization in IVF less likely. Scott Gilbert has an explanation: the cumulus cells are what "hyperactivate" the sperm, better enabling one to fuse with the egg. If this removal of the cumulus is as widespread as some experts suspect, it has caused a lot of additional cycles for the women from whom the eggs were extracted, and it has accelerated the use of ICSI.

Today, ICSI's use has far outpaced male factor infertility. Even the St. Barnabas center, which considers itself conservative in this regard, performed ICSI procedures for four clients and IVF for one the day I was there. Everyone seems to prefer it. "If you see an embryo that has been fertilized after routine IVF, it's like a minefield, there's just little loser sperm all over. They've got their little faces stuck to the outside, and he has to dodge around them," says Chen, referring to Garrisi if he's doing an embryonic biopsy ("loser sperm" can complicate the result). "Our guideline is a very low threshold for ICSI," Garrisi echoes. "If the sperm is normal, we do IVF. If there's any doubt whatsoever, we'll do ICSI. If we're doing genetic testing, we do ICSI. If we have unexplained infertility, we do half ICSI." In short, ICSI is the answer when there's any question. "There's little downside to doing the ICSI for a patient who doesn't need it," he says.

Except, what if there is? And would it be possible to treat "male factor" by treating men?

THE MALE FACTOR

One interesting thing about sperm is their sheer numbers. "If you look at the process of the body making sperm, it's the rapid division of new cells. It's a mark of your cellular health," Sara Naab, one of about 25 "sperm nerds" in the country, explains to me. "A typical man is making 1,500 sperm in a second. Every second. They're cranking out sperm, so these are rapidly, constantly dividing cells. Very few cells in the body do that—the only other cells that divide that fast are cancer cells, which is why cancer treatments are so deadly to fertility" (and hair follicles—also rapidly dividing cells). Thus, a man's ability to produce copious, precocious sperm is a measure of health.

Naab has become an expert in this field not as an academic but as an entrepreneur: she and her husband launched Trak, the first FDA-approved at-home sperm counting device. She wants men to take more of an interest in their health, and in sperm count as the vehicle. Diabetes, heart disease, obesity—"Anything that happens to your body will impact those rapidly dividing cells. They need oxygen, they need all those nutrients." Alcohol, drugs, and smoking can lower counts. So can antidepressants, pesticides, antibiotics, and, perhaps surprisingly, testosterone treatment (though you wouldn't learn that from a "Low T" campaign). Hard-core cyclists can have misshapen sperm—a friend's husband fixed this completely by switching to a "butt pad" seat.

"Men can also have hormonal imbalances. And that's a major cause of infertility, just like in women," says Naab. "For women, high levels of sugar in their diet can lead to problems. It's the same in men." One problem with a high glycemic diet is the surplus of aromatase, which causes too much testosterone to convert to estrogen. At Boston University, a couples study called PRESTO found that even one can of sugary soda a day reduced fertility by one-third in men and one-quarter in women, explains Lauren Wise, one of the researchers. Energy drinks had an even greater impact.[10] Sperm can also take a hit on the storage side after perfect production. They have a very narrow comfort zone, temperature-wise, which is why the testes hang outside the body. But skinny jeans, a laptop, bike shorts—"You could have a low count because you're cooking your balls," says Naab.

This phrasing is actually why we met, at a conference called Fertility Planit (tagline: *Everything you need to create your family*). I was taking a last pass through a hallway of vendors displaying things like growth medium, egg-freezing machines, and a DIY inseminator wand called "The Stork." Then I saw the shot glasses: "Don't Cook Your Balls," they instructed. Naab handed me one and showed me her device, a mini centrifuge that resembles a squat coffee grinder. She was the only one, vendor, speaker, or otherwise, who said anything about male fertility.

The gadget fit in her palm—a round, slate-gray plastic case, powered by two AA batteries. She called that part "the engine." A droplet-sized sample goes in the pupil-like center of the "prop," a dark, slender blade that snaps onto the engine, where it spins at about 6,500 rotations per minute for six and a half minutes under the locked Lucite lid. The spinning basically accelerates gravity, separating out the sperm cells ("the densest cells in the body," she tells me), which are then driven into a clear chamber, creating a visible "pellet" along a ruler that indicates the count. It's essentially a miniature, portable, user-friendly version of the centrifuge professional labs use to separate red blood cells from plasma.

Naab's husband, an engineer, patented the technology with a partner, and the three decided to launch their own company. But they were not yet sure which bodily fluid the device would test, or for what. "When we started talking about fertility and men's fertility, I said, is this even a thing?" Naab had dealt with her own fertility problems when the couple decided to start a family—now they are juggling four kids and a start-up. "I thought, Do men have fertility problems? It didn't even register in my brain."

So Naab, who has a degree in library science, started researching and talking to experts. And she applied some logic: of course men must have fertility problems! In fact, research suggests they account for about half of all infertility.[11] But "people are not doing research because IVF is basically a cure."

One of those experts, Paul Turek, a California-based urologist, has the same mixed feelings about IVF. For the chance it gives men who had, say, survived cancer, to father a child: "Three cheers!" he tells me. But "IVF also was a terrible thing for men's health. Because it has shuttled men who are infertile straight to IVF, and what has been forsaken in that shuttling is the opportunity to take care of them. Because it has become very clear that fertility is a biomarker of health." In 2009, Turek and a team published a study connecting low sperm count to increased cancer risk.[12] "That was incredibly earthshaking basic science research," he says. In 2016, he participated in meetings at the NIH devoted to the subject of male fertility—whether it is declining worldwide, which some studies suggest, and what that reveals about men's health.

In general, however, the focus of fertility clinics is women, and it's on their bodies that the "treatment" is delivered. After all, reproductive endocrinologists are OB/GYNs who went through an extra fellowship, likely at a fertility center. In the United States, they number around 3,000, while there are two or three hundred urologists with training in men's hormones and fertility, says Turek. Male infertility is also not recognized as a subspecialty—there's no board certification like there is for reproductive endocrinologists. Says Naab: "A general urology clinic is not going to have someone really versed in fertility. Most of them will know the plumbing, they're surgeons so they're good with plumbing, but not good at understanding hormonal imbalances."

That is to say, they are not looking at sperm count as a vital sign. It is just a fact. "When I see a man in the office with fertility problems and his sperm count is low, I look at him very differently," says Turek, who has boutique practices (where patients pay out of pocket) in LA and San Francisco. "I give him a 200-question questionnaire, I ask a lot of questions about what he eats, his lifestyle, what his stressors are. People say the fifth vital sign is pain? No more! My fifth vital sign is waist circumference." Turek also screens for Y chromosome deletion (a relatively recent blood test) and other physical and genetic factors. But most men aren't given this kind of attention. He tells me about one study that found that just 18 to 20 percent of infertile men in the United States get a urologic evaluation for the diagnosis of infertility. "Which means that 100 percent are getting a semen analysis, but 80 percent don't get any care," says Turek.

This assumption that low sperm counts just are, that they can't be fixed, is entrenched in medicine. "I came to this field when half of infertility was unexplained, and that has carried through two generations," he says. "The gynecologists happen to have the perfect technology for things you can't fix, which is IVF. It's a cultural problem, not an individual problem, so I've been trying to teach gynecologists that semen analysis is a biomarker of health, and maybe the first referral is to a specialist to get the guy checked out." Turek says in European countries with nationalized health care, this is the norm. "Because it's cheaper! It's cheaper for the system to evaluate the man first. It's one-tenth of the price of evaluating the woman. It's a win-win." Plus, it might save the woman needless procedures, I point out. And maybe make a healthier baby as well. "Yeah, it's a win-win-win-win!" he says.

For example, one common, little-known problem for men is called varicocele. These are dilated veins in the scrotum that heat up the testicles—cooking those balls—Turek explains, and they account for 35 to 40 percent of primary infertility in men. "It's just an anatomical problem of blood going the wrong way," says Turek, something that started happening to humanoids around the time we stood up, something that happens to guys around puberty, often the fit, active ones. Typically a man with unknown varicocele will present with a low sperm count, unexplained, and his partner will be recommended for IUI. Turek's team crunched the numbers and found that surgical repair of varicocele is about the same cost as three rounds of IUI. If the sperm count is low enough to recommend IVF, "then varicocele repair is cheaper hands down than IVF," he says. And that's assuming three cycles (three months of injections, ultrasounds, and procedures for the woman). Repairing that vein, on the other hand, takes one hour. Recovery is a day or two on the couch and some Vicodin.

Staring at Naab's device in the conference hall, it struck me that it resembles the classic hard plastic pack of birth control pills. And this idea, that men have systems that need regular checking—that they have an equal share of fertility issues, that they could simply quit soda or switch to cargo pants or have a minor surgery and save their partners hours upon hours of invasive needles and ultrasound wands, the risks of hormone exposures, and the "dish effect"—this may be as revolutionary as the Pill.

And to Turek's point, that IVF is not really health care in the traditional sense of the word, but rather a technological fix—that it shunts men from actual care—why wouldn't this hold true for women as well?

Two days before Holly, who wanted to use her first name only, was scheduled for her first intrauterine insemination, "Snowzilla" clawed its way from northern Virginia to New York City. On Sunday, January 23, 2016, Holly's home of Reston, Virginia, was under 29 inches of snow. The clinic had stationed doctors in nearby hotels so none of its patients would have to forgo a cycle come Monday. As the storm subsided, Holly and her husband actually heard the welcome sounds of a city plow, but it didn't come all the way down their cul-de-sac. So the day before her 9 a.m. appointment, Holly spent six hours digging out their driveway, coaxing her husband to help for part of the day, though he wanted to just reschedule. Not Holly. She had put in her time for this date. Given the diagnosis of "unexplained infertility" at age 32, she was not going to let Mother Nature give her any more grief. She woke up before dawn the next morning and shoveled for another two hours.

In preparation for the insemination, she had endured "every side effect they listed, and then some," from the drug Clomid. She'd gone back and forth to the clinic, 24 miles away, at least five times for vaginal ultrasounds to check on the follicles. Then she took the "trigger shot" of the hormone hCG, which prompts ovulation. In Holly, it triggered more. "It's pretty terrible. I lose my shit, just pumping those hormones into my body. I cry, I get light-headed, really emotional."

For all of her 20s, Holly hadn't even wanted kids, but then one day around the time she turned 30 something in her switched. Like many women, she went off the Pill and started casually trying. "For the first year, we weren't necessarily in a hurry. So we just lived our lives as normal." But knowing the conventional wisdom that a year without birth control or a pregnancy can mean infertility, she went to her OB/GYN to ask some questions. (For women over 35, the conventional wisdom on that window is six months.)

Her doctor performed a hysterosalpingogram, which confirmed her fallopian tubes were clear. They took blood to check her hormone levels—all within range. Even though her periods were a bit irregular she appeared to be ovulating—she had been checking herself with a store-bought kit for several months. Her OB also looked at something many do not: she tested Holly's husband's sperm count. It was a little low.

Even though Holly looked fine and her husband's count signaled it could be the problem, her doctor suggested she take Clomid. "It was terrible. I had nausea, hot flashes, nightmares, paranoia. I started mixing up my left and right, I was bloated and had an upset stomach," she told me. She quit after a month. She also stopped seeing her doctor—the only OB/GYN she'd ever gone to. "I don't know if I trusted her. I just feel like she didn't answer my questions. I would say, Why isn't my period regular? And she would say, 'I don't know, maybe you should go see a specialist,'" said Holly.

Another year went by, and she found a new OB/GYN who was well rated. "She was really lovely, and she had us do tests again, because it had been more than a year." Again, Holly's tests came back fine. Her husband didn't want another sperm count, so they put it off. When Holly told the new doctor that her periods were irregular, the doctor also suggested Clomid. "I told her about side effects, but she asked me to try again. She said this is really the next step." Holly did two more cycles under her care.

Clomid is typically taken on days three through seven of the menstrual cycle (with day one being the first day of a period). "So the day you get your period you call the clinic and tell them 'Today is day one,'" Holly told me. Then on day three, blood work and a vaginal ultrasound in the office, then five days of Clomid. "I had hot flashes those five days" along with the laundry list, she said. "And oh, I was super emotional. How could I forget that one? It was to the point where for a week I would cry every day about something. I would say, 'I'm so sorry, I don't know why I'm crying, it's the Clomid.'"

Since her doctor had recommended this as a remedy for the irregular periods, which made it difficult to tell when ovulation would occur, Holly "just assumed that Clomid was going to make me ovulate on time," so she and her husband followed the rule to have sex every other day starting on day 12. "But I was probably ovulating later, and it turned out I was traveling on the days when I was ovulating." The second month back on Clomid she had to travel to Turkey for work. "There were nights when I was completely drenched and would have to take all my clothes off. The whole plane ride back I was having hot flashes."

This is when her doctor labeled her with "unexplained infertility." This diagnosis, which typically portends invasive medical procedures, is not defined by test results or symptoms, but rather by time and math. "Let's say you have a couple who has not conceived for one year, statistically their per-cycle pregnancy rate drops from 15 to 20 percent down to 1 or 2 percent per month," says Serena Chen, the fertility specialist in New Jersey. In other words, the label is really more of a prognostication than a diagnosis, and the decision to treat is theoretically a gamble with better odds. "It's playing the numbers game," says Chen. "We're not treating people who are sterile. We're just treating people who have suboptimal fertility—often people could get pregnant on their own, and what we're trying to do is shorten the time to conceive." If that hypothetical couple who hasn't conceived for a year were to try for another year, on their own, they have a 30 percent chance of conceiving at some point. "But with Clomid IUI we can get a 10 to 12 percent rate per month [thus a 32 percent rate in three months]. With IVF you can go significantly higher," says Chen. "So both are shortening the time to conceive and increasing the per-cycle pregnancy rate."

For her part, Chen is focused on the health of her patients as well as making babies, which she says was not part of her training. "Something I really enjoy about what I do is that even if we don't do all these high-tech treatments, we improve their lives and educate them about their body, their health. And because this process is so stressful, the idea of becoming healthier is really empowering to a lot of my patients." So maybe they quit smoking, lose a few pounds, eat more vegetables, get more sleep. "Just to be generally healthier makes a huge difference" in having a higher pregnancy success rate, she says. "I think hopefully today they're teaching that in med school, but it's definitely not something I learned."

Still, Chen has little hesitation about using all of the tools at her disposal. "The treatments we do are very, very low risk. It's true, when I see a couple with unexplained infertility, I say everything looks fine, you can keep trying, or here are the options." But she adds, "What people don't realize is there's a cost to waiting, to doing nothing. There's a lot of data showing that the stress of infertility is just as high as the stress of having cancer or the death of a loved one. People are suffering, they have a tremendous amount of stress and anxiety and divorce and lost days from work."

When it comes to doing nothing or doing something, we in the United States are not only a culture of doing something, we're a culture of doing more. As Chen shows me around her clinic, across the street from Garrisi's lab, she points out the five ultrasound rooms where patients preparing for IVF will "come in and take their bottoms off" and get a read on their follicles. "We do more monitoring here than in any other country," she says. Three visuals the first week, then almost every day of the second week up until the eggs are extracted, even though in Europe they may only get scanned once a week. Why? Number one, "patients want to be monitored," says Chen. They're taking multiple injections, going through a surgical procedure. "They like the hands-on approach." Chen also mentions revenue, referring to the fee-for-service system that incentivizes more billable procedures, but she also believes that close watching results in better outcomes. The typical IVF cycle requires a tightly orchestrated sequence of medications: the patient is given what's called a gonadotropin-releasing hormone (GnRH) analogue, which signals the hypothalamus to stop signaling the pituitary. "That prevents premature ovulation and allows us to control the cycle and retrieve more eggs," says Chen. The next step is to stimulate the ovaries with gonadotropins (follicle-stimulating hormone and luteinizing hormone) and monitor the developing follicles to determine the optimal moment for the "trigger" shot of human chorionic gonadotropin and for egg retrieval. "If you're not adjusting the medications or not starting the medications when you should, then you might have to cancel the cycle," says Chen.

The assisted reproductive cycle is a huge physical, emotional, and often financial investment. But the return isn't that great. The CDC compiled data from nearly 500 clinics and reported that in 2015, just 23 percent of 186,000 cycles with non-donor eggs resulted in a live birth (with donor eggs the success rate was 39 percent). That's an incomplete number because it doesn't account for other treatments and IUI.[13] So for every successful IVF/ICSI birth there are two or three unsuccessful transfers, conferring an unknown amount of risk. Another limitation is that the number is an average across the population of patients. One woman could become pregnant and carry that pregnancy to term after one cycle, while another could only do so after six cycles, and another could go through several cycles, or several miscarriages, and call it quits. Miriam Zoll, author of the memoir *Cracked Open*, went through three unsuccessful cycles, including a miscarriage. A friend of hers went through *eighteen*. Both wound up adopting.

"In this field we're very good at making babies," Chen tells me, "but we're very bad at answering questions of why."

FERTILITY TREATMENT VERSUS TREATMENT

Danielle Miller is a physician in Lancaster, Pennsylvania. She has a busy primary care practice and a reputation throughout the region for helping women in particular. "If you show up to a physician and you say you have chest pain or abdominal pain, people don't generally guess what's wrong with you and give you a prescription and send you home. There is some investigation into what is going on," she says. Chest pain or abdominal pain could mean any number of things. Likewise, infertility can have many different causes. "But in women's health there's so little regard for correcting the underlying abnormalities or for trying to figure out what's going on." Instead, says Miller, "covering up the symptoms, removing the organs, or bypassing normal functions is generally the treatment protocol for most problems."

Miller specialized in family practice but went outside conventional training to learn what's known broadly as restorative reproductive medicine, which is based on close monitoring of hormone levels and cervical fluid and other cyclical biomarkers to make a diagnosis and tailor treatment specifically to an individual. This medical counterpart to charting one's menstrual cycle was pioneered by Thomas Hilgers of the Creighton Model as fertility medicine that would be available to women adhering to Catholic teachings. "It's a way of approaching reproductive care that would cooperate with the woman's cycle and if possible restore her normal reproductive functioning," says Rachel Peragallo Urrutia, an OB/GYN in Cary, North Carolina, who also takes this approach. "By contrast, with IVF you suppress the woman's normal cycle and give her lots of medicines to give her a 'super' cycle."

The field is medical yet it exists on the margins of mainstream medicine, and "part of the reason is the level of research available in this field is low and poor quality," says Urrutia, also a researcher, though she mentions two large studies that found that 50 percent of patients who engaged in restorative care for a year had successful pregnancies. Another reason is that the protocols go by different names—NaPro, Neo, FEMM. Many providers (though not Urrutia) are Catholic physicians who sign an "ethics statement" that they won't provide abortion services or referrals, that they will support local "crisis pregnancy centers," and that they will only assist reproduction for hetero, married couples. "Of course, there are women who are interested in these type of treatments who are not Catholic, because they don't want to go through IVF," says Urrutia.

Miller is not Catholic and prefers to stay "apolitical." Patients find her by word of mouth, many after having undergone basic infertility testing or treatment, some traveling 90 miles or more to see her. "Nine times out of ten they'll tell me they have 'undiagnosed infertility,'" she says. The terms "undiagnosed" and "unexplained" are interchangeable (there's some debate over which term is more scientific) and it infuriates Miller that her peers rarely take the inquiry any further.[14] "We as a medical community, by and large, are completely unprepared to meet the needs of women having a reproductive issue—or men, for that matter."

Aside from testing to detect a blocked fallopian tube or some other structural issue, the formula seems to be to put the patient (back) on the

Pill (so the practitioner can synchronize treatment to the next cycle), then try Clomid, and then refer for fertility treatment. "I'm not saying these things don't serve a role," she says, but the patient generally "doesn't want to undergo painful procedures, with embryos on ice for decades, that may or may not result in a complicated pregnancy, that costs the price of mortgaging a home or not being able to buy a home," she says. "This is not what people want." She's become known in her community and beyond for offering an effective alternative.

For Miller, this unconventional, largely unrecognized branch of medicine offered a protocol to diagnose and treat patients that medical school did not. "I've heard it so many times in assisted reproductive technology that the workup and diagnosis and treatment doesn't matter because it's recommended the patient undergo IVF anyway," says Miller. One of the first skills every medical student learns is to listen to the patient, she points out. "How is it that the vast majority of us don't do that, especially in the case of reproductive health? And so I believe restorative reproductive medicine is the only approach that even offers that basic infrastructure to the patient-doctor relationship."

Diagnosis "is not difficult. It's just complicated. If you understand the complexities, it's easy," says Miller. Most infertility (if it's not structural) is caused by a hormonal imbalance, polycystic ovarian syndrome (which is often tied to a blood sugar imbalance), or endometriosis, which involves inflammatory and immunological processes, and which "most primary care physicians and OB/GYNs don't know how to treat." The hormonal imbalance could be what's called hypothalamic amenorrhea, when the brain has quit signaling the ovaries—it can happen as a result of not eating enough, exercising too much, a tumor, or even stress, and it's usually reversible. A similar thing can happen to women on birth control for extended years, where "the period goes into hiding," says Miller. But it could also be the more stealth "ovulatory disturbance" that Jerilynn Prior talks about. A person can still be having periods but not ovulating. And the store-bought ovulation kits, which measure the surge of luteinizing hormone that precedes ovulation (not that ovulation will actually occur), can miss it.

In 2001, Kirstin Karchmer, a Chinese medicine doctor, founded the Texas Center for Reproductive Acupuncture in Austin. "We were the first and biggest reproductive acupuncture center in the nation," she tells me over tea in downtown Austin, though they offer the full spectrum of modalities, from East to West, all the way to IVF. She reports high success rates—a very low number of miscarriages, a very high percentage of pregnancies, and comparatively fewer NICU admissions for the babies that are born as a result. Based on the decade she spent treating thousands of women there, she created the app Conceivable in 2015, which starts where they do in the clinic: getting as much detail as possible about one's menstrual cycle.

"I took care of seven thousand infertile women. Women would walk into my clinic, and their cycles would be all over the place: long, short, heavy, scanty, clotty, PMS, no PMS." Her treatment protocol is a combination of acupuncture, Chinese herbs, diet, and lifestyle recommendations. "After about three or four months [the cycles] would start to take a very distinct shape. And when they started to take a distinct shape, the women started to get pregnant. After thousands of these, I thought, hmm, that's where the magic is." This is also borne out in the data: PMS, cramping, and clotting are all associated with infertility. They don't singularly cause infertility, but they're indicative of underlying problems. "The reality is your menstrual cycle is an extremely unique barometer of your health," says Karchmer.

Like Miller, her approach is to diagnose the source of the problem and bring the body back into health, which brings the menstrual cycle into regulation. "When a woman walks into the clinic, what I say is, 'I'm not here to get you pregnant. My job is to get you as healthy as possible, and if I do that I can't help but improve your fertility.'"

There are no randomized controlled trials comparing the success rates of women who seek conventional IVF versus restorative reproductive medicine versus Chinese medicine versus shamanism. But the practitioners who are stretching beyond the lab model seem more comfortable answering the question of *why*.

Daniel Kalish, a chiropractic doctor who developed a method of hormonal assessment, breaks it down into three stressors that throw the cycle off: emotional stress, blood sugar dysfunction, and inflammation, he told Lisa Hendrickson-Jack on her Fertility Friday podcast. This lines up exactly with Miller's explanation, and Kalish further illuminated the mechanism: any of those stressors can cause the hormone cortisol to spike, which disrupts the hypothalamic-pituitary-adrenal axis, which drives down thyroid function and throws off progesterone and estrogen. "So if enough stress accumulates between those things, then female hormones drop like a rock and women can't get pregnant," he said. "And you know, in all these years, in testing female hormones, I've never had a case where the female hormones dysfunction all on their own in isolation from the rest of the body. The ovaries are the victim in this, the ovaries are responding with abnormal hormonal output because of emotional, dietary, or inflammatory stress. It's not the other way around."

In other words, the explanation is health. The explanation is untreated metabolic and autoimmune disorders. It's also our cruddy diets, the pesticides and plastics showing up in our blood and even our brains, and the scraping by on two jobs or working 12 hours a day at one. The long commutes and lack of community. The misogyny and racism and sexual trauma. The explanation is our lives. "The natural tendency, which is a very powerful tendency in nature, is for women to get pregnant really easily. So it's really a matter of what are the brakes on that process? We remove the brakes, get women healthy over all—brain, gut, and toxin-related health comes back—and then the pregnancies happen almost effortlessly," said Kalish.

Karchmer observed virtually the same thing. "In seven thousand cases, their cycles got better. Their follicle-stimulating hormone improves, their estradiol levels improve, their progesterone levels come up, their clotting and cramping and PMS improves," and many get pregnant.

Reproductive technology gets the job done, too, of course. But it's an override rather than a restorative. "When a woman is having a hard time getting pregnant and goes directly into IVF, she's missing an opportunity to experience optimal health," says Karchmer.

I talked to a patient of Miller's, Amber, who had gone through a miscarriage, an ectopic pregnancy, and four IUI cycles at a fertility clinic before her first visit. Miller diagnosed a metabolic disorder and a nutrient deficiency and recommended dietary changes and supplements. Amber began eating differently and walking her new dog. She ultimately needed surgery to remove adhesions left over from emergency surgery for the ectopic pregnancy, but she did finally get pregnant. She told me that by then, she had dropped three pants sizes. "Once I started eating better, I started feeling better," she said. Miller "was finally putting the pieces together. Once we found out all this other stuff, she was like, 'OK, well, let's focus on getting you pregnant now.'"

In all of Holly's visits to two different OB/GYNs and a renowned DC fertility clinic, nobody had taken much interest in her irregular period. Might it have helped?

Stress may cause infertility, and the stress that infertility itself causes is real. Even though Holly had just turned 33, she was really feeling the pressure, especially after three failed attempts to conceive with Clomid. So when she heard from her husband that one of his coworkers, who had been diagnosed around the same time, had gone to Shady Grove, a prominent DC fertility clinic with multiple centers, and got pregnant after two cycles, "I was like, 'Let's go!'" said Holly.

The doctor was able to see the couple right away and wanted to run all the tests again, on both Holly and her husband. Now they had yet another confirmation that, on paper at least, Holly was fine, hence her infertility was "unexplained." Her husband's count was on the low side but "fine," according to the reproductive endocrinologist. "Based on the test results and our age, he felt more than 80 percent confident that within three cycles we'd be pregnant. We were like, great! I'll be pregnant by April." The plan was to start with an intrauterine insemination, which meant they'd stimulate Holly's ovaries again and then give the sperm a ride right up into the uterus. The doctor suggested Clomid. Holly cried.

Still, she went through with it, sweating through hot flashes in the snowstorm. The morning of the appointment, after the hours of shoveling, they were able to get their car out. Her husband had deposited his contribution in a plastic cup. Holly held it under her winter coat, next to her chest, to keep it warm on the slow ride to the clinic.

But in the exam room there was a problem: "They said his count was too low, so they actually had him do another sample there. And combined it was only 2 million. They wanted 7 or 8 million." These numbers are too low for natural conception but doable in IUI. As she lay in the stirrups having another ultrasound, they told her there was another problem: the Clomid had made the lining of her uterus very thin, "which is not uncommon," they told her. This is probably why frozen embryos result in more pregnancies (with non-donor eggs): the ovarian-stimulating drugs make the womb less hospitable. If doctors freeze the eggs and wait a month for the uterus to rebound, they have better success.

On the bright side, the doctor told Holly she did have two mature follicles, and her husband's numbers were "on the cusp." So they forged ahead.

The next day and for two weeks after that, she inserted progesterone pills vaginally twice a day—"really not fun," she says. "It doesn't hurt, but they leak, it's uncomfortable and annoying." Along with that normal IUI protocol, she also had to insert estrogen pills twice a day, to bulk up the lining. Those two weeks were also difficult because of the waiting. And this time, like the others before it, nothing happened. "So that cycle was probably just a waste," she told me. "On my end my lining was thin, and on his end the sperm count was low."

I tell Chen about Holly's case. She rants about IUI, which insurance companies often mandate couples try at least six times before they will cover IVF, even when there is a diagnosis of endometriosis or PCOS or low sperm count. Even when the doctor's prescription is for IVF, not IUI. The success rate for IUI highly correlates with age, so does it make sense for a 41-year-old to have to go through six rounds of IUI, spending precious time on something with such a low success rate? Would Holly have been better off just going straight to IVF? Gina Bartasi, CEO of the health tech start-up Progyny, crunched the numbers on this and advised a Silicon Valley company that it would save $9 million if it allowed its beneficiaries to access IVF as needed. Chen also rails against the insurers for discriminating against lesbian couples—she cites a lawsuit pending against a New Jersey mandate that insurance need only cover infertility treatments for women under 35 if they've had "two years of unprotected sexual intercourse."[15]

Holly and her husband did try three more IUI cycles, which were partially covered by their insurance. Instead of Clomid she injected the follicle-stimulating hormone Gonal-F for those. During one round she had too many mature follicles—ten, all in all, too high of a chance of multiples, so they had to cancel the insemination. During the second, she tried a different drug, letrozole, an aromatase inhibitor, mostly prescribed for breast cancer. There were fewer side effects but she only had one mature follicle (what a woman would normally have), and her husband's sample clocked in at 2 million. It didn't work. April came and went. The last cycle they did, in June, she felt was their "best shot." He hit 6 million. She had two mature eggs. Her lining looked great. It still didn't work.

At that point, her husband said he was done. He couldn't watch her go through another round. But Holly was not. "I was just not ready to be done. Up until last summer I'd been a little ambivalent about biological versus adoption, but after putting my body through this and all the time and energy and thinking about it every day, I don't know, I just want this biological child," she told me in this midst of these heavy discussions.

There's always an office visit at Shady Grove after three failed cycles, and Holly had a lot of questions. For one, she was looking back at the history and wondering whether her husband's sperm count was perhaps too low all along. In fact, maybe it was the explanation for her "unexplained" condition. At the next appointment, she broached the issue. The doctor told them with her husband's count they had a 5 to 10 percent chance of success with each cycle, "which he didn't think was too low, but we do! Especially for the side effects I go through," Holly wrote to me the next day via email. Also, even a 10 percent chance per cycle does not add up to 80 percent in three months, as he had quoted them at the first visit. She felt a bit taken.

Finally, after seven cycles on her end, her husband made an appointment with a male infertility specialist, which the Shady Grove doctor "didn't think would help."

Holly is young. For many women who may be diagnosed with "unexplained infertility," the explanation is really just perimenopause. "The natural fertility decline that occurs for both women and men is being medicalized and discussed in framework of something that needs intervention and fixing," says Miriam Zoll. "The attitude is, come down to the clinic, you don't want that menopause stopping you from having a baby." She argues that it's giving false hope, and sends older women down an ethically slippery path. Between ages 40 and 44, the success rates for IVF with non-donor eggs (that is, the percentage of cycles that result in a live birth) dive from 14 percent to 3 percent.[16] At that point, the best chance one has is with donor eggs, and the next step would be to find a surrogate.

FERTILITY BENEFITS

In 2014, tech giants Facebook and Apple announced they would pay for female employees to freeze their eggs. When it made news, Citigroup and J.P. Morgan were already offering it, Microsoft was covering it up to a certain amount, and Google was considering it—it joined the party in early 2015.

And there are actually egg-freezing parties, thrown by companies like EggBanxx, with free cocktails, DJs, and enthusiastic marketing. As the writer Robin Marantz Henig, who attended one, put it, "EggBanxx had billed the event as an evening of 'The Three F's: Fun, Fertility, and Freezing'—no F's left over for 'Failure Rates.'" The event also had the subtext of another F—feminism. "We are only trying to educate and empower women; that's why I'm up here," EggBanxx sales and marketing manager Leahjane Lavin told the room.[17]

While some questioned Facebook's motives—do they just want women to work more?—most feminist thought leaders hailed the move as giving women more choice. In *Time*, Jessica Bennett wrote that this might be "our generation's Pill—a way to circumvent a biological glass ceiling that, even as we make social and professional progress, does not budge."[18]

Egg freezing does seem to offer that control. "You've stopped time," says Chen. "Those eggs are no longer aging. It's as if you've pressed the pause button." On the other hand, the chances that an egg frozen now will result in a live birth down the road are very low, estimated between 2 and 12 percent, according to the American Society for Reproductive Medicine, and that's for someone who "chills out," as it's often called, before age 38.[19] It's also really pricey—even Facebook's "lifetime surrogacy reimbursement" of up to $20,000 would not cover the fees for two rounds and years of storage. Bennett and many others are hopeful that science and the market will work out these kinks. Chen argues it should be covered by insurance rather than categorized as an elective procedure like plastic surgery. "Egg freezing for age is not unreasonable in a society where every year you delay childbearing means that you have a better chance of getting more education, you have a better chance of getting a good career, and there are studies showing a direct correlation with delayed childbearing and higher lifetime income," she says. "Even though it's too soon to say how successful the procedure down the line will be—for women who return, thaw, and begin the process of IVF—it's almost like an insurance policy," wrote Bennett. "And if your boss is offering it up to you for free, what do you have to lose?"

What women stand to lose in freezing their eggs is the very thing they are trying to preserve: their fertility. First, because women who have frozen their eggs may delay pregnancy and find that time actually didn't stop. Brigitte Adams, who froze eggs at age 39 and founded the online forum Eggsurance, told the *New York Times* that freezing gave her "incredible calmness." But five years later, only one of those eggs made an embryo, and implantation failed. "I have no more eggs to try," she posted on the Eggsurance blog. "I have no more eggs to retrieve. I have no energy to try again."[20] The other complicating factor is that the egg donation procedures may affect a woman's chances of a natural conception.

Many women going through IVF or egg donation begin a cycle weeks prior with injections of a GnRH agonist like Lupron, which interrupts communication between the hypothalamus, pituitary, and ovaries, ultimately shutting down the ovarian cycle. (Chen tells me that leading clinics are more likely using GnRH antagonists now, which act on the hypothalamus more directly, thus requiring fewer injections and causing fewer side effects. But they are more expensive.) The purpose is to stop ovulation, and the side effects mirror those of a challenging menopause: hot flashes, headaches, mood swings, vaginal dryness, the list goes on. The effects can persist for months, until the woman's pituitary and ovaries come back online, but in a small number of women, they never seem to.

Women considering egg freezing may want to look to egg donors' experiences. Raquel Cool donated when she was 27, in 2010. In 2012, she and two other donors founded the site We Are Egg Donors, which also has a private, vetted Facebook page with 500 members. Many posts are about ovarian hyperstimulation syndrome (OHSS), which Cool herself experienced after 30 eggs were extracted. "I had a moderate case. I could barely get out of bed for eleven days, I had eight pounds of fluid accumulating in my abdomen," she told me.

Fertility drugs act on the brain and endocrine system. "There's a common misconception among physicians and among women that if you manipulate reproductive hormones that it's only going to affect the reproductive organs. What they're not recognizing is that hormones circulate throughout body and brain and those receptors exist throughout the body, they're in every organ system," says Chandler Marrs. "So when you manipulate the reproductive system you are going to have effects everywhere there are receptors."

One thing that happens in OHSS is that a protein called vascular endothelial growth factor (VEGF) accumulates in the blood. VEGF makes blood vessels more permeable, allowing fluid to seep out. That fluid can collect in a woman's abdomen or around her lungs, which impedes breathing. Since the blood is losing fluid, it also becomes thicker, increasing the chance of a clot or stroke. The reduced blood flow can damage a woman's organs.

According to Canadian guidelines on managing the syndrome, up to one-third of women whose ovaries are stimulated will experience a mild version of OHSS. Physicians can preempt it by closely monitoring patients—a windfall of developing eggs, visible via ultrasound, is a red flag. But it's also a conflict of interest. The decision to taper off stimulating hormones and cancel a cycle means an investment without return. "When fertility doctors make decisions about how many eggs to stimulate and what to do if there are too many, they have to weigh the needs of both donor and recipient—and the interests of the patients are sometimes at odds. More eggs give the recipient a better shot at pregnancy. But too many eggs increase the donor's chance of suffering from OHSS," wrote Alison Motluk in one of the few magazine articles on the subject, in the Canadian publication *Maisonneuve*.[21]

The 2010 documentary *Eggsploitation* features four women, three of whom suffered serious complications of OHSS—one had a stroke, another lost an ovary, and another, who produced 60 eggs, nearly bled to death from a punctured artery. Each was dismissed when she notified the clinic of troubling symptoms. Donors also report developing polycystic ovarian syndrome and endometriosis following retrieval; others don't get their periods back and are essentially perimenopausal. Out of eighteen women Motluk interviewed, five reported permanent changes in their menstrual cycles following donation, which tracks with Canada's Donor Sibling Registry survey, in which a quarter of donors experienced menstrual changes or new infertility. "Might ovarian stimulation alter a woman's menstrual cycle, independent of normal aging? If so, how often do those alterations lead to treatments, like endometrial ablations and hysterectomies, that will render her infertile?" Motluk asks.

A woman I'll call Mary donated eggs twice during grad school in Boston. "My housemates remember me injecting the hormones for two weeks," she told me. "Apparently I had superstar follicles and responded really well to the medication, but I was fine. I got my period back no problem." Three months later the clinic asked if she wanted to do another round. "I was trying to fast-track grad school, and my student loans weren't covering my summer semesters, and I had never really traveled and wanted to do summer semester abroad." She did travel through Eastern Europe, and when she was in Prague met a *Sassy* magazine writer doing a story on women traveling alone. "I told her, 'My girls paid for this trip.'"

But her donation was also a political act. She knew older women who were struggling to get pregnant. She knew that gay couples needed donor eggs. "And somewhere in my head it was related to 'It's my body; I'm going to choose how to use it.' I think I conflated it a little bit with being a bisexually identified feminist."

After the second donation, there were problems. She remembers feeling dizzy and nauseous after the procedure. "I was so poor back then, the clinic didn't want to let me leave without a taxi, but I had no money for a taxi. So my friend met me and we took a taxi to the nearest T station." Two months later she still hadn't gotten her period back, but the clinic told her that was normal and released her from care. A year later, still no period. She was 26 and having hot flashes, comparing notes with her mother. Her primary care doctor told her about a study at Mass General Hospital for women with low estrogen, but when she went to enroll, they couldn't take her because her baseline estrogen was *too* low. "The diagnosis was perimenopause."

Mary spent the next dozen years trying to regulate her hormones. Regular blood tests showed that her estrogen and progesterone, which would normally fluctuate during the cycle, stagnated at near-menopausal levels. One physician, whom she saw only once, told her while he was examining her that she had "the vagina of an old woman." Though she would occasionally spot, her consistent diagnosis was amenorrhea, the medical term for an absent menstrual cycle.

Clearly in need of specialized care, she found herself in medical purgatory. OB/GYNs would scratch their heads and refer her to reproductive endocrinologists, whose office waiting rooms would be full of expectant women. They, too, would tell her they weren't sure how to help. "Reproductive endocrinologists don't want to work with you unless reproduction means wanting to have a kid," she told me.

Finally, she found an endocrinologist who took her case, who regulated her estrogen and progesterone, and who one day asked her if she wanted to have kids. She was 38. The question hit her like whiplash. "He was the first doctor who told me that I could get pregnant," she said. All those years she was telling prospective partners that she was physically unable. "Then it struck me. I would have to do exactly what the women who I had given my eggs to had done. I would have to go through what I went through when I donated, but for myself." She did go through it, but gave up after one cycle.

She continues to struggle with her thyroid, fatigue, dry skin, and more intimate issues, and there's no playbook for how she should handle menopause. "Now I'm this weird anomaly because I've been on hormones for 20 years, nobody knows what to do with me. At some point we have to make a decision to let me go menopausal, but the risk to my bones is so great that I'll probably need to take hormones longer than if I'd kept producing them on my own. Even the level I'm taking is still lower than the lowest estrogen the body makes during menopause. There's no study to help someone like me."

None of her physicians ever suggested that her ongoing problems might have stemmed from the egg retrieval, though the timing is conspicuous. Her medical records repeatedly state, "No significant surgical history."

THE GESTATIONAL FALLACY

If the IVF path doesn't lead to a baby, it may lead to surrogacy, at which point the prospective parents outsource the injections, ultrasounds, and transfers to a woman willing to carry their genetic embryo within her body. This adds layers of ethical and legal complications. In one case, a woman I interviewed had agreed to be a "gestational surrogate" for friends without pay. While lying on her back in stirrups, sedated for the insertion, the doctor sought her consent to transfer three embryos, telling her the chance that they'd all "take" was less than 1 percent. They all took. Her friends didn't want three babies. She was personally against abortion. She reluctantly agreed to "reduce" and carried twins to term, enduring a grueling pregnancy.

At the time, the *New York Times Magazine* had just run a piece about how this new trend in reproductive technology—the ability to fertilize egg and sperm and implant into a third party—had removed both the ick factor and the gamble of a surrogacy arrangement, because the baby inside wouldn't be genetically tied to the woman carrying it. There would be no chance that she'd change her mind and want to keep "her" baby, because contractually, the baby isn't in any way hers.

The woman with twins lived in a state where surrogacy isn't legal, and thus had to persuade a judge to let the biological parents adopt the twins after they were born. This floored me at the time. The babies weren't hers, she didn't want them! I met with sociologist Barbara Katz Rothman and asked her how this could be true. "That's right. It is an adoption," she said flatly. I corrected her, No, no, we're talking about *gestational* surrogacy. "That is so beside the point," she scoffed.

But the surrogate has no genetic connection; the surrogate is not the mother, I said. Wrong, she said. "If you are pregnant with a baby, you are the mother of the baby that you're carrying. End of discussion. The nutrients, the blood supply, the sounds, the sweep of the body. That's not somebody standing in for somebody else to that baby. That's the only mother that baby has." At the time, my grandmother gustily agreed. When she carried my twin aunts she somehow only gained four pounds. "They were eating me, basically. You're going to tell a woman that her body is feeding these babies and they're not hers?" she said.

This idea of separating mother from fetus comes up again and again in reproductive medicine, in obstetrics, and in abortion politics. We cut the cord as fast as we can. But this is problematic, for both mother and child. At its core, it is a dismissal of the intricate biology that weaves the two together as the fetus grows, as labor progresses, and even months after birth. The political ramifications of this notion are obvious: if fetuses, embryos, and fertilized eggs have separate legal rights, a woman becomes an incubator. She loses her right to terminate a pregnancy. It also means that almost anything can be done to her body in the name of protecting the fetus.

For the bulk of Western thought, it was believed that the sperm was the seed, and that women were just the place to plant it. "Think of the homunculus, the nesting dolls, the idea that what makes a person a person is the seed from which it grows," said Katz Rothman. "I think the notion that a woman is pregnant and it's not really her baby is too dangerous an idea to let out of the box." If gestational surrogacy eliminates maternity rights, does it also erode the carrier's reproductive rights—her bodily integrity?

Add to this question that the women who have access to reproductive technology and the women who are supplying their eggs and wombs in its service are divided along racial and class lines. Black women are more likely to experience infertility but less likely to receive treatment, and young women and poor women are more likely to be donors. Meanwhile, we've created a discount economy in the global South, where surrogate "dorms" in India are full of expecting women awaiting their scheduled C-sections to remove mostly white, Western babies.

On the other hand, what of people's right to create a family? "The current conversation seems to be about access to this technology, it's not about exploitation of egg donors," says Raquel Cool. "I'd really like to see advocacy in terms of both access but also what does the ethical procurement of eggs or hiring a surrogate look like?" Sci-fi science may indeed work out these dilemmas—Henry Greely predicts that in the next few decades labs will be able to create eggs from our own skin cells. For now, however, creating a family may put a third party at risk, may cause lifelong harm, and may cause harm to parents and kids. Is this really the "reproductive choice" that the women's movement fought for? Are we comfortable with where these technological workarounds are taking us?

A week after Mary told me her story about donating her eggs, she called to say she was about to shred 15 years' worth of medical records but thought maybe I could use them. "But if you want them you need to come get them," she said. She had carried them from home to office and she wanted the load off her shoulders. She was done. I hopped on the subway and she handed them to me in a bright pink reusable shopping bag. We chatted for a minute and then she apologetically rushed me back out. This was baggage she wanted to purge.

Egg freezing promises to "stop the biological clock," to freeze time. Instead, what the process did for Mary and countless other donors was more like a mistake of time travel, a reproductive time warp. Her ovaries were prematurely aged. She still finds the ordeal difficult to talk about. "There's some self-loathing that I sold my body," she told me.

Isn't some degree of collective self-loathing inevitable when the female body is framed as an obstacle? When the glass ceiling is women's own wombs? When we are willing to defend almost any medical technology in the name of choice? What if instead girls grew up in a culture that acknowledges, wow, the female body does this amazing thing, and it's a limited-time offer. As Nancy London, one of the original authors of *Our Bodies, Ourselves,* told *New York* magazine: The '70s were liberating, allowing women to participate in so much of life that had been off limits, "but then we had to find out that biology is not some patriarchal concept created to keep us barefoot and pregnant. To mother is part of our nature. To toss that out the window and say, 'Hey, that's not for me,' and then at 50 to say, 'Oops, forgot to have a baby'—something is not processed in our thinking."[22]

To be sure, mothering is not in everybody's nature. But maybe we as a culture, and women as a social movement, need to make some choices about what we advocate for. An egg-freezing benefit seems like a hollow victory. What if our health care system was more geared toward getting women healthy so our fertility functioned better, so we left the needle-pipette conception for when it's really medically necessary? What if we had such decent maternity leave policies and affordable childcare that women felt it feasible to have a family *while* building their careers, while their bodies were inclined toward it, so fewer women would go through this in the first place? Instead, we have embraced high-tech medical solutions for what are really social problems. We are running a race designed by and for men and literally taking steroids to compete.

The fertility clinicians I talked to didn't give much thought to the cultural side of things. But the history of fertility medicine speaks to the possible consequences. Toward the end of my visit at St. Barnabas, we were standing around the island—Garrisi, Chen, the med student, and myself—while an embryologist pulled a five-day-old embryo from one of the incubators and handed it off to a physician, who was waiting in an adjacent room with the intended recipient.

Garrisi was giving some historical context, speaking of the earliest egg extractions, which were done without ultrasound. For a time, in the 1980s, intrepid surgeons were passing thick, long needles *through* the bladder to reach the ovary, he said. The med student visibly cringed; Chen's jaw dropped. "Those bleed like stink!" she said. Garrisi talked about the development of ICSI, the early attempts to get past the zona pellucida, first with acid. (It caused abnormal fertilization and poor development, "because it turns out the agent we used to make the hole affected the egg. We didn't realize how sensitive it was at that time.") For a time they tried friction to create an opening, which worked but let too many sperm in. The scientist Gianpiero Palermo, at Cornell, who ultimately slipped a needle straight through the zona pellucida, says it happened by pure accident.

"Just so you know, Jennifer, this was kind of crazy to think instead of looking at these embryos in the dish, we're actually going to try to physically manipulate them. It was really radical at the time," Chen offered. "Yeah, it was . . . I'm not going to say reckless," Garrisi hesitated, "but we didn't know what we didn't know."

3: PELVIC TENSION

MEGAN ASSAF STARTED shaping polymer clay into uteruses in 2006, several years after she turned her massage therapy practice toward the organ. It was important to her that they be to scale, the same weight and shape as the real organ in different phases of life, so she made them in three sizes: ovulating, menstruating, and menopausal. Pointing out the difference was part of her intent: the menstruating uterus is about twice as large, and that much heavier, than an ovulating one, which is in turn much larger than the menopausal uterus.

To this day, four times a year, Assaf shapes and bakes batches of wombs, fulfilling orders from around the world.

When she's not sculpting, she's with clients. "I move uteruses into place," she explains. A uterus, she goes on, can be out of place—tipped back and leaning against organs, or even folded onto itself, potentially restricting blood flow, causing pelvic floor tension and nerve pain, and disrupting other organ function, among other problems.

The early anatomists and physicians believed in the "wandering womb," a vector of disease and madness that traveled around the female body wreaking havoc on organs as improbable as the lungs. Modern medicine rejected this wholly. Assaf is suggesting a truth buried in the myth. Her evidence is the thousands of women she's treated, as well as her own body.

"When I first started menstruating, I had really bad periods," she tells me. "I felt like I was being turned inside out. I would throw up. I would miss school." This went on for years, from the time she was 11. At around age 15, the pain got so bad that Assaf was hospitalized. Surgeons did exploratory surgery and found ovarian cysts that had been rupturing. Today, they might have diagnosed her with polycystic ovarian syndrome. If she had been in a large teaching hospital with a particularly savvy surgeon, he or she might have identified it as endometriosis. But this, too, wasn't widely known back then.

The ER physicians treated her pain with narcotics, but that was hardly sustainable. Her OB/GYN put her on birth control pills, but they didn't help. "Then they said, well, it's all in your head, so they threw me on antidepressants." In college she consulted a homeopath and a naturopath and started to see a psychotherapist, "because maybe it was all in my head." She sought out an internist. "I really tried to take charge of my health."

By her 20s, her excruciating period was bringing on such severe digestive problems that she couldn't keep any food down for a week and a half out of every month. She had seemingly untreatable vaginal infections, for which she would take round after round of antibiotics, to no avail. Nobody had an answer. Her love life suffered. Everything suffered. "By my late 20s, I was feeling hopeless. I knew deep down inside that I was going to have a hysterectomy if I didn't get organized."

Then, in a week of synchronicity, she heard about uterine massage from three different sources. She looked it up online and nodded her head as she read through the long list of common symptoms of an out-of-place womb. "A ridiculously long list," she recalls. She had every one. She was 27.

The nearest practitioner was four and a half hours away, in San Francisco. "My boyfriend and I got in the truck and we drove on up." Assaf lay down on a massage table. "Then [the practitioner] went and found my uterus, and do you know where my uterus was? It was folded in half, upside down, and stuck behind the descending colon on the left. How the hell are you supposed to menstruate with it in that position? You can't."

The visit was pivotal for Assaf, both biomechanically as well as spiritually. When the treatment was over, she sat up, lowered her feet to the floor, and stood up. "I was in my body," she says. "I walked down the hallway to go to pee, because I had to pee right away. And I was skipping. And I observed myself skipping like a little person would skip on their way to school, and I remember feeling this unbearable lightness of being, and it was honest to god unbearable, because I hadn't remembered feeling that light and joyful since I was a kid."

The treatment wasn't a miracle cure. Her uterus had to empty "massive amounts" of stagnant old blood that had been pooling for years, she says, which took a few rough cycles. But soon, the debilitating cramps no longer came with her period, and it became lighter, smoother. It took several more months to heal her colon, which she believes her uterus had been crimping, but eventually her digestive problems eased up as well, as did the previously intractable bacterial vaginosis. She now had a physiological explanation for that, too: the constant contact between her womb and colon was causing a breakdown of the tissues, a cross-contamination essentially, introducing bacteria from her intestine into her uterus.

She sought out training to learn the technique that had been used on her, which led her to Rosita Arvigo, who studied abdominal massage with traditional healers in Belize. "If you look historically around the world you will find that there were many cultures who had a version of uterus massage, and it was part of their standard care for women," Assaf says. Even "old timey" American doctors, like her house-calling grandfather, she says, knew the importance of uterine alignment for fertility and posture and digestion. This also worked in the reverse: midwives on the island of Java would intentionally tilt women's uteruses backward to *prevent* pregnancy. An anthropologist visiting at the turn of the last century found that half of the women were retroflexed, but the midwives assured him that "they could restore the uterus to its normal position by massage whenever a woman wanted a child."[1] Assaf admits that in this century, at least in the United States, uterus moving is "pretty out there."

Still, she sees the kind of dramatic healing she experienced mirrored in her clients. And she believes this work has another dimension. "What I experience as a practitioner is that here's a channel of energy in the woman that opens up from the pelvis all the way out to the top of her head, and it's like this life force rises," says Assaf. "A lot of women just tell me, 'I feel really calm, I feel really centered. I feel like me again.'"

The clients who come to Assaf are usually "at the end of the line": women who've already been to a dozen (or more) doctors, women who've had procedures or surgeries without relief, women who have reached the point when they'll "try anything." Most of the time, says Assaf, the position of the uterus is a piece of the puzzle. Occasionally, it is the puzzle.

"SOMETHING HAS TO HOLD THESE BONES TOGETHER"

The number of women in North America suffering from some form of chronic pelvic pain is staggering: it is estimated that one in four women, at some point in their lives, will deal with it. And it generally takes many years and doctor visits before they come upon any relief.[2] To better understand why, I meet with Isa Herrera, a New York City–based pelvic floor physical therapist, whose name comes up when anybody is talking about the subspecialty—it did not exist when she was training in the 1990s, and she's one of its pioneers. Herrera is built like a gymnast, and she can lay into the medical establishment as if doing so were a practiced mat routine. "I got 30 minutes [of training] on pelvic anatomy," she tells me, "I had to go and research this myself."

She is excited to show me the new plastic pelvic model she had just ordered for the classes she's teaching. Overlaid in the basin of the skeletal pelvis is the deep pink pelvic floor, the web of muscles that weave together like a basket between the hip bones. Not part of the model are the organs and several ligaments—the round ligament, which wraps from the back of the uterus around the bladder, its arms weaving into the musculature beneath the labia; the broad ligament, a large sheet that wraps from front to back and attaches to the sidewalls of the pelvis; the uterosacral ligaments, which hang as if on a hook from the back of the pelvis to the cervix and upper vagina, and which join with the cardinal ligament, which branches from the base of the broad ligament, suspending the cervix and vagina to the pelvic sidewalls. The pubocervical ligaments run from the cervix to the front of the pelvis. Then there are the extensive branches of nerves that stem from the sacrum throughout the pelvic and abdominal cavity, and the blood vessels and arteries that pass through the uterus and enervate the entire region. Each has a complicated relationship to the pelvic floor.

Herrera teaches the three *S*s for pelvic floor function: sexual, sphincteric, and supportive. "Remember, one of the primary focuses of this is stability," she tells me. "Something has to hold these bones together!" Herrera flips the model over to show me how the muscles also wrap around and between the vagina and anus and vast internal clitoral tissue—picture a bird with its wings extended, almost ready for flight. The "clitoris" that we typically think of is just the bird's head; meanwhile there's ten times as much erogenous tissue under the labia and around the vagina. (This gives lie to Freud's "inferior" clitoral orgasm—the female orgasm is both clitoral and vaginal and engages the uterus as well. More on this anatomy in chapter 4.) "I had to have my husband drill a hole for the vagina. Can you believe they sent me a female pelvic model without a vagina?"

The vagina is in fact a key entry point for the physical therapy that frequently helps patients who come to Herrera because of stubborn, life-altering, sometimes debilitating pain that can make sex, urination, wearing underwear, even sitting, torture. Sometimes women come to her on crutches because walking is too much. For many, she explains, the pain is originating from tension deep in the muscles of the pelvic floor. "They can pull, they can go into spasm, they can go into trigger points, they can develop scar tissue," she says, pointing to the woven muscular basket in the pelvic model. The sinews of muscle help to illustrate how a pull in one place can translate across the pelvic area. Herrera moves uteruses, too. All organs need to move within a certain range, she says, but the uterus can move in such a way that it pulls on the pelvic floor. If enough tension forms, the entire structure can become "stuck and tight," she says. "Women could have pain in the labia, the vagina, the bone, the anus, the glutes, the sacrum, the sacroiliac joint . . ."

The weave of muscle, ligament, nerve, and blood supply is extremely complex, says Herrera—just the lines of the musculature in the models she's holding are difficult to follow visually from end to end. Similarly, there is often not a clear line between a person's pain and its source. Megan Assaf describes the potential for pain transference this way: "The whole belly sits in a big balloon called a peritoneal sac," made of connective tissue, or fascia, "and the ligaments are actually highly specialized extensions of the peritoneal sac," like the stem of the flower it's cradling. So the uterus—the flower—can move and impact the surrounding structures, or a section of muscle can tighten in one place, creating a problem across the belly.

Writing in *ELLE* magazine several years back, Veronica Manchester described the relief she found from what felt like a chronic urinary tract infection from pelvic floor therapy.[3] Same story for Chloe Angyal, who penned an essay in Salon about her journey with pelvic pain in the form of tender letters to her younger self, who winced through sex for nearly a decade: "Dear Chloe, Tomorrow is your first day of vagina therapy. After five years of painful sex, after half a dozen stumped NPs and OBGYNs, after one doctor who prescribed you a numbing cream to use during sex, for god's sake, one gynecologist did you a mitzvah and recommended a physical therapy practice that specializes in 'pelvic pain.' It's not covered by health insurance, of course. Also, you don't have health insurance."[4]

The impetus for tension-related pain can also be specific and identifiable: inadequate support on the perineum (or an intentional cut) during childbirth; adhesions left after a cesarean, where layers of connective tissue may be stuck to each other or stuck to an organ. Pregnancy in general stretches the muscles and ligaments, so the pelvic floor can tighten in an effort to compensate (in France, for example, postpartum physical therapy is universal). Women can even develop trigger points from doing Kegels (Dr. Arnold Kegel was a man, by the way), or from a misguided yoga instructor focused on *bandhas*. Some 30 percent of female runners, Herrera tells me, have vaginal pain, often as a result of nerve compression in their hips. "It's all connected," she says.

The trauma of a violent assault can also cause physical scarring, but the psychological impact of any abuse can create real physical injury as well. "With sexual trauma, what I notice is a complete squeezing down, a complete shutdown of the muscles," says Herrera. "Because why would you ever let anybody in again?" Research shows a clear connection between physical abuse history and pain, says Jessica Drummond, founder of the Integrative Women's Health Institute and a physical therapist. For her, this connection raises a larger question about the broader impact of a #metoo culture where "there's a sort of lack of sensation of safety that a lot of women carry around with them," she says. "I've seen this clinically for over 18 years."

A person's propensity toward pain can be imprinted early in life, Drummond goes on. "We have some understanding that the hypothalamic-pituitary-adrenal axis, which is your stress buffering system, has a window of development in early childhood, where if people don't feel secure, they're being abused, or they have an unstable life situation, that system doesn't develop as efficiently or effectively as in others," she says. "Pain is kind of the output of a whole lot of inputs into the brain, and some people have a more robust capacity to handle more inputs into the brain before they experience pain."

And pain, it turns out, can behave almost like a contagion, spreading from one organ to another, sensitizing the central nervous system, which helps explain why once someone has one pain condition they're more likely to develop another.

In 2011, the National Academy of Medicine (then the Institute of Medicine) released a report finding that four in ten American adults live with chronic pain disorders, costing the country more than $500 billion.[5] It also noted two important facts about this: pain disorders mostly (and some solely) affect women, and conditions like endometriosis, interstitial cystitis, vulvodynia, migraines, irritable bowel syndrome, and fibromyalgia are often happening simultaneously in the same body. That same year, the National Institutes of Health formally recognized chronic overlapping pain conditions (COPC), but up until 2014 it devoted less than 1 percent of its budget to studying the phenomenon.[6]

"Researchers used to think that the majority of people who had any one of these conditions would just have one disorder," says Christin Veasley, who led the National Vulvodynia Association and went on to found the Chronic Pain Research Alliance, which has been lobbying for more research. She and other patient advocates noticed that there was a solid minority who had several at once. "At the time they were considered the psych group, because there obviously had to be something wrong with them to have all these conditions. But as research went on, what we actually learned is it's more common for people, especially women, to have multiple diagnoses, and the longer you have any one of these conditions, the more likely you are to develop multiple conditions."

The medical community has made almost no progress in definitively saying what causes most of the disorders; treatment is trial and error—and very few treatments are evidence based or FDA approved. "It's all diagnoses of exclusion. You don't have infection, you don't have cancer, you don't have a skin disorder, but you have pain in this part of your body and we don't know why, and that's pretty much the diagnosis for the majority of these conditions," says Veasley.

With pelvic pain, the evolution of terminology tells much of the story. Vulvodynia is now the official term for vulvar pain, most often of a burning or stabbing nature, of at least three months' duration *without clear identifiable cause*, according to the consensus of three professional organizations in 2015.[7] The old term "vestibulitis" referred to an inflammation ("itis"), but it turns out there is often no inflammation. "Vaginismus" is a holdover term from the dark days of early gynecology—it referred to patriarchy's nightmare of the vagina swelling to the point that it would capture and strangle anything that had been inserted. "Interstitial cystitis" now goes by "painful bladder syndrome," because again, there may be pain even though nothing is detectably wrong with the bladder.

"In general, the research in vulvodynia is inconclusive," says Maureen Basha, a physiologist at Louisiana State University. "There are different camps of people looking at different pathways that might be involved, but nothing is coming out as a singular problem." Some are finding associations with pelvic floor tension, but it's not clear if that develops as a result of an underlying cause or whether it's primary. Other research suggests vulvodynia has an immune component, other studies an inflammatory component, and still others have shown it can develop from repeated yeast infections.

Drummond says pelvic pain is one of the most challenging problems to treat. "Women will often have what's called terrible triplets," she says, "endometriosis *and* interstitial cystitis *and* vulvodynia, and a lot of times on top of that they'll have a functional bowel issue." The overlap makes sense, she explains, because the physiology all meet in the pelvis. "There's a lot of organs from a lot of different systems"—pelvic floor muscles, connective tissue and ligaments, the digestive system, the bladder, the urogenital system, and the reproductive system—"so there's a lot of organ crosstalk there. It's very rare that someone has a really clean case of just one thing," she says, which also makes symptoms harder to study.

More than challenging to research, the medical system has no centralized way of treating pelvic pain. When you go to the gastroenterologist with your bowel symptoms, he's unlikely to ask about headaches or jaw pain. And patient expectations are in similar silos: What if you went to your dentist with jaw pain and she asked about your genitals? And yet it turns out the jaw and the vulva, for example, are frequently yoked in suffering. In one of the only long-term research studies looking at these overlapping conditions, 78 percent of women with vulvodynia also had symptoms or diagnoses of orofacial pain, including temporomandibular disorder (TMD).[8]

Pain is also modulated by the endocrine system. And here women are at another disadvantage—our bodies are full of estrogen receptors, and the past century has seen an explosion of endocrine disruptors in the air we breathe, the food we eat, and the water we drink. Aviva Romm, a Yale-trained physician known online as the Natural MD, points out there's a direct connection between estrogen and how stress manifests, and she believes that connection is related to the prevalence of pain, autoimmune disease, and thyroid dysfunction in women. "Women are more likely to have physical symptoms than men as a result of stress. That's not because we're the weaker sex, it's because we're wired differently."

Complicating matters even further, hormone therapy is often the recommended treatment for any pain related to the menstrual cycle. "One hundred percent of women on hormonal contraception have lower amounts of estrogen and testosterone," says Andrew Goldstein, an OB/GYN leader in treating vulvodynia who sees patients from around the world. "That's by definition, that's how they work. They suppress ovarian function." The vulva, meanwhile, is hormonally sensitive. "Certain parts of the vulva are very, very dependent on testosterone," he says, especially the opening of the vagina, or vestibule.

But not everyone will have problems on the Pill. Goldstein believes there's a genetic explanation and led a study that suggests a connection between pain and sexual dysfunction and a person's genetic code of their androgen receptors.[9] "You may have some dryness, you may have low libido, you may not get as aroused as easily, you may have difficulty achieving orgasm," he says. Or if you're particularly sensitive, "frankly, you can barely have sex."

Goldstein is of the mind that vulvar pain and vulvodynia (nomenclature he helped revise in 2015) generally have a cause that is knowable—not always, but often. And yet his biggest beef with his OB/GYN colleagues—he speaks several times a year at professional conferences—is that they don't investigate. So women come to him having been diagnosed "a million times" with yeast infections or bacterial vaginosis, treated for both "a thousand ways" without improvement, then put on steroids without a clear diagnosis, "which isn't good," and then put on antidepressants "either because their doctors have been told that's the treatment or because they think these women are crazy and anxious. That's a very typical scenario." Goldstein sends a lot of women to pelvic floor physical therapy. He also prescribes hormones, injects Botox, and performs vestibulectomy surgery, which he argues is only appropriate for the very tiny number of women born with hundreds of times too many nerve endings around their vagina.

Herrera entered the field after getting the brush-off firsthand when the birth of her only child left her with problems—her doctor told her to just have a glass of wine and try to relax. "I want to get people to understand that pelvic pain is a physical issue," she says. She teaches OB/GYNs, Pilates instructors, midwives, doulas, and massage therapists. They don't learn pelvic floor anatomy in their training, either, she says. For her book *Ending Female Pain: A Woman's Manual,* she spent four months researching and writing the two pages on the internal clitoris because so few textbooks get it right. Maureen Basha, who teaches medical students, called out the same discrepancy: for the male, "it's full on. You get all of the anatomy and a full description of the sexual response," she says. "Then you get to the woman, and you get a picture of the uterus and vagina and external genitalia, and it jumps right to pregnancy. It's amazing, every single book!" she says. "We know the anatomy of the clitoris, why don't you have it in a medical physiology textbook?" Says Herrera: "Is it ignorance, or is it sexism? I think it's a combination."

A DISEASE OF INVERSION

If ignorance of female anatomy has painful consequences for women, so does ignorance of pathology. Endometriosis is estimated to affect about

6 million women and costs the country billions of dollars, and yet it claims few research dollars. There is still no lab test to confirm endometriosis; the only sure diagnosis requires exploratory surgery.

Endometriosis is often talked about as a disease of inversion: tissue that is supposed to be on the inside of the uterus somehow gets outside of it, attaching perhaps to the bladder, intestines, ligaments, or all of the above, where it starts up its own satellite operation, responding to the hormonal cycle the same way the womb does. That is, the rogue tissue bleeds. That blood has nowhere to go, so it collects, irritates, and forms scar tissue. If enough forms over enough time, one is said to have a "frozen pelvis."

Endometriosis doesn't look one way or behave one way. The growths can be tiny, barely noticeable to the naked eye, or they can be so large that they overtake the organ they've glommed onto. "Endometriosis has different appearances," says Jeffrey Braverman, an OB/GYN and endometriosis specialist who treats women across the world from his New York office. "There are white lesions, purple lesions, brown lesions, there are even lesions that sometimes you can only see with a special fluorescent lamp." They also come in the red, pink, yellow, and blue variety. They have names like "chocolate cysts" and "powderburns."

In some women, these growths can cause horrific period pain, or horrific pain all the time, or no pain at all. There might be intense bleeding, digestive problems, fatigue, bladder problems, or lower back or hip pain, often in combination, he says. "These women are being bounced around from doctor to doctor, thinking it's back pain, a slipped disc, irritable bowel syndrome, interstitial cystitis, I mean, they get all these diagnoses. It's endometriosis." "Endo" lesions are referred to as "benign," which in medicine simply means they are not cancerous. But the pain that the disease causes some women, like Megan Assaf, is excruciating, isolating, and exhausting. It also causes infertility.

Endometriosis wasn't named in the medical literature until around the turn of the twentieth century, though some have suggested that women branded with "hysteria" may have in fact been suffering from the condition, also referred to as "suffocation" or "strangulation" of the womb.[10] In 1927, John Sampson, a physician in Albany, New York, proposed the origin: "retrograde" or "reflux" menstrual flow, which he believed backed out through the fallopian tubes and spilled into the abdomen, where shed endometrial cells remained and proliferated. This theory was incomplete—all women seem to have some reflux, but the stem cells of endometriosis sufferers alone cause that overflow to grow. And how would endometriosis get as far as a woman's lungs or brain, where lesions have been found? The "how" of endo is still a point of great controversy.

In any case, this theoretical origin meant that endometriosis fell under the purview of gynecology and stayed there—a disease of the womb. And yet, it turns out that while the tissue of endometriosis appears *similar* to that of the endometrium, it is different "in dozens of profound ways."[11] It generates blood, but it also releases what are called inflammatory cytokines into the fluid that surrounds all the abdominal organs, causing inflammation throughout the abdominal cavity, including in the uterus itself. As researchers have dug further into the cellular habits of endometriosis, they've come to see it not as a reproductive disease per se but as a more systemic disease, possibly autoimmune, with impacts on the reproductive system. A woman with endometriosis will have a certain "immune profile," explains Braverman, and women with endometriosis are more likely to have other autoimmune conditions—Hashimoto's thyroiditis, multiple sclerosis, asthma, rheumatoid arthritis, and celiac disease, to name a few.

The immune and inflammatory mechanisms explain why some 40 percent of women with endometriosis have fertility trouble—trouble getting pregnant, trouble staying pregnant—and they're even more likely to have late pregnancy complications like preeclampsia, preterm birth, and stillbirth, says Braverman. "What's happening is that the inflammatory component or underlying autoimmune component—either can be triggered by endometriosis—interferes with the normal maternal immune mechanisms that typically generate tolerance for the paternal genetics of the embryo." In a healthy woman, pregnancy will modulate her immune system so that it doesn't attack the pregnancy, he says. "In women with endo, that mechanism of tolerance doesn't work." This inflammatory environment is also damaging to the mitochondria of a woman's eggs, he says, which can interrupt the cell's ability to divide once fertilized.

Ten years ago, Braverman had a typical OB/GYN practice on Long Island. But he had patients with recurring miscarriages whom he'd refer to fertility specialists, without success. He was haunted by them. (He has seven kids.) His OB/GYN training left him unprepared to figure this out, he says, so he spent two years studying immunology and brought on a PhD immunologist to work in his practice. They began to do immunological workups on seemingly healthy women who couldn't get or stay pregnant, and what they found was that a high proportion looked almost identical to the profiles of women with symptomatic endometriosis. The "healthy" women had no pain, but their bodies were rejecting pregnancy after pregnancy, even when they'd gone to fertility centers and taken the extra step of genetic testing to ensure a normal embryo (an egg with damaged mitochondria can still produce an embryo that presents with healthy genetics). Braverman started to treat these women for endometriosis, and they began to have successful pregnancies.

"I became so confident that this was a way to diagnose it, I began referring these cases to top endometriosis surgical specialists. And they said, 'What, are you crazy? They have no symptoms.'" But he persisted, and his patients were desperate for answers, so the surgeons obliged. "We began uncovering case after case," he says. He started describing these women as having "silent endometriosis."

For his patients with silent endo who want to get pregnant, one of the first steps of treatment is surgery to remove as many lesions as possible, to "debulk" the inflammatory tissue to reduce the inflammation. "The correct surgery—and really only a few people around the country do it well—is excision," says Braverman. This means cutting out the tissue by hand with "cold" scissors, rather than energy-based instruments that cauterize tissue, and it takes a lot of skill. It's also not the standard treatment, he says. Most OB/GYNs will use laser or heat. "If you don't excise it, you leave behind a lot of tissue that can make these inflammatory cytokines and a lot of these women still don't get better."

OB/GYNs are surgeons, I point out. Why isn't excision the treatment of choice? "Well, I've been through the training myself," he says. "Gynecologists can do hysterectomies, we can take out an ovary." But when it comes to dissection around critical structures like the uterus or diaphragm or bowel, "that's not our training," he says. Cancer surgeons and general surgeons develop these skills, but to tackle endometriosis you need a deep knowledge of the pelvic crossroads as well as the ability to recognize the lesions in their many varied forms, he says. It takes years to master. "There's too many mixtures of fields where nobody is an expert." And even if women find an expert, the surgery may not be covered by insurance.

Endo is one of the most underdiagnosed and misdiagnosed chronic diseases. According to the Endometriosis Foundation of America, sufferers go an average of ten years without knowing what's causing their symptoms (and that's down from 15 years, says Drummond). Many are not diagnosed until their late 20s or 30s, though the tissue probably starts growing at puberty.

These growths are stimulated by estrogen, but the tissue also produces a crafty enzyme that can grab another hormone and convert it into estrogen—so they are self-sustaining. This explains why hormonal treatment doesn't always help. Endometriosis's receptivity to estrogen is one reason some researchers believe it became so common in the twentieth century—our chemical inheritance of the Industrial Revolution, pesticides and plastics and preservatives, are estrogen mimickers. In one study, scientists exposed female rhesus monkeys to dioxin over a period of years. They found a direct correlation between the level of exposure and the incidence of endometriosis: the more toxin, the more endo.[12]

It's difficult to say whether the disease is more prevalent today than it was 50 or 100 years ago because it was and is so underdiagnosed and untracked. Estimates range from 2 to 10 percent of reproductive-age women. Most experts lean toward the higher number: "So if you have a high school class of 20 or 30 girls, 2 or 3 girls will have it," says Drummond. I scanned the women in my life—plenty I know have bad periods or chronic digestive problems or bladder issues or back pain, but I could only think of a couple as having been diagnosed with endo, which made me wonder.

So I posted on Facebook, asking the hive about endometriosis and infertility. Figures emerged from the past, including a soprano and an alto from the small high school girls choir I sang in. Charlotte, the soprano, was finally pregnant after much intervention, and Ellen, the alto, had just adopted a baby boy. I gathered from previous posts that both were intimately familiar with pregnancy loss.

Ellen's story is painfully illustrative of how endo can silently wreak havoc on your life plans. When we talked, I asked her when her problems began. First there were bladder spasms, which went on for years. Then the diagnosis of interstitial cystitis, which turned out to be wrong, though she went through years of painful tests and treatments for it. Then there was a second-trimester miscarriage, then the discovery of ovarian cysts, and the surgery that finally revealed endometriosis. But then she paused and moved backward in time. "The beginning *beginning* was probably when I first got my period. It was really intensely heavy," she said. "I was so anemic I had to have iron shots in my butt."

Other problems started early, even before puberty. Stomachaches, chronic headaches, pain, then a case of mononucleosis and symptoms that never seemed to go away. Doctors sent her from our midsize New England town to Boston, where some very progressive doctors did an immunological workup. By age 15 she was diagnosed with chronic fatigue and fibromyalgia, both in the autoimmune big tent.

She told me she managed all this over the years with a collection of doctors, physical therapists, acupuncturists, nutritionists, and energy workers. "I've tried it all—east, west, north, south." Sometimes her health would get better, sometimes it would get worse. Nobody ever mentioned endometriosis. Until one day when abdominal pain sent her to the emergency room. She had a ruptured cyst on her ovary that required immediate surgery. When she woke up, the gynecologist explained that she had found endo. Lots of it, everywhere, "the worst she'd ever seen." Lesions had wrapped around Ellen's bladder and colon, the cyst had engulfed her right ovary, fusing it to her bladder. "I cleaned out as much as possible," the doctor told her. At age 35, actively trying to get pregnant, Ellen was diagnosed with stage 4 endometriosis.

Ellen had been to so many health care providers—so many—in some of the most respected institutions. Yet she went undiagnosed until age 35. "The unfortunate truth is that endo is probably underdiagnosed across the board, because we don't have great tools as gynecologists for diagnosing it. And part of that really has to do with the need for more research," says Amina White, associate professor of OB/GYN at the University of North Carolina. The other part, she says, is that there's no great way to treat it. "So at this point surgery is still the gold standard method of diagnosis and treatment, and even then, after you've diagnosed it surgically, and you've attempted to remove all the implants that you can see with your eyes, it remains a microscopic process, so there are always cells left behind that you cannot see." She goes on, "Should somebody have ten surgeries over the course of their life? Well, that's not a great option, and yet that sort of remains the gold standard."

She and Braverman both bring up the dictum of first do no harm, thus the preference is to treat the symptoms. "You can simply treat the painful periods by suppressing the cycle" with birth control pills, says White. But does it actually prevent endo from growing, or does it just make the disease less painful (if it works at all)? "There's at least some thought that perhaps suppressing the cycle keeps endometriosis from growing more than it would if you didn't suppress, but there actually isn't really strong research showing that in fact that is the case," she says.

And what about when that young woman wants to get pregnant? "The question is how useful is something like hormonal suppression for someone who is suffering from endo and infertility, because you can't suppress the cycle and get pregnant. You can't do both." And there's the potential for that hormonal suppression to cause problems of its own. White works with Rachel Peragallo Urrutia at Reply OB/GYN & Fertility, the Cary, North Carolina, clinic that follows a "cooperative and restorative" model of care, whether the patient wants to get pregnant, avoid pregnancy, or just get better. "I think there are a lot of potential uses for fertility awareness in routine GYN practice," says White.

It turns out Braverman, White, Danielle Miller in Pennsylvania, and maybe other progressive doctors out there have an additional approach that isn't "gold standard," but that seems to be helping. They look at other ways of reducing inflammation: diet and lifestyle changes, supplements, and stress management.

"We recommend trying to reduce inflammatory foods and substances and exposures, and even trying some anti-inflammatory supplements," says White, though she makes clear that there's no conclusive research. Braverman points out that the immune profiles of women with endometriosis are almost identical to those with celiac disease—people who cannot break down the protein in wheat and other grains. "Even if they don't have celiac disease we find that they have a high sensitivity to gluten," he says. "A lot of them didn't know they had sensitivity until I took them off gluten, and they feel so much better." Like many evolving practices, he hired a health coach to work with patients.

He's also put together a regimen of anti-inflammatory supplements and a probiotic. "We found that the gut flora in women with endometriosis are damaged," he tells me. Jessica Drummond also focuses "first and foremost" on healing the gut, "because otherwise you're triggering inflammation where most of the immune system is." Braverman cautions, "These are not panaceas, but we've been having success for years." He believes these adjustments are reducing the inflammatory cytokines that damage a woman's eggs and promote miscarriage.

Drummond teaches these very concepts to health professionals interested in a more "functional" approach. One way she connects to medical doctors is to point out that historically the advice to young women diagnosed with endo was that they get pregnant—in quieting the immune system and hormonal cycle, pregnancy seems to offer a reprieve. It can temporarily ameliorate other autoimmune diseases as well, like rheumatoid arthritis and multiple sclerosis. Drummond also has seen pregnancy relieve women's vulvodynia symptoms and points to evidence that this too may have an immune component. She also just wrote up a case study of a woman whose irritable bowel syndrome and vulvar pain resolved with diet, supplements, and stress reduction.

It's possible that this is the future for endo sufferers. It's also possible that the physical manipulation that therapists like Assaf and Herrera do can break up the lesions and keep "frozen pelvis" at bay. "I don't like the word 'frozen' because if you have the right person you can get it to move," Herrera told me. "I always feel that endo is 100 percent of the time helped with pelvic therapy, it's just that nobody knows about it."

For Ellen, who had been seeing holistic practitioners along with MDs her whole life, who was already eating well and meditating, and who was 37 and felt the biological clock ticking faster, the next step was IVF. She and her husband were living in Boston at the time, and they went to a renowned center. She filled out the forms, answered questions about her health, and the lead physician laid out the protocol: there would be three cycles.

In the first, Ellen didn't respond to the drugs, so they had to keep increasing the dosage. She ended up on the maximum, had two mature follicles, and they were able to extract two eggs. One fertilized and implanted. "I was very briefly pregnant," she tells me. "Very briefly."

The couple took a year-long break. "I just wasn't sure I wanted to do it all again," she says. They saw two other specialists, to see if they had any different recommendations. But everybody seemed to follow the same protocol based on age, so they returned to the original practice.

Ellen went through the second cycle, suffered the side effects, the trips back and forth to the clinic for tests, the hope and anticipation. An ultrasound showed she had two mature follicles, so they prepped her for the surgical retrieval. When she woke up, the news wasn't good. "I had nothing, no eggs at all. I remember coming out of retrieval, out of anesthesia, and I was like, did I dream that? Zero eggs. To go through all of that and to have zero is sort of unimaginable." They went through the third cycle: one follicle, one egg extracted, successfully fertilized in vitro, incubated for five days, transferred to Ellen's uterus, no pregnancy.

Looking back on all this, Ellen recalls that the protocol felt very formulaic. "It was based on my age," says Ellen. "My age and my quote, unquote 'health.'" The fact that she had several autoimmune diseases, including stage 4 endometriosis, didn't factor in.

But halfway through the treatments, Ellen was at the clinic having an ultrasound to check the follicles, and something seemed to click for the doctor. "It was an awful moment," she says. "He sort of barges in and he looks at the screen and he's like, 'Oh, yeah, your ovaries are done.'" At that point, the endometriosis wasn't something she'd given much thought to. "I didn't know much about it. And I'm there in the stirrups, and he's saying, 'It's a horrible disease. It's an awful disease.'" It was not something she'd thought about as a disease, because up until that moment none of the doctors had presented it that way. Now, suddenly, it was the explanation for her fertility problems, "that it had aged my reproductive system significantly."

"Women are going into these centers, especially the top centers, thinking that they're going to get the best of care," says Braverman. "And they make the good embryos. They have the best labs, that's most of what they do. But when they get into a complex situation, an immunological situation—not just endometriosis, but other underlying, undiagnosed autoimmune diseases—if these aren't worked up and treated, these women go through a vicious cycle of failure, failure, failure, income depletion, and then they essentially quit." In Massachusetts, insurance covered most of Ellen's costs. In New York, women come to him having spent $100,000.

Braverman also takes issue with the idea that a woman's ovaries are "done." "We have hundreds of women who were told their eggs are no good, 'you need donor eggs,' and then they fail with donor eggs." It's true that by a certain age, a woman's follicles stop priming eggs for release, which is called "low ovarian reserve" and is part of the natural decline of fertility. "Numbers you can't get back, but you can improve the quality of the eggs by fixing the environment they're made in," he says. The inflammatory environment damages them, as does insulin resistance, which is a hallmark of the disease known as polycystic ovarian syndrome. He mentions that PCOS and endo often run together, and some researchers believe it too belongs in the autoimmune bucket, because the disease is also marked by antibodies and inflammation.[13]

PCOS is what Charlotte, the soprano, didn't know she had until a year of IUI attempts resulted in failure and miscarriage at age 38. It was her acupuncturist who first suggested it, based on her symptoms and a reading of her menstrual charts, and she worried Charlotte was at high risk for ovarian hyperstimulation syndrome if she underwent IVF, which is exactly what happened. "I had something like 50 follicles. I was in tons of pain. I had to go on blood thinners because my estrogen was so high I was at risk for a stroke," she told me. After a break, she tried IVF again, this time on a protocol modified for PCOS and low thyroid, which lab tests had also confirmed. Charlotte had read up on the immunological properties of the disease and also voluntarily gave up gluten, sugar, and dairy. That cycle resulted in a healthy pregnancy, and a very smiley baby who occasionally lights up my newsfeed. I remarked that her clinic, in western Massachusetts, sounded particularly evolved. "It took a lot of my own advocacy, honestly," she said.

DELIVERING THE UTERUS

On Valentine's Day 2018, Lena Dunham published an article in *Vogue* about deciding on—that is, admitting herself to the hospital and demanding—a hysterectomy at age 31. She had jousted with endometriosis for a decade, enduring excruciating, mind-numbing pain, and had tried everything she had the resources to try. She was done, even though she'd always known she wanted kids. "But I know something else, too, and I know it as intensely as I know I want a baby: that something is wrong with my uterus. I can feel it, deeply specific yet unverified, despite so many tests and so much medical dialogue," she wrote.

She awakes from the surgery with "doctors eager to tell me I was right. My uterus is worse than anyone could have imagined. It's the Chinatown Chanel purse of nightmares, full of both subtle and glaring flaws . . . The only beautiful detail is that the organ—which is meant to be shaped like a lightbulb—was shaped like a heart."[14]

Hysterectomy is the second most common surgery in the United States, after the cesarean section, and like C-sections, hysterectomy rates vary widely depending on where a woman lives and the color of her skin, and how many procedures are necessary is a point of controversy. Women in the Southeast and black women across the country are much more likely to have a hysterectomy, and it's not because they have more risk factors: a large study that controlled for such things as fibroids and obesity still found black women were 3.5 times more likely to have the surgery.[15] Fibroids are the number one reason for the operation, but with a skilled surgeon these can almost always be removed—the procedure is called myomectomy—and there are non-surgical ways to shrink them.

Endometriosis is another common reason for hysterectomy, but unless it is performed by a surgeon skilled in also removing endo lesions, the symptoms are likely to remain (and even then, they still return for a significant minority). Younger women face the difficult choice of whether to remove the ovaries, which is associated with less recurrence, and hope to trade endometriosis for menopause (and increased risk of heart disease, sexual dysfunction, dementia, and osteoporosis).[16] Cancer—the one reason everybody agrees requires surgery—only accounts for about 10 percent of hysterectomies.

In May 2017, I met Tracie Long in pre-op the morning of her hysterectomy. When I arrived, she was on a gurney looking a little ashen after the multiple attempts it took the IV nurse to get a vein. She was also nervous. Her doctor, Myron Luthringer, said hello, and then rhetorically,

"So, tell me what we're doing today." "Robotic-assisted vaginal hysterectomy. Keeping my ovaries," Long said firmly. It was 6:40 a.m., a damp, early spring morning in Syracuse, New York. Luthringer stood in his blue scrubs and cap leaning next to a whiteboard that had the same info written in green marker, answered a few last-minute questions, and went through the standard immediate complications—other organs or structures he could damage once inside, bleeding, infection—and what she could expect when she woke up. Then the anesthesiologist arrived. "Are you ready?" he asked. "As ready as I'm going to be," she said.

Long was 41, the hysterectomy was a last resort to remove a permanent birth control device called Essure that she and Luthringer felt had damaged her uterus and was causing pelvic pain and a multitude of health problems (more on this device in chapter 4). She was hopeful that it would alleviate her symptoms and restore intimacy with her husband.[17]

I talked to several surgeons in order to understand what exactly happens to the anatomy during this common surgery. Ahmed Al-Niaimi, a surgeon and professor at the University of Wisconsin who trained in general surgery, OB/GYN, and gynecologic oncology, generously agreed to give me a detailed lesson. We meet in his office, and he draws several diagrams on a notepad. Then he puts on a video of a robotic laparoscopic hysterectomy he had performed, pausing frequently to narrate what's happening.

A surgeon will start by "killing" the uterine arteries and vessels, which cuts off the uterus's blood supply, he explains. Next, the taut ligaments that encase the uterus are one by one decommissioned: the round ligament, then the broad and cardinal ligaments, the uterosacral and pubocervical ligaments. At this point, the only connection remaining is the top of the vagina, which rings the cervix. This part of the surgery is called the colpotomy. I watch as the electrified instrument burns through this anatomy, as the uterus turns a dull gray.

Once cut free, the surgeon will "deliver" the uterus (if it's a vaginal hysterectomy) and finally sew the top of the vagina into a "cuff." Al-Niaimi emphasizes how this last part requires the surgeon to "take our time, because that's where the thick tissues are." The uterosacral ligament is the strongest in the human body, he says, it's what holds the uterus up when it is growing a baby or babies. This ligament is embedded into both the top of the vagina and the cervix, and it's possible for the surgeon to preserve the former section of it and then further tighten it to provide "apical support" to the vagina, so that there's less likelihood of prolapse. "I've had extremely great outcomes from that," Luthringer told me. The surgeon needs to go "slowly, slowly," to do this, says Al-Niaimi.

It's not clear how many other surgeons do this. Since 2014, it has been recommended by the American Association of Gynecologic Laparoscopists (AAGL), the association of minimally invasive gynecological surgeons.[18] And it's not clear that robotic surgery improves outcomes (a promotional video for the da Vinci Surgical System, which has dominated the market for two decades, reassures: "Today, you don't have to have your mother's hysterectomy").[19] One rare but devastating complication is when the vaginal cuff separates, called dehiscence. A 2011 review article of 13,000 hysterectomies found that this was three to nine times *less* likely to happen if the cuff was sutured by hand transvaginally, as opposed to laparoscopically or robotically.[20]

James Robinson, a Washington, DC, gynecological surgeon who's on the board of the AAGL, tells me that if a woman is having an abdominal hysterectomy, which was standard until the early 2000s, "the approach to that actually cuts right across those uterosacral ligaments, so they got severed, so you lost that support. It also shortened the vagina by a couple centimeters, and then they used to take out everybody's ovaries too, so people went into menopause, they got hot flashes, night sweats, they had pain with sex because their vagina was too short. It was a pretty miserable procedure." One-third to one-half of hysterectomies are still abdominal (the CDC only tracks in-hospital procedures, but researchers estimate that 100,000 to 200,000 per year are occurring in ambulatory surgical centers, and most of those are laparoscopic), and in 40 to 50 percent of procedures, doctors still remove the ovaries.[21]

When I ask Al-Niaimi about the risks and aftereffects of the surgery, he focuses on the risks of the surgery itself—anesthesia complications, infection, and organ injury. I press about the anatomical and physiological impacts. "One of the biggest things you might have is impact on self-image and function," where a woman "feels like less of a woman, so sexual health is a problem, intimacy is a problem, there's always a fear that she's not quote, unquote 'good enough' for her partner." But this, he believes, is not the physical reality, it is psychological. "There are a lot of myths that the cervix is important for orgasm. These have been shown not to be true," he tells me.

I point out that many women can feel their cervix during intercourse, and that without the cervix, the "vaginal cuff" makes the vagina a fixed length—wouldn't that logically have an impact? He nods. "We intuitively think there's less vaginal lengthening [after the surgery], but we actually haven't quantified that in research."

As for what else happens internally, Al-Niaimi runs down the scenarios: the small intestine may take up the space left by the uterus, or the bladder may shift backward and the colon may shift forward, and they may fuse to each other. The rectum, normally held back by the uterosacral ligaments, may bulge into the back of the vagina. The top of the vagina may scar unevenly, says Al-Niaimi, pulling it to the left or the right. "I'd say about 15 to 20 percent of patients do complain about some pain in the pelvis after" due to scarring. He agrees it's not a procedure to be taken lightly. "Every hysterectomy should have a reason. But I can tell you that not all 600,000 [that are performed each year in the United States] have a legitimate reason."

According to the physical therapists I talked to, the physical effects of this pelvic reshuffling may take months or years to manifest. Those can be incontinence, prolapse, difficulty moving one's bowels, reduced mobility, pain, and loss of sexual response or sensation or orgasm, or pain with penetration. With the broad and round ligaments severed, "you're cutting out the rubber band that connects the pelvic bones on the inside, and you're also cutting out the support structure that keeps the small intestines from falling down," says Megan Assaf. The hip bones can actually begin to drift apart, which can impact a woman's gait. The severed arteries and vessels can diminish blood flow to the vagina, clitoris, and ovaries. Nerves can be damaged, causing pain.

Assaf likens the effects to "a loose jigsaw." She typically sees women five to seven years post-hysterectomy—instead of moving the uterus, she moves the organs that have fallen in its place, and she teaches her clients techniques they can do on their own each day to give themselves some lift. "The women I see come to me because something didn't go right with the hysterectomy, or something didn't go right with the way it healed, or they're having symptoms from the side effects of having the cornerstone taken out of their building," says Assaf.

The way Assaf and Herrera talk about this is entirely different than the way GYN surgeons tend to talk about it. Paul MacKoul and Natalya Danilyants run the Center for Innovative Gyn Care, a boutique practice with three locations in Maryland. "The research clearly shows there are no side effects from removing the uterus outside from fertility. So people don't have issues from sexual function or pelvic floor function or any of those things," Danilyants assures me. MacKoul agrees: A supracervical hysterectomy, which leaves the cervix and the ovaries, "has no effect on ligaments or vaginal length or vaginal width or the cervix," he says. "If you did a pelvic exam on that patient you wouldn't know she had a hysterectomy."

Rosanne Kho, a GYN surgeon at the Cleveland Clinic who promotes vaginal hysterectomy (including removal of the cervix), says if she has patients who are concerned about what's going to happen to their sex life, "I can feel comfortable looking them in the eyes to say that there is no evidence that hysterectomy will impair your sexual health and function if it's done for the correct reason."

But when I talked to Tracie Long six months after her hysterectomy, she was having problems. "Sex is still painful," she said. "I feel as if my vaginal canal is shorter." Researchers note that some 20 percent of those who undergo the procedure report sexual dysfunction in follow-up studies.[22]

Among surgeons the cervix remains controversial. Robinson used to leave it intact about half the time, he says, but now he almost always removes the entire organ (leaving the ovaries). "There's good evidence to tell us that leaving the cervix does not improve pelvic support, like we historically thought it might, does not improve sexual function, like we historically thought it might," and increases risk of endometriosis and abnormal bleeding. "There's not an insignificant rate of people coming back to have their cervix removed," he says. Other sources, like the AAGL, say the research is inconclusive.

It's difficult to reconcile these perspectives—a hysterectomy either destroys a woman's pelvic integrity and sexuality or it's a big nothing? But others say the research is very limited. Hardly any studies follow women more than two years from their hysterectomy. Jenny Higgins of the University of Wisconsin points out, "The uterus is involved in orgasm. It moves up, it balloons, it contracts, it causes the vagina to tent and balloon." This is aided by the broad ligament, which swells and tightens, drawing the uterus up and lengthening the vagina.[23] "I think we have a very narrow view of what's involved in women's orgasm and women's sexual functioning in general and tend to measure things like coital frequency when we do research. So we know much less than we should about how hysterectomy affects women's sexuality, but it does." Twenty million women in the United States have had hysterectomies, but research on how this has affected them long term is minimal. Higgins goes on: "If there were some equivalent surgery on that large a proportion of men involving the seminal vessel or any part of the man's sexual functioning or ability to orgasm, we'd have come up with tons of alternative therapies."

The non-surgical therapies have their own drawbacks: the long-acting GnRH agonist Lupron Depot that is used to shrink fibroids and to treat endometriosis induces a menopausal state with attendant side effects. In uterine artery or fibroid embolization, a radiologist shoots tiny pellets of plastic into the arteries that feed the uterus, such that the fibroids are cut off from their blood supply. This works a lot of the time, though occasionally too much of the blood supply is cut off, and women can lose ovarian function (and thus enter menopause) and sexual function, and a number go on to need hysterectomies to remove an anemic uterus.[24] Uterine ablation uses heat to cauterize the endometrium, inside the uterus—a frequent side effect is pain, since the ovulatory cycle carries on but the endometrial lining can't be shed. It's also not an option for those wanting to conceive. About 20 percent of women have hysterectomies following ablation.[25]

If the ovaries are removed what follows is "surgical" or "sudden" menopause. These glands normally remain active even after menopause, producing androgens that impact bone and muscle health, mood, libido, and energy levels. The Mayo Clinic studied about 1,200 women who had both ovaries removed before reaching natural menopause and followed them for 25 to 30 years. The researchers found that they had an increased risk of Parkinson's, cognitive impairment, and symptoms of depression and anxiety.[26] The overwhelming research consensus is that women suffer a net loss of health and longevity when their ovaries are removed.[27]

"Even if the ovaries are not removed, often within a few years ovarian function significantly or dramatically can decline anyway," Jessica Drummond points out, because their main blood supply has been cut off, and because the uterus generated hormones that fed back to the pituitary, which signaled the ovaries. The communication loop is gone. According to Eve Agee, a medical anthropologist by training and author of *The Uterine Health Companion*, the uterus, once thought to be merely a passive receptacle of hormones, actually produces an array of chemicals that benefit women beyond fertility, including some 60 kinds of prostaglandins and enzymes, which have anti-inflammatory properties, among them: prostacyclin, which prevents blood clotting; endorphins, which probably have an immune function when they're not countering the pain of childbirth; and "vast amounts of anandamide," a compound similar to those found in marijuana and dark chocolate.[28] So the loss is both anatomical and physiological.

"Early menopause and fast menopause is just no fun," says Drummond. "My biggest problem with hysterectomy is that I think women really aren't well informed about the fact that it's not extraordinarily effective in removing pain. So you've gone through this massive procedure that has hormonal effects, that has bone effects, that has cardiovascular effects, that has brain effects, and it's only modestly effective in terms of the symptoms. Now if you have cancer, that's a different story, but most of the time we don't look at cost-benefit. It's just 'take the organ out.'"

MODERN HYSTERIA

Many women I talked to felt they had little alternative but a hysterectomy. I met 27-year-old Nikki Powis via Facebook. She had suffered with endometriosis since her period began and was also diagnosed with irritable bowel syndrome. The Pill, Depo-Provera, surgeries, psych meds, nothing helped. "I think probably since I was 18 I had asked for a hysterectomy at every single gynecological visit," she said. The doctors all protested that she might want kids. Eventually she found one who was willing—he performed an old-fashioned abdominal hysterectomy, taking out everything but her cervix "for muscular integrity." He had suggested leaving one ovary, but she didn't want to risk returning for another surgery. "I feel lucky that I found him because he did exactly what I wanted," she told me. Still, several months post-op she was struggling with pain and bloating and said she couldn't tolerate the hormones, so she's going through menopause. Via Skype, she showed me the maternity pants she was wearing—she looked several months pregnant.

I met another woman, Holly S., who was dealing with chronic hip pain following a car accident. Nothing seemed to help, nobody had any answers, and she was worried about getting hooked on pain pills. But then a new OB/GYN found a cyst on her ovary and suggested a hysterectomy might help. "We both knew we didn't know for sure where the pain was coming from," she said, tearing up. "But she seemed to really care about the pain I was in. And I was looking for anybody to get rid of it." At age 40, Holly had a hysterectomy, including both ovaries and her cervix. "The recovery was a lot harder than everyone had said," she told me. She became depressed. The hip pain did not go away; in fact it became worse following the surgery. She went on disability. She walks slowly, slightly bent, and takes opioids that knock her out.

A big reason women turn to hysterectomy is blood. Fibroids can cause bleeding so heavy that women become anemic and need fainting couches. And the perimenopausal years can make the bleeding unpredictable and intense. Santina Smith travels between the Bahamas and the United States for work and remembers lying on airport floors because she'd get so light-headed—her belly was so distended with fibroids that she looked six months pregnant. When she was younger, her physician was laissez-faire about the growths, but as the years wore on she grew 11 pounds of them. By that point the hysterectomy felt inevitable.

The attitude of inevitability, particularly in the black community, irked Tanika Gray, who founded the White Dress Project to start a conversation about fibroids, which have plagued her family. "It was just kind of like a way of life when I started listening to women's stories. It was just like, yeah, we got fibroids. Yeah, my mother had a hysterectomy,

I'll probably have to have one," she says. "I just felt that was wrong." She also came across a lot of silence. "It's very hush hush, very taboo, and when I think about it, I really think despite cultural socioeconomic status and race, I really think as women we're taught you just don't talk about issues below the belt," she says. "I think we've let that grow into how we think about our health."

The problem with silence is that women don't know that they have options. "A provider speaks to their level of expertise," says Gray. Before she found a surgeon to remove her fibroids by myomectomy—she had 27—she was offered a hysterectomy and told to get a surrogate if she wanted kids. "We always tell our community members, it's so, so, so, so important to get a second, third, fourth opinion," she says. "This is where loyalty has to go out the window."

For every woman who willingly sought out the surgery, or readily agreed to it, there seems to be an equal number of women who went under the knife expecting surgery *on* the organ, but not the loss of it. Nora Coffey, who founded the advocacy group Hysterectomy Educational Resources and Services (HERS) in 1982 and still answers its 24-hour hotline, is one. She thought she was having an ovarian cyst removed and biopsied but woke up to learn that the surgeon had taken her ovaries and uterus even though they were not cancerous. This was in 1978, but women still call the hotline and post on Facebook with similar stories of waking up with organs removed instead of treated. The standard consent form allows for the possibility. Coffey coined the verb "to hysterectomize." She also uses the word "castration" for ovary removal, which is provocative but anatomically fair.

The skill of the surgeon seems to be a factor in what happens while women are unconscious—like endometriosis, fibroids require skill. These swirls of muscle can be easy to pop out or snip off or they can be embedded deep in the inner musculature of the uterus. They can be the size of a grape or the size of a baby, and there can be 3 or there can be 20 (and the fee is the same regardless of how long the operation takes). It's not always clear from ultrasound what a surgeon is going to find in the moment. And in that moment, preserving the organ may be out of their depth.

"If you have to take something out of the uterus, you need to be capable of repairing the uterus," says James Robinson, the DC-based OB/GYN and leader in minimally invasive gynecological surgery. The uterus has very vascular areas, so blood loss becomes a concern if a surgeon can't work quickly enough. He echoes Braverman's critique that surgery is not the emphasis of OB/GYN training. For all other surgical specialties, the training is five years. OB/GYN is four years, with at least half the time spent on obstetrics. "So how much time do you actually spend doing surgery? Most of the surgery you're doing is C-sections," says Robinson, which realistically leaves a year and a half to become competent in every other surgery, from removing cysts, fibroids, and endometriosis to repairing prolapses, cystoceles, rectoceles, and fistulas. That's 18 months for gynecological surgical specialists compared to five years for every other surgical specialty. "Unfortunately, when people come out of an OB/GYN residency they probably don't have a ton of surgical experience," he says.

Ten years ago, Robinson created one of a handful of minimally invasive gynecologic surgery (MIGS) fellowships around the country, in which OB/GYNs train an additional two or three years. Today there are 30 such fellowships, which is progress.

While surgical skill matters, doesn't it also matter how we as a culture, and medicine as an institution, value the female sex organs? Powis was discouraged from hysterectomy because she might want children; Holly S. was offered it because she'd already had three; did Gray's race play into her doctor's recommendations? If the organ serves only the function of procreation, then logically we'll do everything we can to preserve it or we'll be quick to discard it depending on the woman—and what kind of babies she'd produce. This was made explicit in the early twentieth century, as medicine organized and surgery advanced, and the eugenics movement won laws mandating sterilization of the "mentally unfit," with women of color disproportionately represented among those sterilized. Even after these laws were eliminated, tens of thousands of women were unwitting recipients of what came to be known as the Mississippi appendectomy, well into the 1970s. Today, one in three black women will have had a hysterectomy by age 50.[29] When Harriet Washington published *Medical Apartheid* in 2006, one in three women *over age 18* had had the operation in Mississippi.[30]

The way we've viewed the uterus is not unlike the dichotomous way white patriarchy has viewed women: pure, virtuous, able to breed, or promiscuous, diseased, the source of "hysteria." As several historians have pointed out, gynecology emerged as a surgical specialty right along with feminism's "first wave" in the nineteenth century. Some, like radical feminist theologian Mary Daly, argued it was a direct response: "The purpose and intent of gynecology was/is not healing in a deep sense but violent enforcement of the sexual caste system," she wrote in her 1978 book *Gyn/Ecology*, noting the rise of clitoridectomy ten years after the first women's rights convention in 1848 and the "gynecological craze" of ovary removal as the suffrage movement gathered steam.[31] Physicians advocated removing the gonads for hysteria, nymphomania, masturbation, and a new disease, "ovariomania." "It was not long since disorders of the uterus had been held responsible for almost every ailment," wrote the historian Harvey Graham. "This line of thought was familiar and it was all too easy to apply it to the ovaries."[32]

To be fair, many pioneering surgeons were treating women with symptoms so grave that they willingly participated in surgery without anesthesia. These surgeons removed tumors of several pounds, drained several pints of fluid from cysts, and removed ovaries in the hopes that induced menopause would improve conditions for women for whom they could not yet successfully remove enormous uterine fibroids or a diseased uterus—surgery was not yet that advanced.[33] But other surgical subjects were institutionalized or enslaved, and consent was not theirs to give. And some women endured multiple experimental surgeries, like the enslaved patients of J. Marion Sims, lauded as "the father of gynecology" (more on this in chapter 4).

The nation's first successful hysterectomy was performed in 1853, but the odds of post-op survival were unfavorable well into the early twentieth century. By the 1940s, however, they improved to 99 to 1. "In recent years, in fact, hysterectomy has become safe enough to be abused," wrote Graham in 1951.[34]

By the 1970s, as feminism's second wave was in full bloom, hospitals began documenting an upsurge in hysterectomies, which some were marketing as "hysterilizations."[35] Physicians like Connecticut OB/GYN Dr. Ralph C. Wright were openly advocating prophylactic hysterectomy.

After childbearing, "the uterus becomes a useless, bleeding, symptom-producing, potentially cancer-bearing organ . . . To sterilize a woman [through tubal ligation] and allow her to keep a useless and potentially lethal organ is incompatible with modern gynecological concepts," he argued in the journal *Obstetrics & Gynecology* in 1969.[36] In 1977, the vice president of the AMA told Congress that this major surgery was a reasonable contraceptive for women with "pregnophobic" anxiety.[37] In the 1980s, women could pick up *The Woman Doctor's Medical Guide for Women* by Barbara Edelstein, MD, and read, "Your uterus is nothing but a big, unresponsive blob."[38]

The OB/GYN community's current rhetoric is now less disparaging and rather emphasizes the "minimally invasive" nature of the twenty-first-century hysterectomy: it can be done with two quarter-sized incisions in the belly button or removed through the vagina with no external scars whatsoever. "A vaginal hysterectomy done correctly is an elegant, neat procedure with excellent safety and very quick recovery," blogged OB/GYN Jennifer Gunter.[39] A father-son team in New Jersey created the "One Kilo Club," "an exclusive international association of pelvic surgeons" who could boast removing that much worth of uterus/fibroid laparoscopically.[40] There is no professional movement to reduce the number of hysterectomies, only to reduce the size and number of incisions. But as I'll explore in the next chapter, this singular focus on "minimally invasive" has brought a new risk to surgical patients.

If the uterus is the cornerstone of the pelvis, does hysterectomy hold a similar place in American gynecology? Rates of the surgery in North America are more than twice the rates in most European countries.[41] A scientist at Columbia University who studies the biomechanics of the human cervix told me that her European colleagues are jealous of how easy it is for Americans to get lab specimens. As one critical OB/GYN put in her 1989 book, "The uterus is the only part of the human anatomy that lacks a constituency determined to preserve it."[42] For the most part, hysterectomy is a solution American women have been content enough with.

This issue did capture the attention of the feminist health movement of the '70s and '80s. "There was the legitimate sense that the predominantly male medical profession and predominantly male OB/GYN specialty did not respect women's bodies, bodily integrity, or the importance of women keeping their organs intact," says Cindy Pearson, executive director of the National Women's Health Network. Activism led to congressional hearings on hysterectomies in 1976 and again in 1993, and to activists demanding more research.

"I remember when I was on staff of National Black Women's Health Project, we had to go to NIH and FDA and say why the hell are you not studying fibroids?" says Loretta Ross. The answer she recalls is that "it simply hadn't emerged as a research priority" ("and it still hasn't, as a matter of fact, 25 years later," she quips). She didn't buy that. "It's a question of which population has the problem, isn't it? . . . If the problem doesn't manifest predominantly among white people, it doesn't become a problem, does it?" Pearson points out that by the '90s, "we were able to grab resources in health agencies and insist that they devote a fair share to us and our questions," which led to the availability of non-surgical alternatives like embolization and ablation. Still, nobody can explain why so many North American wombs are riddled with fibrous masses.

What if that research led us to uncomfortable answers about our culture and society? One thing we know about fibroids is that they run on estrogen, and estrogen is cheap modern fuel: diets high in sugar and simple carbs stimulate it, fat stores it, and environmental pollutants mimic it. The cheapest foods are high in all of those, so it would stand to reason that the obese-making diet of American poverty may exacerbate it. Endocrine disruptors also abound in cosmetics and hair relaxers, the latter of which is often posited as a reason for the prevalence of fibroids among black women. But there's another potent endocrine disruptor that's even more ubiquitous: racism.

The stress of racism—distinct from money stress or relationship stress or family stress—has been well established as having multiple health impacts—"weathering," as it is now called. One study looked at the connection to fibroids and found a direct relationship: the more racism black women experienced, the more fibroids they had.[43] The authors considered the possibility that the stress of fibroids could lead to unhealthy behaviors, like drinking and poor diet, which could increase their number or size. But when they controlled for such habits, the association persisted. Meanwhile coping skills and vigorous exercise seemed to mitigate the association, which they concluded suggests a "stress mechanism."

If the stress of racism stimulates fibroids, what does the stress of other "isms" do? While money may stress our psyches, discrimination stresses our souls. Sitting with Isa Herrera and her pelvic model, there came a point in the conversation when the anatomy and physiology became secondary. "Why do women grow things?" she asked in a voice soft and full of maternal concern. "I think it's because there's a void. There's a lack of support."

Megan Assaf asked me right away if I wanted her to stick to the clinical realm, because otherwise she'd venture into the spiritual. I invited her to tell all—we don't have all the scientific answers, so it can't hurt to consider ancient beliefs. "The womb is a second heart," she said early on in our conversation. "It's very much connected to the upper heart in a woman. And when we have our uterus in a state of health and balance and connectivity to our upper heart, as women we're centered, we're grounded, we're present, we're embodied, we have access to our strength, to our clarity, we have access to the direction of our creativity." The fact that women were diagnosed with "hysteria" for centuries in the West, the fact that all manner of disease was blamed on the womb, that the womb was seen as controlling the woman, is exactly what you'd expect from patriarchy, she said. "Who can blame them? This is a superpower organ."

What about women who've had hysterectomies? I asked. Certainly there are artists, leaders, powerful women who have let the organ go because it was sapping them of strength, and nobody offered them a better alternative. Assaf said just because the organ is gone doesn't mean the "energy body" went with it—kind of like a phantom limb. Most can still access this energy body, she says. In the spiritual realm, anything is possible. Or perhaps it's more helpful to think of the womb as a metaphor.

So Assaf makes her clay womb models, hoping for a sort of voodoo when they land in women's hands, that by holding a surrogate of the "second heart" women will forge a better bond with their own.

4: GYN EXCEPTIONALISM

NATALIE MAY WANTS to show me the "beautiful" German stainless-steel, size-small speculum she was gifted. We're standing in the hallway of a medical school in Connecticut where she has spent the better part of a Wednesday in early November teaching two groups of future nurse practitioners the art of breast and pelvic exams, using her own breasts and pelvis—and speculum, which she pulls out of her shoulder bag for me to admire. May, 21, is a gynecological teaching associate, or GTA, as well as a student at nearby Wesleyan. "We're sort of a parody of ourselves," she says of the various forms of reproductive justice activism—and political activism in general—on campus. "This is something I can do with my body."

The GTAs teach foremost that exams "should not be painful," but rather "thorough, comfortable, and respectful." They've rewritten the script in many other ways: "Language is really important. This is not a bed, it's a table. This is not a sheet, it's a drape. These are not stirrups—this isn't a saddle," Hana Koniuta, another GTA, tells a coed group of four during the morning session. Rather than having a patient lie flat, the table should be tilted at 45 or 60 degrees, she instructs. For teaching purposes, Koniuta adjusts hers to 90 degrees.

A pelvic exam is actually several different exams: visual inspection, "bimanual" exam, speculum exam, and sometimes rectal exam. In the bimanual, the provider inserts two fingers into the vagina and with the other hand on the abdomen palpates the uterus and ovaries. Koniuta walks each of her students through the bimanual with her woolly socked feet in the *footrests*, blue drape strategically covering her legs, leaving her vulva in view. She suggests they stand up for better leverage. "But try not to loom over your patient," she tells the one male student. "Remember to tuck your fingers so you don't accidentally touch the clitoris." She tells him when he's reached her cervix, when he's found an ovary. Clinicians should always check in, she tells the students. "Say 'Let me know if anything is painful or tender.'" Reassure the patient that "Everything looks healthy and normal" if it is. But never say *I'm going to look/touch/feel*. She asks the students to brainstorm clinical words instead: *assess*, *examine*, *inspect*, *visualize*.

The pelvic exam—with its cold table, crinkly paper, and impending metal—has in many ways been a defining event of the female experience as well as the history of medicine. For the patient, it is an exam of supreme vulnerability, potentially triggering, generally unpleasant. In *Mad Men*, Peggy Olson submits to an exam in order to get the Pill; the doctor warns, while the speculum is inside her, that "easy women don't find husbands." In *Girls*, Hannah's doctor asks her, "Is that painful?" Hannah responds: "Yeah, but only in the way it's supposed to be." Surveys of female-born trans men suggest they avoid gynecological appointments altogether.

The annual pelvic chore may also be largely unnecessary. In 2012, the Veterans Administration reviewed all the available evidence on routine annual bimanual pelvic exams and found zero benefit and the potential to lead to overdiagnosis and unnecessary treatment, as well as pain, discomfort, anxiety, fear, or embarrassment in the moment.[1] As a result, the American College of Physicians (the professional group for internists) recommended against it in 2014, citing the research. The American College of Obstetricians and Gynecologists (ACOG), meanwhile, has stood by the annual exam, citing "expert opinion."[2] Surveys of U.S. gynecologists show that most still offer it, and most women expect it.[3]

In her book *Public Privates*, artist, scholar, and former GTA Terri Kapsalis wrote about the gynecological exam as performative, structured "to both produce and reflect proper performances of womanliness," and also as a synecdoche of the doctor-patient relationship writ large. Historically, resident physicians practiced on the bodies of women who were anesthetized. By nature, these patients were quiet, compliant. They also weren't able to give consent or feedback, so the physicians weren't taught to ask. An entitlement to enter the body was baked in to the routine.

In the 1970s, women began "taking back their bodies," specifically by taking the speculum into their own hands, viewing their cervix with a mirror, and showing the trick to others. The gynecologist's office was deemed ground zero for patriarchy, and an early feminist health goal was to keep women out of it. For a time, "self-help" groups flourished, and a nationwide Federation of Feminist Women's Health Centers grew, offering a women-run alternative for basic gynecological care. The GTA model was pioneered by a male physician in Iowa, Robert Kretzschmar, in the early '70s, but "the women's movement undoubtedly influenced this model," wrote Kapsalis. "In fact, many early GTAs were directly associated with [self-help] groups and clinics and believed their new position . . . could allow them to bring their alternative knowledge to the heart of the beast."[4]

Today, most medical schools employ GTAs. The practice of pelvic exams on unconscious, unconsenting patients is officially discouraged by ACOG, though it still happens enough that a researcher wrote in 2018 that "the practice is alive and well."[5]

May and Koniuta work for Praxis Clinical, a company founded by former Yale GTA Alexandra Duncan in 2014, when she was just 23. While the work is well paid, at around $75 an hour, for most it is a passion project. "It's helping people be good to other people's bodies," May told me. Duncan discovered GTAs while she was a student at NYU volunteering as a doula. "I was like, Yes, I want to take my pants off for science!" Yale essentially handed its in-house program over to Duncan, and now Praxis trains every single medical and nursing student at Yale, along with several other colleges in the area. Duncan emphasizes that the form of teaching is as important as the content. "A lot of the power in this model is that the person on the table is the source of knowledge and authority. You have to look at the person whose body it is—they're the expert."

Praxis is unique among programs, I'm told, because the teachers work solo—nobody "uses" their body to teach but them. This is Duncan's signature contribution to the pedagogy, and the GTAs seem to prefer it. Many programs, like the one in New York City, use the "team teaching" model, where two GTAs switch off playing the roles of patient and provider.

The GTAs also teach an exhaustive breast exam—it's so thorough that Koniuta mentions muscles and lymph nodes I've never heard of. The exam extends from the elbow to under the clavicle to three levels of pressure on the breast itself. Nobody in the room has ever had a breast exam like this. "You know more than we do!" one of the students marvels. Then the subject of self-checks comes up—"during this time you can talk to your patient about self breast examinations if you choose to promote that, though I know it's controversial now," she says. The students groan and mumble under their breath. "I don't know why," says one out loud.

In 2009, the recommendations on breast cancer screening changed: routine mammograms were no longer recommended for women under age 50 or over age 74, and for the ages in between they were recommended every two years rather than annually. Another recommendation was that clinicians should no longer teach the self breast exam. The origin of these new guidelines was the U.S. Preventive Services Task Force (USPSTF), an independent group of volunteer researchers and clinicians that evaluates preventative medicine practices like screenings based on epidemiological evidence.[6]

When the task force looked at breast cancer screening, they found that too-frequent mammograms led to the problem of overdiagnosis. Ned Calonge was head of the task force when it changed its recommendation. "You have to screen somewhere between 1,000 and 2,000" to save one life, he told me. "It's hard to visualize 1,000 women." He went straight to a male analogy: the football field, filled with women on every inch of Astroturf. "That's the number of women you have to screen every year for ten years to save one of them [compared to if you didn't screen them]. That's the benefit." Meanwhile, half of them will have abnormal mammograms and go down the treatment path. Some will get biopsies, surgeries, and radiation; some will have severe complications.[7] One 2015 study comparing geographic areas with high screening rates to low screening rates found that the former counties had more diagnoses but no fewer deaths.[8] Nobody in the exam room in Connecticut speaks up for this point.

The task force also found "insufficient" evidence to support the clinical breast exam itself. The National Cancer Society now recommends against it. This also doesn't come up in Connecticut.

George Sawaya, an OB/GYN and professor at the University of California, San Francisco, served on the USPSTF for several years. The task force, he tells me, trained him "to think equally about the harms of prevention as much as the benefits." In spite of the "early detection saves lives" mantra and pink ribbons donning everything from cat litter to the NFL, every test, every screening tool has more than just the potential to detect a dangerous cancer and save a life. It also has the potential to trigger unnecessary harms, injuries, even deaths.

The squinting eye of the USPSTF has looked at screening tools across the medical spectrum, and several within women's health. It turns out that Pap tests also have a lower harm threshold than originally imagined: the recommendation since 2003 for women aged 21 to 65 is to test every three to five years depending on one's age and whether the test is combined with an HPV test.[9] And the recommended protocol for treatment has become more conservative—studies show that cone biopsies and LEEP procedures (common treatments to remove lesions) make pregnancy complications twice as likely, including premature birth.[10] The scarring can have other impacts. I know one woman who couldn't have orgasms for a year after having a procedure.

Still, the Pap test—now combined with the HPV test—is an effective prevention tool. If someone gets tested at the recommended intervals, cervical cancer has almost zero chance of spreading. The number of cervical cancer deaths that still occur around the world are primarily in populations without access to screening or treatment.

The routine bimanual pelvic exam, on the other hand . . . Even before he joined the task force, George Sawaya wondered about the annual pelvic. He knew of no evidence to support it. At the time, he was a resident and wanted to study it. "I was met with a lot of resistance from colleagues, because it was a bit of a sacred cow, it was kind of the foundation of what we do as gynecologists," he says. Yet he remained curious. "Anything that is unquestionable needs to be questioned, almost by definition."

As a clinician, he would see patients "being led down these paths of fear and unnecessary surgery." In 2010, some 63 million pelvic exams were done each year in the United States, at an estimated cost of $2.6 billion.[11] One of the purported reasons there are so many is to detect uterine fibroids and ovarian cysts. "I just felt there was this unseen epidemic of women who were having lots of interventions and lots of follow-up tests and lots of unnecessary surgeries with complications, and I couldn't quite figure out what the endgame was, other that this is just something we do all the time."

Speculum exams have been documented as far back as the ancient Hebrews, but the bimanual pelvic was first described for a Western medical audience in the 1890s, according to Sawaya. Still, these exams were for diagnostic purposes; for many decades, modesty precluded male physicians from visualizing anything below the waist—a famous woodcut shows a male doctor kneeling before a standing woman with his hand underneath her skirt and his eyes deliberately looking away. When did the hands-on pelvic exam make the jump to preventative health?

Nobody I asked knew the origins of this practice. Sawaya's guess was that it grew out of well-meaning logic: "Ovarian cancer is awful, it's a terrible, terrible disease. It doesn't take a rocket scientist to say, You know what would be a good idea—instead of waiting for the cancer to show up, why don't we try to find it?" Perhaps it followed on Dr. George Papanicolaou's test to detect changes in cervical cells that indicate possible cancer—earning the "Pap" name—which by the 1940s women were encouraged to get yearly.

But it turns out the recommendation of a yearly check preceded the Pap: it was Howard Kelly, the first professor of OB/GYN at Johns Hopkins University and a prolific author of medical articles and texts in the twentieth century, who suggested it for all women who've had children until age 55 (presumably menopause?) in his seminal 1908 monograph *Medical Gynecology*. This was a handbook for the aspiring "general practitioner who intends to practice gynecology" and included everything from sample office floor plans, recommendations on waiting room decor, and personnel ("a cheerful, kindly wife, a pleasant secretary, and even a bright-faced maid are all assets of much value in helping to hold a nervous impatient patient") to best clinical practices ("metal instruments are best sterilized in a fish kettle").[12]

Kelly advocated a conservative practice with limited, judicious use of surgery. He emphasized that the exam begin with a detailed history-taking, sensitive to the patient's mental state. "If the patient is nervous and distressed, a few routine questions directed in a kindly, reassuring manner will serve to give her time to collect herself and set her at ease," or if she has a lot on her mind, "it will be best to let her talk freely at first."[13]

The physical exam that followed was to be comprehensive: breasts, abdomen, vagina, and rectum. "The physician must never forget that a large percentage of his patients have other ailments than those which are covered by gynecology." The bimanual exam, he wrote, "reveals the exact position of the uterine body." Kelly instructed the practitioner to "displace" the uterus to examine the tubes and ovaries, to test for the mobility of the organs, and to discover any enlargements. "The question must be asked and answered whether the uterus has its normal play, and whether or not the ovaries are free." Lack of play could indicate adhesions or cancer. His instructions echo many of the directives I hear in the GTA session—check the Bartholin's glands for discharge (an indication of gonorrhea), check for rectocele or cystocele (collapse of the vaginal wall separating the rectum or bladder, respectively), check for pain or masses.

I have to thank Ronald Cyr, a retired OB/GYN from Toronto and an amateur historian, for introducing me to Kelly.[14] "When I trained in Toronto during the 1970s, the classic texts were all written by Kelly's trainees and their descendants (Williams for OB, Te Linde for GYN surgery). We were also taught to do complete exams on all patients, lest we miss something: 'if you don't put your finger in it, you'll put your foot in it' was the slogan of one of my professors," he wrote over email. "The 'thoroughness' argument has undoubtedly been used by doctors with ulterior motives to justify unprofessional or illegal behavior; in other cases, the 'thoroughness' is prompted by a need to tick all the boxes on the exam chart in order to bill the insurance company for a higher-level visit than might otherwise be justified. The fee-for-service system does lend itself to daily conflicts of interest."

Kelly was well intentioned, but screening for ovarian cancer unfortunately doesn't work. Physicians have tried screening with a blood test, with ultrasound, and with a bimanual pelvic exam, but all fail to reliably detect cancer. Studies show no benefit and plenty of harm. Yet the pelvic exam remains a GYN staple. After the VA ran the numbers and the internists and OB/GYNs released conflicting recommendations, everyone was hoping the USPSTF would settle the debate. But in 2017 it concluded there is "insufficient" evidence to make a recommendation either way.[15]

Barbara Levy, vice president of health policy at ACOG, told the *Washington Post* in 2015 that "a lack of evidence does not equal lack of benefit." Some suspect the organization advocates for the exam for the practical reasons cited by Cyr—insurance companies are currently mandated to cover the annual well-woman GYN visit, and it's harder and harder for practices to make ends meet. Carolyn Westhoff, a Columbia OB/GYN who authored a 2011 journal article asking "Do New Guidelines and Technology Make the Routine Pelvic Examination Obsolete?," told the *Post* that some of her colleagues needled her—"Carolyn, are you trying to put us all out of business?" In her article, Westhoff referred to the annual pelvic as "ritual" and wrote that it "may partly explain why U.S. rates of ovarian cystectomy and hysterectomy are more than twice as high as rates in European countries."[16]

Meanwhile, Levy argued in favor of the annual exam on the basis of patient-doctor bonding: "It opens the door and is a time of intimacy between the patient and care provider" in which the patient might be more likely to share taboo or embarrassing concerns, she told the *Post.* Sawaya quotes this statement when he lectures on the topic at hospitals—he tells me he finds it "creepy." "I almost titled my grand rounds presentation 'Excuse me, but your hand is in my vagina.'"

Sawaya studied the impacts of these recommendations on patients: among a group of 450 women, 80 percent initially said they would opt for an exam if one was offered. Conventional wisdom is that women find them reassuring. But when half of those women were given the American College of Physicians' recommendation against routine exams, that number dropped to 39 percent (the other half were given the ACOG recommendation, and still eight in ten continued to opt for the exam).[17]

I was curious how GTA programs have adapted to the conflicting recommendations. They are using their own bodies to teach an invasive exam that all med students learn but not all will use clinically, and which it turns out should be imposed far less frequently across exam rooms. To my surprise, Praxis's founder, Alexandra Duncan, is sympatico with ACOG and even more candid about her rationale. "I'm biased in favor of bimanual exams," she says, laughing at how that sounds. "They're my favorite." She says the learning curve is steep, but "once you've done enough and hit that tipping point, you get very good at it. You can get a lot of very useful information from those exams."

Furthermore, she is "still very much in favor of getting the bimanual every time you're at the GYN. In most cases I'm anti–unnecessary procedures that are for the doctors' sake. But this is one of those ones where I think I'd be in favor of people continuing to get and receive those. They're not more invasive than anything that's already happening there," she says. "If providers aren't practicing them, how are they supposed to have that understanding?"

Julie Carlson, formerly a GTA in New York and a producer of the documentary *At Your Cervix*, is now a nurse-midwife who performs exams clinically (they remain an important diagnostic tool). She disagrees with Duncan. If patients don't need clinicians' hands in their vaginas, those hands shouldn't be there. The original purpose of the GTA, after all, was to protect patients from being reduced to training mannequins—and GTAs can be utilized to help providers keep up their skills.

And GTAs really are taking a hit for vaginas everywhere. While the intent is that their students go on to be gentle, humble clinicians, the work of teaching on one's own body can be physically and emotionally trying. Natalie May tells me that most of the time she ends a training day elated, but occasionally, especially when she first started teaching, she would have a "sad" or "weird" feeling after. "But also it's such a physical job that you could be feeling off and it's actually just because you had something poking around your cervix like seven times in a row." One of the most senior GTAs, Victoria, recalls working for Yale many years ago, when the GTAs would teach in pairs. She dreaded working with one colleague in particular. "You just gritted your teeth and got through it." Koniuta tells me that once a student who was "really bad at following my instructions" jabbed her cervix so forcefully during the bimanual that she passed out momentarily.

Most medical schools now have in-house clinical teaching associates programs—they are beginning to hire male associates to teach proper prostate exam—but participants may be "teaching associates" in name only. "They are not necessarily the kinds of programs where the GTAs are occupying the space of teacher," says Carlson, calling it the "mute model format," in which a faculty instructor "is teaching how to do the exam on a body that has no voice, and so [the students] are not learning how to interact with the patient." Duncan is similarly concerned about other programs. Has the feminist GTA model been co-opted?

"Any good health care provider is going to say that the patient is the teacher," says Carlson. A good, thorough story is often what leads to an accurate diagnosis—more so than the MRI, X-ray, or lab work. "So if a health care provider student isn't learning how to interact with the patient to 1) get their story and 2) create an environment that's empowering and comfortable, then they won't ever get the story because someone is just going to check out and disassociate, particularly during a GYN exam, particularly if they're a survivor of sexual violence, which so many women are." She cites a 2003 study of med students in Philadelphia that found they had less commitment to patient autonomy after they'd finished their GYN rotation.[18]

In general, the GTAs love the work and feel it's important. "It's really gratifying to know that future practitioners have had this experience," says Koniuta, "and it will hopefully translate into really positive experiences for women in terms of preventative care."

GYNECOLOGY'S BIRTH STORY

In the twenty-first century, every field of medicine has had to reckon with the twin problems of overdiagnosis and overtreatment. In men's health, routine blood screening for the prostate-specific antigen (PSA) is no longer recommended by the USPSTF, though most physicians still offer it. In orthopedics, numerous clinical trials have found that spinal fusion and knee surgery offer *no benefit* over physical therapy.[19] In dermatology, skin spots are overbiopsied and overtreated, particularly in the elderly.[20] We know the story with antibiotics—their overuse has bred scary superbugs. The nonprofit National Academy of Medicine has been on top of this phenomenon for 20 years and estimates that health care excess costs about $750 billion.[21]

OB/GYN isn't exceptional in this regard, but the surgeries tend to be major: hysterectomies, removal of ovaries, cesarean sections.

Women who are diagnosed with cancer in one breast are increasingly choosing prophylactic mastectomy of the healthy breast, though there is no evidence that it is beneficial.[22] And women who discover they are carriers of a genetic BRCA mutation, which indicates they are at a higher risk for breast and ovarian cancer, are increasingly electing prophylactic removal of breasts and ovaries. The USPSTF notes a "moderate" cancer prevention benefit here as well as harms.

Like the annual pelvic exam, one can understand these practices originating and persisting from a well-meaning logic. But the preemptive removal of organs is a trend that affects women alone, and we often fail to fully account for the trade-off of benefits to harms. Do we ever suggest men remove their testicles "just as a precaution?" performance artist and BRCA carrier Cyndi Freeman jokes onstage. "Come on, if we just take off everything that makes me a woman then I'll, like, finally be able to live forever!"

The tendency to cut out or into female sex organs, which disproportionately affects women of color, also fits neatly into the history of obstetrics and gynecology.

Obstetrics as we know it is a very new profession—the term *obstetrician* wasn't introduced until the mid-nineteenth century, derived from the old Latin word for midwives, "obstetrix."[23] Up until then, the business of attending women in childbirth was called midwifery. Men wanting to insert themselves in the birth chamber were called "man midwives"; male physicians and barber surgeons were only rarely called in. According to historians Richard and Dorothy Wertz, *obstetrician* "had the advantage of sounding like other honorable professions, such as 'electrician' or 'geometrician,' in which men variously understood and dominated nature."[24]

It was in many ways a hostile male takeover of a female domain, as well as a white male takeover of a profession comprised largely of indigenous, black, and immigrant women. In the beginning, norms of modesty and morality slowed down the incursion. It took a century in America for male obstetricians to gain a foothold—the practice was first resisted by the "popular" health movement of the mid-1800s as well as the growing women's movement.

But by the turn of the twentieth century, the politics shifted. Doctors had organized into societies and begun publishing in journals, gaining the respect of the elites. "Between 1900 and 1930, midwives were almost totally eliminated from the land—outlawed in many states, harassed by local medical authorities in other places. There was no feminist constituency to resist the trend," wrote Barbara Ehrenreich and Deirdre English in their 1978 history of patriarchy in medicine, *For Her Own Good*. "Middle-class feminists had no sisterly feelings for the 'dirty' immigrant midwife. They had long decided to play by the rules laid down by the medical profession and channel their feminist energies into getting more women into (regular) medical schools."[25]

This transfer of power did not immediately result in better outcomes. In many cases, it made births more complicated and dangerous. Besides forceps, male doctors had little to offer over midwives, and far less accumulated knowledge and expertise. The main complication of pregnancy was protracted labor, and for centuries midwives had kept women upright to facilitate easier deliveries—women labored mobile and gave birth standing, squatting, or sitting on birth stools, of which there are records going back to antiquity. "By the turn of the twentieth century, birth chairs were reduced to delivery tables with stirrups, steel shoulder clamps, ankle and wrist restraints, and sterile field guards that separated the mother from the birth of her child," wrote the historian Amanda Carson Banks.[26]

This sterility did not prevent infection because the patient was not the source: physicians didn't wash their hands until the late 1800s, and proper antiseptic technique remained a problem into the twentieth century. Unlike a midwife who attended just one woman in her own home, hospital-based physicians moved from patient to patient. "He could and did carry to parturient women laudable pus from his surgical cases, droplets from scarlet fever cases, and putrefaction from the corpses he dissected," wrote one historian.[27] "Childbed fever"—infection—was a man-made epidemic. It caused half of maternal deaths in the 1920s.[28] The records of eighteenth- and nineteenth-century midwives in America and Europe show that their outcomes were actually very good for the pre-surgical, pre-antibiotic era; when U.S. public health inquiries looked into maternal and infant mortality in cities, they found it highest among doctors in hospitals.[29]

Still, the medicine men triumphed.

Midwives' scope of practice had been broad—they treated children's ailments, served families in death, used herbs to treat menstrual problems and miscarriage and also to induce abortions. The physician-led movement to outlaw abortion in the nineteenth century was motivated more by professional interest than any moral claim (more on this in chapter 7). "With the elimination of the midwife, all women—not just those of the upper class—fell under the biological hegemony of the medical profession," wrote Ehrenreich and English. "In the same stroke, women lost their last autonomous role as healers. The only roles left for women in the medical system were as employees, customers, and 'material.'"[30] Today, women make up the majority of medical students and practicing OB/GYNs, and midwives returned with the late 1960s and '70s counterculture and feminist movements. But the power dynamic and turf wars continue.

The history of gynecology follows a somewhat different trajectory. It obviously grows out of midwifery and obstetrics, but for a critical period in its development it is contiguous with the history of general surgery. That period starts in middle of the nineteenth century, when surgical pioneers advanced the profession on female bodies with gynecological operations. One of those pioneers was James Marion Sims, often called "the father of gynecology."

Sims is credited with refining the speculum along with the repair of vesicovaginal fistula—a tear between the bladder and vagina caused by protracted labor that renders a woman incontinent, infection-prone, smelly, and socially ostracized. He is also credited with founding the first women's hospital in the United States, in New York, in 1855—a "brilliant achievement" that "carried the fame of American surgery throughout the world." These are the words on the plaque accompanying his bronze statue, which in 2018 was relocated to Brooklyn from its perch on Fifth Avenue at the edge of Central Park. This origin story is a lie of omission, according to historian Deirdre Cooper Owens. The *first* hospital was the one he founded a decade earlier in Mount Meigs, Alabama, where he performed surgeries on enslaved women who also served as his assistants.

"Sims was a master brander," says Cooper Owens, author of the 2017 book *Medical Bondage: Race, Gender, and the Origins of American Gynecology*. Cooper Owens doesn't dispute Sims's status as pioneer, but she corrects the historical record to recognize his work in the Deep South and the women who made it possible: Betsy, Anarcha, Lucy, and six other enslaved women whose names we don't know. Sims relocated to Alabama after two patients in his care died in his home state of South Carolina, which put a damper on his practice. "Part of the nineteenth-century medical world that's infused with ideas of masculinity but also entrepreneurship is that you're not just trying to heal people, but you're also trying to establish a name for your career that can give you financial reward," she tells me.

Anarcha, Betsy, and Lucy had all developed fistulas resulting from childbirth, which Sims went about trying to correct. Over the course of five years, Anarcha was subjected to some 30 surgeries before the one that finally repaired the injury. Sims's technique now honed, he applied it on the other women successfully and published the case studies in a medical journal, winning international fame. Sims refashioned the speculum, calling it the "Sims speculum," and coined the "Sims position" for the side-lying, knees-to-chest position he put his patients in for the procedure. His career redeemed, Sims packed up for New York to found the hospital that would be etched in history.

But Sims was just one of many patriarchs of gynecology with similar bios. "Most pioneering surgeries" in American gynecology "happened during interactions between white southern doctors and their black slave patients," wrote Cooper Owens.[31] François Marie Prevost was a French-born physician credited with perfecting the cesarean section in Louisiana. He, too, practiced on enslaved women there, and before that in Haiti (a fact rarely mentioned in his biographies). Ephraim McDowell became famous for the first early successful ovariotomy on Jane Todd Crawford, a white woman; less known is that he experimented on four enslaved black women with ovarian tumors over the course of a decade. Henry Campbell, who helped found the American Gynecological Society in 1876, served as president of the American Medical Association, and edited the South's first medical journal, operated exclusively on enslaved women in Augusta, Georgia.[32]

In the North, physicians, including Sims, relied on poor immigrant women, mostly Irish, for experimental surgeries. Though anesthesia became available around the time that Sims and others were practicing, it was not used. "Black women and those whom blackness was sometimes mapped onto, such as the Irish, were seen as willing and strong servants for white medical men, impervious to physical pain and unafraid of surgeries," wrote Cooper Owens.[33] This belief in the biological difference of race was also used to dismiss the Americans' work. British surgeon James Johnson derided McDowell as a "backwoods Kentuckian" and doubted his achievements. "All of the women operated upon in Kentucky, except one, were negresses . . . [and they] will bear cutting with nearly, if not quite, as much impunity as dogs and rabbits."[34]

Cooper Owens doesn't use the word "torture" to describe this experimentation, though others have. These men had an interest in healing, because women's value was tied to their ability to reproduce. Still, she argues, we have to recognize the foundations of obstetrics and gynecology as born of racist ideology and rooted in the institution of slavery, where male doctors not only had power over female bodies but literally *owned* them. "Slavery's importance to their research could neither be denied nor ignored; it was at the heart of their practice and scholarship, even if these doctors did not explicitly identify the institution as the linchpin of their intellectual work," she wrote.[35]

Cooper Owens writes these women back into gynecology's origin story, arguing that they deserve credit not only for what their bodies went through but also for their knowledge and skilled work as Sims's assistants. "In a very real sense, these women know more about obstetric fistula repair than anybody else. They're being taught by the man who is pioneering this surgery," she points out. If Sims is the father of gynecology, "they are the rightful mothers of this branch of medicine."

By the late nineteenth century, gynecology was "a vibrant new specialty," says Ronald Cyr, "whereas nothing much was happening in obstetrics, except new types of forceps." The cesarean was still too fatal to become routine, "so ambitious young doctors swarmed to GYN, abandoning OB . . . They created a new specialty that divorced itself from boring, 'watch the hole' man-midwifery."[36]

In Europe, England, and Ireland, obstetrics and gynecology combined much earlier, probably because they still shared the market with midwives, who remained primary attendants. Today, OB/GYNs in Europe function as high-risk consultants rather than frontline providers. In the United States, where midwives had been stamped out or driven underground, the divorce between OB and GYN stuck for several decades. What reunited them was mutual professional interest. Obstetrics, according to the 1932 White House Conference on Child and Health Protection, was "not attractive" as a profession, with tedious hours and small fees, and it "received scant respect from the public at large."[37] Meanwhile, gynecologists wanted to be more than a "mere branch of general surgery," and general surgeons wanted them to stay out of the upper abdomen.[38]

Obstetrics was fashioning itself as more surgical anyway: prominent physicians of the 1920s and '30s were advocating for routine forceps and episiotomy, while the cesarean section—and abdominal surgery in general—was becoming safer and more viable as an alternate delivery route. In the early years, an emergency cesarean was performed by general surgeons or gynecologists, not the attending obstetrician. Leaders proposed separating the departments of gynecology from general surgery and combining it with obstetrics. By the end of World War II, most medical schools had done so.[39] By merging the two specialties, both would expand their scope of practice, and obstetricians could enjoy the prestige of surgery.

In the early days, neither specialty alone was enough to keep a solo practitioner busy or fulfilled. But in the following decades, the surgical repertoire grew along with the technology to intervene in the birth process. Meanwhile, leaders continued to have an interest in OB/GYNs serving as generalists, as Kelly had. In the 1990s, the profession had a small crisis: the Clintons' health reform plan would have required patients to get a referral from a primary care physician to see an OB/GYN. In response, ACOG launched a "primary care initiative" and successfully recategorized the specialty, which meant residency training shifted toward more primary care. This sparked a debate about whether surgical training would suffer.[40]

The debate continues. A 2014 survey of directors of fellowships in pelvic reconstructive surgery and gynecologic oncology—these are for OB/GYNs who want to become advanced surgical specialists—found that fewer than half could independently perform a hysterectomy.[41] In other words, these OB/GYNs had graduated med school and residency yet couldn't be left alone in the operating room. A 2015 survey of practicing gynecologists expressed concern about this. "We are training poorly prepared OB/GYNs who are not capable of handling a variety of clinical problems, and who are not truly surgically independent and competent when they finish residency," one respondent commented.

Sarah Cohen, a gynecologic surgeon at Brigham and Women's hospital in Boston, cited the above surveys in a 2016 article titled "Is Surgical Training in Ob/Gyn Residency Adequate?" She clarifies that there's no evidence that gynecologists are doing a bad job in the operating room or endangering patients. Rather, these surveys capture the anxieties and desires of newly graduated OB/GYNs: they want more training. In her opinion, their plates may simply be piled too high. "What is unique to our field is that we only have a four-year residency to do both surgical training and obstetrics, and our specialty also expects us to be primary care physicians to some extent as well," she told me. "It's a lot to squeeze into four years."

MINIMALLY INVASIVE

On October 17, 2013, a woman named Amy Reed checked herself into Brigham and Women's hospital in Boston for a routine surgery: she would have her uterus removed along with the fibroids that had been causing her daily misery since her last child, her sixth, had been born. Reed, 40 at the time, was a highly educated patient—more than most. She was an anesthesiologist and critical care doctor at neighboring Beth Israel Deaconess Medical Center, an MD/PhD, and a member of the teaching faculty at Harvard Medical School. She had administered anesthesia to patients having the same operation. She and her husband, Hooman Noorchashm, also a Harvard-affiliated MD/PhD and a cardiothoracic surgeon, knew this was garden-variety surgery and that Reed was in the most capable hands—Brigham and Women's was Noorchashm's employer.

Reed went home that evening. Her youngest child, Ryan, had just turned one. She was still breastfeeding. A week after the operation, her surgeon, Karen Wang, called her. "Are you alone?" she asked. The pathology report on her tissue had come back, and the news wasn't good: leiomyosarcoma, an aggressive form of cancer. Wang was sorry. Reed's phone rang again: it was Michael Muto, the oncologist who had evaluated her and ruled out cancer: He was also sorry she was going through this. She should return for a scan.

Reed called her husband, who was in North Carolina in the middle of assisting in a lung transplant surgery (Harvard had sent him there). A nurse urged him to scrub out because his phone kept buzzing. Reed sounded panicked and scared, but managed to tell him the news. He then received a call from Karen Wang. He asked her, "Did you get it out in one piece?"

The answer was no. Noorchashm wrote down the word Wang used: "morcellated." Actually, he spelled it with an 's', like "morsel."[42] He left the hospital and headed for the airport, where he started Googling. "It took me about thirty minutes to figure it all out," he told me.

Morcellation means cutting up tissue, and OB/GYNs began doing it in the 1990s to achieve more "minimally invasive" hysterectomies. Laparoscopic surgery in general was advancing, reducing risks of infection and blood loss for many abdominal surgeries, like appendectomies, gall bladder removals, and hernias. But fibroids can be large, and large incisions mean weeks of recovery.

What enabled surgeons to remove a large uterus or fibroid through tiny "keyhole" incisions was that they were downsizing it first—removing it one morsel at a time. At first, surgeons did this by hand. But then in 1993, the FDA approved the first power morcellator—basically a hand blender—without a single clinical trial, through what's called the 510(k) process.[43] Devices in this class need only prove they are "substantially equivalent" to a previously approved device, which may have been equivalent to another device, and so on—the root device may never have been clinically tested. Several other companies followed with similar products, including Johnson & Johnson, and very quickly morcellators were being used on tens of thousands of women per year.

Noorchashm didn't have to read more to understand the implications: the cancer cells inside his wife's uterus had just been splattered throughout her abdomen. Noorchashm told me this was the first time either he or Reed had ever heard of the device, or the practice. It was baffling, because they had learned the core surgical principle that you "respect the margins" of potentially cancerous tissue; you would never cut up a tumor or diseased organ—that would spread and "upstage" the cancer.

General surgeons almost always remove masses and organs whole—in the rare cases they do not, the tissue would first be biopsied and even then cut by hand in a containment bag, to minimize the chance of any cells left behind. But the power morcellator was heavily promoted to gynecological surgeons, and they adopted it enthusiastically for what were deemed "benign" surgeries.

For the first couple of weeks following her diagnosis, "Amy was completely devastated," in Noorchashm's words. But they had to figure out what to do. They learned many more details about the morcellator device and practice. For one, the odds that a fibroid would be cancerous were believed to be almost theoretical: 1 in 10,000. Fibroids are by definition benign. Michael Muto, the oncologist, had told Noorchashm that Reed was just very unlucky.[44] But Noorchashm came across a research paper dated November 2012, almost a year before Reed's surgery. It looked at the pathology reports of morcellations at Brigham and Women's hospital, and one of its authors was none other than Muto. The authors reported finding atypical cells in 10 out of 1,091 morcellations, suggesting a risk "much higher than appreciated currently."[45]

One of Noorchashm's first calls, after family, was to a medical school friend, Michael Paasche-Orlow, an internist and epidemiologist at Boston University. Paasche-Orlow and colleagues reviewed the literature and estimated that the rate of leiomyosarcoma in women with troublesome fibroids was closer to 1 in 415. While Reed fought the hungry tumors spreading through her body, Noorchashm was on a warpath: he blasted sharply worded emails to Brigham and Women's, to the media, and to the FDA, which began investigating. The *Wall Street Journal* and *Boston* magazine ran features about the couple's plight.

In April 2014, the FDA issued a warning about power morcellators, estimating that the risk of "seeding and upstaging" a hidden leiomyosarcoma was 1 in 350 surgeries. That means out of 100,000 procedures—hysterectomies or myomectomies—to relieve symptoms of "benign" fibroids, 286 women would essentially get a death sentence. In 2018, another study suggested that the rate of any hidden cancer is even higher—1 in 50.[46] Then there's concern about the impact of spreading "STUMP" cells—stromal tumor of uncertain malignant potential. The emerging evidence has led to lawsuits against manufacturers by women and their families, including Noorchashm.

Following the FDA's warning, Johnson & Johnson pulled its three morcellators from the market. In July 2014, the agency convened a panel to consider further action. Representatives from ACOG and the American Association of Gynecologic Laparoscopists (AAGL) spoke strongly in favor of keeping the device on the market, arguing that the technology allows tens of thousands of women each year to avoid "open" surgery, which carries greater immediate risks. Jubilee Brown of the AAGL presented a "decision analysis model" comparing the risk of leiomyosarcoma (close to the FDA's estimate) to the risk of complications from abdominal surgery and concluded, "More women each year would die from hysterectomy . . . We must not sacrifice our patients in an emotional response to a rare event." When it was Reed's turn to speak, she challenged this directly. "Is this true? No. Laparoscopic surgery is surgery through small incisions. Morcellation is shredding up tissue. They are distinct. Other branches of surgery, thoracic, general surgical oncologists, breast surgeons all operate laparoscopically without morcellation." Noorchashm was less polite: "The gynecologists who don't see this are poorly trained, are not thinking straight, and they don't see the devastation they cause," he said.

One of the few non-GYN panelists, Craig Shriver, a surgeon and director of the Murtha Cancer Center at Walter Reed, said he was "perplexed over the last two decades, watching the introduction of a laparoscopic power morcellation that is totally anathema to . . . my core principles as a cancer surgeon."[47]

The FDA decided on a black-box warning—its strongest action short of a ban. In its wake, UnitedHealth announced it would no longer reimburse for procedures using the power morcellator. The couple had won, sort of. Manual morcellation continues. Some surgeons are using a new device with a containment bag. And power morcellators remain on the market in the United States. All this goes on without objection from ACOG and AAGL. In late 2017, the FDA reiterated its warning and reported that "some groups continue to request that we scale back our recommendations."[48]

The power morcellator came along right around the time that the Accreditation Council for Graduate Medical Education, the board that sets requirements for medical residencies, shifted to require OB/GYNs to spend more time training in primary care. Some believe it also contributed to another trend: the decline of the vaginal hysterectomy, proficiency in which is considered a milestone of surgical skill. The morcellator essentially offered surgeons a shortcut to "minimally invasive" laparoscopic surgery.

Two other devices emerged around the same time, promising less time in the operating room for GYNs and less recovery time for patients: transvaginal mesh—polypropylene implants used to treat incontinence and prolapse—and the permanent contraceptive Essure, both of which have been implicated in thousands of adverse event reports to the FDA, as well as in lawsuits, and both of which were marketed as "minimally invasive" techniques.

Essure was approved in 2002 and hailed by women's health advocates as a non-surgical method of sterilization—something that could be done in a doctor's office and in clinics like Planned Parenthood rather than the operating room. Two tiny metal coils, each wound with a polyester called polyethylene terephthalate, are inserted through the cervix and uterus and into the fallopian tubes. (While the procedure is considered nonsurgical because there is no incision, it still requires sedation and local anesthesia.) The coils are made of stainless steel and a "superelastic" metal called Nitinol, and they expand like little springs to keep them in place while the synthetic fiber stimulates an inflammatory reaction, creating scar tissue that blocks the tubes (and sperm).

Within a few years, women began reporting problems: devices that migrated and punctured other organs, devices that broke apart and did the same, causing pain and bleeding. Some women got pregnant. Others came down with chronic autoimmune illnesses. When one woman started a Facebook page called Essure Problems in 2011, it quickly grew to have thousands of members, and they started making noise. They discovered that Nitinol contains nickel, a known toxin. They learned the device was approved based on a trial of a few hundred women who were followed for just one year, with no control group to see how it compared to tubal ligation.[49]

Noorchashm and Reed, who were both awarded PhDs in immunology, felt kinship with the "E-sisters" and attended an FDA hearing for the device in 2015: "Women are presenting just like you would see in a rheumatologist's office—hair loss, rashes, joint pain, tired," Reed told the panel. She called these "classic symptoms" of an immune system gone haywire. Noorchashm pointed out that "this device is not designed to cure an incurable disease . . . It's a medical device that's completely avoidable. And what I want to know from this panel is what percent harm are you going to accept: 0.1 percent, 1 percent, 5 percent, 10 percent? And how are you going to justify that?"

By the fall of 2018, some 30,000 reports about Essure had been made to the FDA, including 21 deaths believed to be related. In December, Bayer, the maker of the device, finally pulled Essure from the United States, its last remaining market, citing "low sales." On the Essure Problems Facebook page, which at last count had more than 41,000 members, women continue to post pictures of themselves in hospital beds, ready for surgery to remove the device. To become "E-free," the vast majority are getting hysterectomies. Surgeons have found that the device breaks apart if they try to remove it. As one Illinois gynecologist put it to the *Chicago Tribune*, "There's no way to really save the uterus and remove the coil completely."[50]

Mesh is even more difficult to remove once it has been implanted. "It's permanent and irreversible," says Michael "Tom" Margolis, a pelvic surgeon based in the Bay Area who spoke at an FDA hearing on mesh. "It's the herpes of medical devices."

Borrowing from the general surgery practice of using plastic mesh in hernia repairs, these pieces of polypropylene netting were cut specifically to form a "sling" under the urethra (in the case of incontinence) or to be placed between the vagina and bladder or vagina and rectum, or to provide "apical support" at the top of the vagina in the case of pelvic organ prolapse. They came in "kits" with special guides and catheters for vaginal insertion, rather than requiring open abdominal or laparoscopic surgery. The idea was a ready-made surgery, so OB/GYNs could address patients' symptoms themselves, rather than having to refer out to specialized surgeons.

Pelvic mesh was never tested in humans. The first to market was Boston Scientific's ProteGen sling, in 1996. Like the morcellator, this was cleared by the FDA through the 510(k) process, without any clinical trials. That process was supposed to be an "exception," former FDA commissioner David Kessler told documentary filmmakers, but "that exception became the rule," and the majority of medical devices now come to market this way.[51] ProteGen became the "grandmother" device for some 60 other pelvic meshes over the next two decades, which were cleared as "substantially equivalent." Some of these were cleared even *after* grandmother herself was recalled by her manufacturer in 1999, because, the FDA summarized, it was associated with a "higher than expected rate of vaginal erosion" and breakdown of the surgical wound, called dehiscence, and "does not appear to function as intended."[52]

Pelvic mesh, also called tape or sling, was designed to be fast and easy. That's how it was presented to Tammy Jackson, a nurse living in Frankfort, Kentucky. Jackson was 42 and healthy, save for the "leaking" that followed the birth of her "change of life baby" the year prior. She would go to work at the local hospital with an extra change of pants, socks, and underwear because she couldn't keep up with changing pads every hour on a 12-hour shift. She made an appointment with a local urologist she had shadowed years earlier in her training. "Oh, we have this new, simple, outpatient surgery. It's 45 minutes, you'll be back to work within a week or two," she remembers him telling her. This was 2007. She had the surgery, "and then the hell began."

Within days she was back in the hospital with a raging infection, and from then on she had recurring urinary tract infections, bladder infections, and kidney problems. By 2009, she was sitting in a gynecologist's office, complaining of stabbing pain, pelvic cramping, and cramping in her legs. "He said, 'Well maybe you need a hysterectomy. Maybe it's just time, you're going through the change of life." So she had a total hysterectomy, including her ovaries, "because I have cancer in the family."

The hysterectomy didn't help. The pelvic pain remained, and her legs started giving out—she would lose feeling in them while she was driving and had to stop driving long distances. She was fighting fatigue; it was too painful to sit. She hadn't been able to return to work since the surgery. The bladder and kidney infections just kept getting worse. The doctors in Frankfort kept telling her they couldn't find anything wrong. "Maybe you need a hobby, you're just a bored housewife," she recalls one saying. "I literally thought I was going crazy." Finally, her husband drove her the 50 miles to Louisville, where a urology team diagnosed the problem: the mesh had worked its way into her urethra.

In April 2018, Jackson, her husband, and their daughter traveled to New York City to attend the Tribeca Film Festival—she appears in the documentary *The Bleeding Edge*, about the harms of medical devices like Essure, transvaginal mesh, and the da Vinci Surgical System. She had to bring with her an IV pole and antibiotics and sat in her hotel room doing infusions while her family went sightseeing. Her right kidney is currently failing and constantly septic—treating it has required a PICC line, a permanent port in her arm, for the IV antibiotics she takes three times a day, seven days a week. She's become resistant to three different kinds of antibiotics and is running out of options. She's had 20 surgeries since the initial mesh was put in. Her kidneys are functioning at 30 and 60 percent, respectively—she's on the registry for a transplant. "Mesh was my very first surgery, ever. I was so healthy, 120 pounds," she tells me. With her first two children, boys, she was an "active mom," boating, camping, riding bikes, even skydiving. Her daughter, now 12, "has never known me well."

Jackson has retained an attorney and been active with the Mesh Awareness Movement, a group of women around the world who believe this simple outpatient procedure has caused them irreparable damage. Women report severe bleeding, they live in pain and become dependent on painkillers, they need to self-catheterize to pee, they deal with chronic infections. For many, intercourse is unthinkable. "I've talked to hundreds of women who say I have nobody to help me," says Jackson. "You can't be intimate with your husband, so they go outside the marriage; you get divorced, you literally can't work, your whole life is gone. There's been quite a few suicides."

Studies estimate that at least one in ten pelvic mesh patients have serious complications, requiring follow-up surgeries.[53] Once the mesh is in place, scar tissue envelops it, affixing the plastic to nearby tissue or organs. The mesh shrinks as the scar tissue forms and hardens around it. One of the most frequent complications is "erosion"—when the mesh works its way to the surface of the vagina, or into an organ. In 2010, a randomized controlled trial was halted because the mesh caused erosion in 15 percent of recipients.[54] Coming full circle to the early days of gynecological surgery, the device can essentially create a fistula.

When Jackson finally discovered her complication, she remembers the doctors telling her the mesh should come out, but "we've never been trained to take it out, it's not supposed to come out." Margolis is one of a handful of surgeons around the country willing to operate. "You won't get it all out," he tells me. In order to get all the mesh, "you'd have to do the most incredibly morbid procedure, you'd have to remove major organs."

Before transvaginal mesh kits were available, specialist pelvic surgeons would treat incontinence or pelvic organ prolapse with "native tissue repairs," in which they would shorten or reattach ligaments to create the necessary lift. Margolis still offers something called the Burch procedure, in which ligaments are attached to the neck of the bladder. Traditionally, this was achieved by making a large abdominal incision. "Only a few of us in the country ever learned how to do a laparoscopic Burch," Margolis tells me, in which the same procedure is done through small thumbnail incisions, which means less scarring and recovery time. These are difficult, delicate surgeries, and they require great skill. "Let me tell you something, the female pelvis is no place to go dicking around in if you don't know what you're doing," he says. "There are a whole lot of landmines you could step in. And if you step in them *you* don't blow up, the patient does."

The younger surgeons, those who trained in the last 20 years, have likely never done a Burch, he says. They never developed these skills. "Those surgeons were trained on the sling," says Margolis. "And this is really where it becomes a problem of ethics," because instead of referring to a more skilled surgeon, they'll offer the riskier mesh. Daniel Elliott, a urologic surgeon at the Mayo Clinic in Rochester, Minnesota, wrote to the FDA urging the agency to take mesh off the market: "All too frequently, industry knowingly targets less experienced surgeons, knowing these mesh kits have not, and never will be, accepted by more experienced surgeons who are fully aware of their inherent risk without benefit."[55] Yet if the new practice persists long enough, those green surgeons replace the elders, and the profession becomes "deskilled."

In April 2019, the FDA took the rare action of forcing transvaginal mesh designed to treat pelvic organ prolapse off the market. The United States finally joined Australia, Ireland, New Zealand, and the United Kingdom in restricting the kits. Meanwhile, more than 100,000 women are suing mesh manufacturers.[56] In one case against Johnson & Johnson, the plaintiff was awarded $57 million, though the company is appealing and has denied any wrongdoing.[57]

For now, mesh for urinary incontinence remains in use. The investigative journalist Alicia Mundy, who is working on a book about mesh, explains that while these smaller "slings" also have high complication rates, prolapse kits tended to cause more extensive and severe damage because they involved much larger pieces of mesh with multiple "arms" to wrap around organs and complicated surgical directions. "The mesh in the prolapse kits was hard to insert correctly and could cause permanent damage to the bladder, urethra, vagina and critical leg nerves," she says.

Together, power morcellators, Essure, and transvaginal mesh suggest a gruesome trifecta of regulatory failure. Steve Xu, a physician researcher at Northwestern University, looked at some dozen GYN devices approved in recent years and found "significant weaknesses" in the FDA approval and surveillance processes—and these were considered the highest-risk devices, which had gone through the most rigorous application (mesh and the morcellator were approved without clinical trials). "It seems every two or three years we have another controversy in women's health," he told me.

But as much as this pattern points to a failure of government oversight, what responsibility should the profession bear? How much harm *are* we willing to accept?

IS SURGICAL TRAINING ADEQUATE?

In June 2017, Reed lost her battle with cancer, leaving behind Noorchashm and their six children. At this writing he continues to wage a legal battle against the device maker and the physicians involved in Reed's care, and he's taken his fight beyond the device, beyond Brigham and Women's hospital, to the gynecological establishment at large. In several open letters published on Medium, he's argued that morcellation reflects a structural flaw in OB/GYN that goes back to its split from general surgery. Gynecologists, he argues, train "in a cloistered silo, away from cross-disciplinary training with other surgeons." And it's in that isolation, he argues, that they embraced a practice that is anathema to modern surgery.[58]

Of course, for Noorchashm this is personal. But others, even those within gynecology, have raised the issue of surgical training publicly. It's evidently the only surgical specialty that does not require multiple years of general surgical training. And in my investigations of each of these devices, and into pelvic surgery more broadly, the question of skill and training came up again and again.

Margolis argues that transvaginal mesh became routine even though it "defies core surgical doctrines." As he explains to me, surgeries are classified by the sterility of the field: abdominal surgery is considered "clean." An incision inside the vagina, which is home to bacteria that don't belong inside the body, is considered "clean-contaminated" (this cringeworthy term applies to many sites, in both sexes), and the risk of infection is double. Passing an implant through that incision is another level of risk, and Margolis argues it flies in the face of a surgical tenet: "that you are never to implant a synthetic foreign body through any operative field that is by definition contaminated," he says.

Nonetheless, pelvic mesh was widely embraced. Its story follows the pattern of other risky devices and drugs, in which research concluding the product was safe and effective was funded or ghostwritten by the manufacturer (in this case Ethicon),[59] "key opinion leaders" were courted and paid tens of thousands of dollars in speaking fees—one, Vincente Lucente of Allentown, Pennsylvania, admitted in a deposition to accepting $1.7 million over several years,[60] and professional organizations accepted large sums in the form of conference sponsorships.[61] Internal emails and footage of a deposition of one of Ethicon's medical directors reveal that the company had evidence of complications before it launched the product.[62] Doctors were "fed a line," says Margolis.

James Robinson, the previously mentioned gynecologic surgeon in Washington, DC, and board member of the AAGL, was an early adopter of Essure and implanted hundreds, he believes without incident. After attending the FDA hearing, he started removing some. When I interview him, I tell him that the majority of women I had talked to were getting hysterectomies. “That's nuts,” he says. “I'm not saying it's a super simple procedure . . . it's sort of like taking out a fibroid.” The coils not only embed into the fallopian tubes but the corners of the uterus as well, which are rich with blood vessels. If one removes something from the uterus, one needs to be capable of repairing the uterus, says Robinson. I ask him if some extra level of training or expertise is needed to do that. “I think you just need to know how to operate.”

But the majority of surgeons willing to remove Essure continue to recommend full hysterectomies. And the majority of women with bothersome fibroids are not offered myomectomies, in which a surgeon would remove the fibroids but spare the uterus. Instead, 600,000 U.S. women lose their uteruses each year. Isn't part of this due to how little we value the female organs? On his web site academicobgyn.com, Portland, Oregon, physician Nicholas Fogelson wrote under the “criteria for a hysterectomy” that the patient needs to “not be emotionally attached” to the organ. “From a scientific point of view a uterus is a bag of muscle to carry a baby in.”[63]

From a surgical point of view, I ask Robinson if the uterus is really so difficult to repair. That's when he points to residency training: five years of *surgery* for all surgical subspecialties—except gynecology.

Margolis echoes this criticism. “It's inadequate,” he tells me. “Your average OB/GYN resident simply doesn't get enough surgical volume to become a competent surgeon. That is why urogynecology became the fourth subspecialty, because people were getting out of residency training programs not knowing how to do a fucking hysterectomy.” He goes on, “In a four-year training program, you can count on maybe one or two hands the number of months that the OB/GYNs get surgical training in GYN surgery.”

David Jaspan, chair of OB/GYN at Einstein Health Network in Pennsylvania, disputes these criticisms. Yes, residents are doing fewer hysterectomies, but that's because there are more non-surgical alternatives, "which isn't necessarily a bad thing for women's health." He tells me that each year of an OB/GYN's residency is "equal part OB and equal part GYN," plus experience in GYN oncology, reproductive endocrinology, and female pelvic medicine and reconstructive surgery. "There's no argument that it would be great to have more surgical experience," he says, but there's no evidence that it's needed.

Margolis thinks gynecology should return to its surgical roots and split from obstetrics. "I think the perfect GYN surgeon of the future gets one year of obstetrics, two years of general surgery, and three years of all GYN surgery," he says. "Now that's somebody who can operate on my wife, my daughter." Why is general surgery so important? I ask. "That's the core tenets. The basics, the foundation. General surgery is the rebar, the brick and mortar of surgical technique. Every other surgeon—plastic, thoracic, vascular—has a core foundation in general surgery."

Because of the shorter residency and isolation from grueling "blood-and-guts" surgical residencies, gynecology is derided as a "back door" to surgery. "It's not subtle that they [OB/GYNs] are regarded as second-class citizens in the surgery world, they're regarded as not having the skills," one physician told me. "That is a criticism, that is a cultural belief that I've heard ever since I was interested in medicine, for the last 25 years," says Aileen Gariepy, an OB/GYN and researcher at Yale. She always chalked it up to sexism—"a devaluing of women and women's work . . . OB/GYN is at the intersection of a lot of 'isms'"—and she just hasn't found it to be true in her milieu. "I've been operated on by my colleagues," she says. But Ahmed Al-Niaimi, the Wisconsin GYN surgeon, nods when I bring up the question of surgical training. "It's a problem," he says.

Another core surgical tenet that seems to be defied in GYN surgery is what we might call fibroid exceptionalism: a fibroid is the only human tissue mass that is not routinely biopsied before surgery is contemplated. A man with a prostate mass isn't sent directly for a radical prostatectomy. Thyroid tumors, even breast lumps, are biopsied before a surgery. This has not been the standard in gynecology.

"Generally speaking, when you're seeing any mass in any organ or managing it, you would like to know what you're dealing with and for that reason, the biopsy is the way to go," David P. Winchester, medical director of cancer programs at the American College of Surgeons, told the *Wall Street Journal.* The CDC had announced it would convene a panel to determine if OB/GYNs should have new guidelines for preoperative fibroid screening—this was in large part a response to the study that suggested a much higher rate of cancer in symptomatic fibroids than previously thought: 1 in 50. "It is imperative," the authors wrote, "to further advance gynecologic cancer screening techniques."[64]

Perhaps one of the things GYNs could offer if they had more general surgical training is excision of endometriosis, myomectomies that relieve women of fibroids but leave their uterus and pelvic floor intact (without relying on morcellators), and "native tissue" repairs for prolapse and incontinence. But I also wonder if it's possible we're having the wrong conversation. Perhaps the bigger question is whether women should need so many surgeries in the first place.

CLITORAL DAMAGE

One of the most epic arguments in Greek mythology is a lover's quarrel over whether women or men enjoy sex more. Zeus argues it's women; Hera argues it's men. To settle the debate, the immortal couple go to Tiresias, who had experienced sex from both sides of the binary—Hera had transformed him into a woman for several years as punishment for disturbing a pair of copulating snakes. Tiresias sides with Zeus—women's pleasure eclipses men's by *nine times*, he reports. Having lost the argument, Hera punishes Tiresias again, this time by blinding him.[65]

Pity the messenger. In 1976, the faintest reverberations of this row could be felt at the Feminist Women's Health Center in Los Angeles. The "book team" was trying to rush out a self-help manual for women who couldn't access group cervical exploration: it was to include color photos of a healthy cervix throughout the ovulatory cycle, illustrations of the anatomy and of women self-exploring, and a mail-order form for a speculum.

Our Bodies, Ourselves had been out for five years, but the book team felt women needed more focus on the anatomy. And to their knowledge nobody else had yet tried to photograph the cervix. The book was almost ready for the printer, but then someone had suggested that if they were going to have careful drawings of the female anatomy and how to examine it, they ought not to skim over the details of the clitoris. And anyway, they were curious. They sent one woman, Lorraine Rothman, to the UCLA biomedical library. It was supposed to be a "simple little task": look at some anatomy books, write up a summary, photocopy some illustrations. Suzann Gage, who had shown up on the doorstep of the clinic in 1971, having dropped out of art school to join the movement, was illustrating the book. She would draw based on the photocopies "and that would be that," according to Gage.[66]

But Rothman returned empty-handed. She had looked at several books but they all said different things. "Oh, it can't be that difficult," said Carol Downer, the manual's editor and a cofounder of the clinic. Rothman returned to the library. Gage went as well. It *was* that difficult. They checked out a pile of books and brought them back to the clinic so everyone could see for themselves.

The entire book team was summoned and they laid out all the books. Indeed, contradictions abounded. With some notable exceptions, medical texts from the nineteenth and twentieth centuries barely mentioned the clitoris (while the penis was given pages). "They'd show a little bump, maybe, to suggest the glans of the clitoris but they wouldn't show all the parts of it. Women's sexual anatomy was the vagina, and that was it," Gage tells me. "The penis, however, would be rendered in great detail." Surprisingly, the eighteenth-century books featured more female anatomy. "I'd just dig though the stacks and I would pull out the oldest textbooks I could find, the textbooks that seemed the most antiquated, and these were the ones that had the best drawings," says Gage. The women noticed a "deterioration in accuracy and detail in medical illustrations" as the decades progressed.[67] In 1947, the clitoris was deleted from *Gray's Anatomy* entirely. By the 1950s and '60s, several sources followed.[68] Having found little guidance on female sexual response in two centuries of authoritative medical texts, the women doubled down on their investigation: they took off their pants.

They compared themselves to the pictures in the books, they compared themselves to each other; they self-stimulated while others photographed, documenting physical changes. They tried to solve the puzzle. Where did the clitoris begin and end? Was it analogous to the penis, as the ancient Greeks and Masters and Johnson had claimed? Not only were the drawings from the nineteenth or even eighteenth centuries more detailed, they were more accurate. "There were some spectacular drawings, incredibly detailed drawings that we found, many of which were in really old textbooks, some of them from Germany or other countries, done by artists who had done cadaver dissections, and that was where we started to find some detailed drawings of parts of the clitoris that we hadn't found in the modern textbooks," says Gage. It seemed these anatomists just drew what they saw, without an agenda. "But then at some point, there just didn't seem to be any interest in women's anatomy."

The women learned that yes, the penis and clitoris form from the same embryonic tissue, the same "bunch of cells" rearranged depending on chromosomes. The glans was just the tip of the iceberg, so to speak. The clitoris extends well beyond the little nub—picture a bird-like form, with partially extended wings. The nub is the bird's head. The debate over whether women or men enjoy sex more will carry on, but Tiresias seems correct in that there is nine times more clitoral tissue than the little nub that's visible.

A New View of a Woman's Body would take another five years to complete. The chapter on the clitoris grew to 25 pages—the longest in the book—with 33 illustrations by Gage, more than in any other chapter. The authors offered new language to describe the vast internal clitoris: they renamed the "bulbs of the vestibule" (the bird's body) the "clitoral bulbs," noting that they wrap around the vagina and extend into the inner labia, which they renamed the "clitoral lips." They called the wings, which extend back along the pubic bone, the "legs." They located a pad of soft tissue on the front wall of the vagina that surrounds the urethra, "undoubtedly protecting it from direct pressure during sexual activity." Finding this part unnamed, they called it the "urethral sponge." They found analogous tissue on the perineum, and lacking a label they called it the "perineal sponge."[69] While most medical texts showed the clitoris in one dimension (if at all), Gage drew the clitoris from all angles, based on the old dissections and her own live observation.

She also drew the interconnected pelvic floor muscles, ligaments, blood vessels, nerves, and organs. There's a drawing titled "The uterus during sexual arousal" and text describing how it "becomes swollen with blood and balloons upward." In another revolutionary spread, Gage drew a schematic cross section of the internal female clitoris compared to the male penis, marking the analogous tissue with the same squiggly paisley-ish pattern. "The redefinition of the clitoris is no mere semantic quibble. Its significance is apparent when it is realized, for example, that if the perineum is part of our sex organ, an episiotomy is more than a surgical incision. It becomes a mutilation of the clitoris," the women wrote.[70]

But history has not been kind to female pleasure or feminists. *A New View* did not change dictionary definitions or medical texts (or medical practice), which held fast to clitoral minimalism. *Hole's Human Anatomy & Physiology* calls the clitoris "a small projection . . . usually about 2 centimeters long and 0.5 centimeters in diameter." Merriam-Webster calls it "a small erectile female organ." Google's definition: "a small sensitive and erectile part of the female genitals at the anterior end of the vulva."[71]

Just as the anatomically correct clitoris has been ignored, reduced, or erased, so, too, has the team of '70s clitectives. It wasn't until around 2010 that media and blogs picked up on the work of medical researchers in Australia and France, who had mapped out the "clitoral complex" with MRI, dissection, and 3D ultrasound. Artists soon followed. In the years since, the clitoris—borders redefined—has become jewelry, sculpture, stencil, graffiti, urban chalk mural, and even the focus of a ClitArt festival in London.[72] In 2014, the Huffington Post published a terrific mini-site titled "Cliteracy," though it, too, passes over the '70s activist women with their mirrors and specula:

> In 1969, we put a man on the moon.
> In 1982, we invented the Internet.
> In 1998, we discovered the full anatomy of the clitoris.

The "we" in 1998 refers to Helen O'Connell, an Australian urologist and researcher, who broke a decades-long silence in the English-language medical literature with a paper in the *Journal of Urology* that concludes "current anatomical descriptions of female human urethral and genital anatomy are inaccurate."[73] O'Connell's work made several strides for the organ: using dissection, she and her coauthors found it to be much larger in size than typically described—extending from the vulva to the urethra to the vagina and perineum—and these structures share blood and nerve supply "and respond as a unit during sexual stimulation."[74] The term "clitoral complex" is hers.

"The vaginal wall is, in fact, the clitoris," O'Connell told the BBC.[75] O'Connell, to her credit, referenced her feminist forbears, both in her 1998 paper and in another blockbuster paper published in 2005. And the feminists had heavily borrowed from the anatomists. There is a long history of supposed "discoverers" of the clitoris—including one named Columbus.[76]

In 2012, Gawker's sci-fi site io9 announced in a headline, "Until 2009, the Human Clitoris Was an Absolute Mystery," reporting on a study that, for the first time, used 2D and 3D sonography to generate images of the clitoris.[77] Not only was the coverage belated, it ignored O'Connell's work. And so it goes.

Of course, we all deserve to know the precise geography of the clitoris. A 2017 study of some 50,000 U.S. adults found that only 65 percent of heterosexual women reported always or usually having orgasms during sexual contact, compared with 95 percent of heterosexual men and 86 percent of lesbian women.[78] Cue the joke about how the best sex toy might be a map of the clitoris. Its true depth and structure also put to rest the Freudian/feminist argument over the existence of the "vaginal" orgasm: the clitoris is both vulvar and vaginal, so orgasms must be all of the above!

O'Connell raised another problem of poor mapping: "surgery is guided by accurate anatomy," she and coauthors wrote, which "should provide the surgeon with information about how to preserve" the corresponding nerves and blood vessels. "But detailed information is lacking . . . The clitoris is a structure about which few diagrams and minimal description are provided, potentially impacting its preservation during surgery."[79]

During her urological training, O'Connell noticed how her mentors "took special care" when removing a prostate—they gingerly dissected around particular nerves and blood vessels to preserve their function. For women undergoing pelvic surgery, the clitoral nerves and blood supply were "a matter of guesswork."[80] The more researchers explore the clitoral territory, the more contiguous they find its borders with the rest of the pelvic anatomy: The latest contribution comes from Italian endocrinologist Emmanuele Jannini, who set out to explore several remaining controversies, like the existence of the G-spot, and in so doing dispels the myth of the passive vagina (in her famous 1970 essay "The Myth of the Vaginal Orgasm," feminist Anne Koedt wrote that "women need no anesthesia inside the vagina during surgery, thus pointing to the fact that the vagina is in fact not a highly sensitive area"). Jannini and coauthors report that it is actually rich with nerves and flickering with electrical impulses, which create rhythmic contractions upon penetration. "Sexual pleasure cannot be attributed to a single organ," they conclude.

What implications does this have for common gynecological surgeries and increasingly common "vaginal rejuvenation" procedures—labial reductions, G-spot injections, vaginal "tightening"? Anatomically speaking, these are all surgeries on parts of the clitoris, the international definition of female genital mutilation.

5: BIRTH TRAUMA

ON THE MORNING of June 4, 2012, a Monday, Tamara Taitt and Michelle Fonte drove south through the city of Miami to a mirrored government building surrounded by royal palms. They had a meeting with the city's zoning administrator, which they requested through the contractor they'd hired to build a birth center a few miles north on Biscayne Boulevard, in a building for which they'd signed the lease several months prior. They had prepared for the meeting with a binder full of detailed renderings and municipal permits for every other birth center in the state of Florida.

Taitt and Fonte had already begun offering childbirth classes and parent meet-ups and doula services in the building under the auspices of the Gathering Place, but the anchor of the business was to be the birth center—two home-like rooms where clients could labor and give birth under the care of midwives. Before signing the lease, they had checked with the zoning board about red tape and were told the process would be simple. "We're not stupid girls, we had gone to the city to inquire if this use was permitted there. We were told yes," says Fonte. Four months later, they still had no permit for births.

Taitt had trained as a midwife at Miami Dade College after getting her bachelor's at Princeton University, and at the time was on the board of the Midwives Alliance of North America (she is now a licensed midwife). Fonte is a mother of six and had been attending births as a doula for 20 years. They met in May 2009 doing grassroots organizing for midwifery in Florida and by 2012 had become partners in both business and in life. "Even though there are more birth centers in Florida than in any other state, there has never been one within the boundaries of the city of Miami," says Taitt. The women soon learned what that would mean for their venture: the planning and zoning office would make a determination of how to zone the business, because nothing like it had ever existed before within city limits. The contractor suggested they "engage" more with the office, so they requested the meeting, zoning references in hand.

"The administrator never even opened the binder. It sat there between us on the table, sort of mocking us," Taitt recalls. "We were super optimistic about the meeting, but when he didn't even open that binder, I think all the air left the room for us." Just one week later, they received his determination: he put the birth center into the same category as an assisted living or nursing home, called a "community support facility," which their modest house wasn't zoned for, "which was completely ridiculous," says Taitt. A birth center has no permanent residents, no full-time nursing staff, no dining hall. There would never be more than two women birthing there at the same time; if they needed more intensive care, they'd transport to a hospital.

The city of Miami has one of the highest cesarean rates in the country. For about ten years, there have been nearly as many surgical births as vaginal births in Miami-Dade County. In 2014, Consumer Reports put together a national hit list of large hospitals with the highest C-section rates: three out of ten were in Miami. In 2016, South Miami Hospital topped the Consumer Reports list, with 51 percent of *low-risk* first births happening via cesarean. Again, the city was well represented, with Baptist and Jackson hospitals in the top 20. Smaller hospitals have even more astounding rates: in 2016 at Hialeah Hospital it was 64.6 percent—again, for patients deemed low risk—(down from 68 percent in 2015). At Kendall Regional Hospital, the total C-section rate was 62 percent; at Mercy Hospital, 55 percent.[1] There's even a rumored "Miami Cesarean," a combo tummy tuck and baby delivery. As far as I can tell it's urban legend, but the myth's namesake is notable.

Taitt and Fonte wanted to offer a refuge. "There wasn't a place in the community where people could go to find out about birth options," says Fonte.

The two women found the perfect location on a historic stretch of

Biscayne Boulevard, just north of the glitz and west of the sand. The northern stretch of the boulevard, where Taitt and Fonte poured their hopes, was constructed in the '40s and '50s as car culture exploded. "Motor courts" and another new concept called the motel ("motor" + "hotel") sprung up on either side of the road, and many are still standing. The two-story house the Gathering Place occupied was a remnant of art deco–inspired residential development, with linear embossed panels below the windows and a wrought-iron balustrade at the entrance. An enormous mango tree hovered over the back parking lot, and the women put two white rockers on the front porch. They loved the feel of the place, and while they created a peaceful vibe inside, they also wanted to be seen, so they had their logo of three stylized flowers painted as a mural across the building's facade. The large neon motel signs competed for attention, why couldn't they?

The community part of their business took off immediately. "We were offering doula services, breastfeeding support, childbirth education classes in all forms, lots of support groups, and other events for moms and families that were free to low cost," says Taitt. But the permitting process was stuck.

The zoning administrator had said that the women could try to get a "warrant" to allow a community support facility to exist in their differently zoned building, which would allow them to operate the birth center. So they began that process. This meant that every building modification the house had gone through in the previous 50 years needed to satisfy the warrant, from the water main to the former garage on the first floor. "We spent six months doing a microfiche search to find out if the closure of the garage walls had been done with a permit, but there was no evidence that it was," Taitt told me. They were going to have to hire a structural engineer to do renovation forensics. They would need to conduct a traffic impact study. "They started looking at things like how the lines were drawn in the parking lot," says Taitt.

In 2014, the city approved construction plans for an eight-story, multimillion-dollar luxury condo and retail complex in the lot just two doors down. (The developer, it was later revealed, was a Venezuelan oil magnate with close ties to Hugo Chávez.) It was becoming clear to Fonte and Taitt that this was likely a "who you know" situation, and they were clearly out of their league.

Two years went by, then three. They loved their building and the quirky, kitschy neighborhood; their clients loved the centrality, but the business was hemorrhaging money to stay there. "Because we're now paying rent in a building providing services that were never designed to pay any money. So at a point we decided we'd come back to this perhaps, but we needed to get the birth center open because that was the financial cornerstone of all the things we wanted to do," Taitt tells me. The final straw was when they were notified about a complaint to the historic preservation board: the flower mural. "We were like, the writing is on the wall." They stopped pursuing the warrant and began looking for a new space.

In May 2015, the women were driving around North Miami Beach and saw a "for lease" sign and a realtor out showing a modest stucco ranch on a busy avenue. They pulled over and learned that it had previously housed a clinic. They already had the paperwork to be a clinic. "We saw the building, called the city of North Miami [its own smaller municipality], and within 48 hours we got a letter" confirming the birth center could operate there, says Taitt. They made an offer to the landlord and within two weeks had signed the lease. In February 2016, they opened their doors.

Taitt and Fonte called the birth center Magnolia Birth House and had it painted white with black shutters and a large green and buttercream magnolia mural. The Gathering Place still functions within it. The neighborhood is neither on the map for tourists nor of interest to the historic preservation board, yet they still want to be seen. The day I arrived, there were three loud yellow plastic signs spiked into the thin strip of grass between the road and the parking lot, the kind that usually say things like "CHECKS CASHED" or "NO MONEY DOWN!" Instead, these had their phone number and read "MIDWIVES & BIRTH CENTER," "EASY ACCESS PRENATAL CLINIC," "CALL US!" A smaller sign in the window, more in keeping with their clean, modern, lowercase aesthetic, read:

evidence based care.
respectful guidance.

beautiful surroundings.
joyful birthing.
consider a birth center.

When I walked in, Taitt was at the reception desk on hold with an insurance company—a pencil stuck in her twist of dreadlocks—and had been for the previous three hours. Medicaid in Florida is administered by private insurers, called managed care organizations, and Taitt was calmly explaining to this one why it owed the center a facility fee for ten births that had happened there during the previous year, setting it back less than $10,000. This is a large chunk of change for the birth center, and a drop in the bucket for the payer (in this case, taxpayers)—the average facility cost of one uncomplicated hospital birth is at least that much *per birth*. She hung up 30 minutes later, not at all hopeful, and not at all surprised.

"It's a hard life. It's not a lucrative business," says Diana Jolles, a nurse-midwife at El Rio Birth and Women's Health Center in Tucson, Arizona, who also leads government-funded research on birth center outcomes. Her recent study of 3,000 births covered by Medicaid found that, even among the higher-risk population, the outcomes were better for those who used the birth center than those who got traditional hospital care: the cesarean rate for women who went to a birth center was just under 10 percent; the national average is 32 percent.[2]

In two large studies of birth centers in 1989 and 2015, the overall cesarean rate was under 5 percent. "For a lot of years the research has been dismissed—'it's all healthy, low-risk people, that's why your results are better,'" says Jolles. The "low-risk" crew is at lower risk for a C-section—in her study the rate was just 4 percent. "But this last study we published controlled for all those factors, and it showed that actually no, when you look at low-risk people, choosing to go to a hospital for no reason increases the cesarean rate—you're four times more likely to have a cesarean just because you went to the hospital."

Birth centers help mitigate a phenomenon called unwarranted variation in care, in which a procedure happens 90 percent of the time in one hospital but only 20 percent of the time in another. This has been recognized as a modern health care problem by academic medical centers like

Dartmouth for years, but most of the medical literature documenting it focuses on orthopedic, cardiac, and end-of-life procedures—not women's health or maternity care, says Jolles. "It means that instead of the care being based on the need of the patient, the care is based on the system," she explains. "So if you take a healthy, low-risk woman and they walk into a hospital with five operating rooms and a neonatal intensive care unit [NICU], their chance of having an operation and the baby being admitted to the unit is significantly higher than when a healthy woman walks into a birth center." In other words, the system with the OR and NICU needs to use the OR and the NICU. A birth center has squat bars and birth tubs. If women truly need surgery, they transfer to the hospital.

But even if a birth center has an easier time opening than Taitt and Fonte had, it is universally more challenging to keep the doors open. "One thing is that Medicaid, the payer of over 40 percent of the births in the U.S., is not cooperating with reimbursing birth centers," says Jolles. (In Florida it covers 50 percent of all births.[3]) This phenomenon of payers stiffing providers happens among private insurers as well, and across specialties, but birth centers are usually "mom-and-pop shops," she says, with the least ability to absorb the losses. "So it's really hard. Forty percent of everything we bill is not collected. We're giving away a lot of care."

WHAT TO REJECT WHEN YOU'RE EXPECTING

Tuesday, December 13, 2011, 5:54 a.m.: Jill Arnold, single mom and creator of the blog The Unnecesarean, posts the 2010 cesarean rates of all hospitals in the state of Minnesota, based on calculations she's made from raw data not easily obtained. The week before, on Sunday, December 4, at 5:00 a.m., she had posted the rates of Illinois hospitals. A month before that, on November 6, at 4:00 a.m., it had been Florida's turn: that year the citywide rate in Miami was 49 percent.[4] From 2009 to 2013, the national cesarean rate peaked and plateaued just shy of one-third of all births—Arnold was crunching numbers from atop this plateau.[5]

This was becoming a pre-dawn ritual for her: first figuring out whether and to whom hospitals were reporting such information, then clicking deep into the web sites of whatever entity had the data: for Minnesota it was on the state's Hospital Association's web site, for Illinois it was several clicks into the state's Department of Health; Florida's data was provided to the state's Agency for Health Care Administration. From there she might be looking up diagnosis-related group (DRG) codes to tease out cesarean procedures, then she'd factor the denominator from which to determine the total proportion of C-sections performed at each hospital, and from there she would do basic math.

"I would sit at my kitchen table," Arnold tells me, the sky dark, her kids sleeping, a French press full of strong coffee nearby. "I don't even know how many hours it took. It was one of these projects that once I got started on, I couldn't stop." Arnold had just moved solo with her two small daughters to Bentonville, Arkansas, from Southern California, where she'd been working in communications for San Diego State University.

"It was crazy, Jennifer. I had no money at the time . . . I just thought somebody needs to do this. Somebody needs to show everyone how terrible the state of reporting of maternity care data is." Arnold was hoping someone would notice that a bleary-eyed single mom was doing more from her kitchen table than PhDs with million-dollar grants or salaried statisticians at departments of health. "It wasn't set up to be this amazing, standardized, clean database," says Arnold. "It was a snapshot of how inconsistent and unavailable necessary data is."

Individual hospital cesarean rates are important information for consumers, and taken in aggregate they are a measure of health care quality: a perfect example of "unwarranted variation in care" or, simply, "overtreatment." Arnold began posting these rates on TheUnnecesarean.com, a blog she'd started in 2008 to vent and connect with other women angry about their treatment in childbirth, as she'd been about her own during the birth of her first daughter.

The Unnecesarean grew to be one of the most widely read blogs in its niche, generating 5 million page views at its height, and it was part of a thriving online community of birth activists—there was Stand and Deliver, Mothering Dot Commune, and a profusion of groups on Facebook. There were women who'd felt railroaded into labor inductions; women who'd had things done to them during labor that they hadn't wanted or had explicitly refused: vaginal exams, waters artificially broken, episiotomies. And there were women who felt bullied or flat out forced into surgical deliveries—"unnecesareans"—who were dealing with the physical, psychological, and emotional fallout. By 2011, Arnold tells me, she was tiring of her role as trauma moderator and felt healed enough to turn her own energy toward external work. In February 2012, she launched Cesareanrates.com.

"At that point I'd compiled the largest registry of C-section data ever," she says. She presented this data at a patient summit organized by Consumer Reports in November of that year. She was surprised to learn they had allotted her an hour—as much as a keynote speaker. Consumer Reports had in fact begun to take an interest in evaluating U.S. maternity care as they do cars and appliances, and had recently published the provocatively titled "What to Reject When You're Expecting." (Among the top ten: medically unnecessary C-section, C-section after previous cesarean delivery, and early elective birth, either by induction or C-section.) Consumer Reports met with Arnold, licensed her data, and hired her as a consultant.

Thus began a series of Consumer Reports publications scrutinizing hospitals and their practices, like "What Hospitals Don't Want You to Know About C-sections" (2014), "Hospitals to Avoid if You Don't Want a C-section," and regularly updated "What to Reject . . ." These reports did not mince or sugarcoat words. "Over the past few decades, the U.S. healthcare system has developed into a labor-and-delivery machine, often operating according to its own timetable rather than the less predictable schedule of mothers and babies," the group stated. "Keeping things chugging along are technological interventions that can be lifesaving in some situations but also interfere with healthy physiological processes and increase risk when used inappropriately."[6]

Consumer Reports called out large hospitals like Baptist South Miami, which topped the charts with a 59 percent C-section rate in 2015.[7] Jack Ziffer, chief physician executive of Baptist, which owns other hospitals, claimed the rate was attributable to "various factors" like "advanced age of the mother, high blood pressure, gestational diabetes, as well as maternal request."[8] Consumer Reports challenged such common responses and showed that hospitals with similar patient populations could still have vastly different cesarean rates. "Too often the medical establishment blames mothers. 'They must be older, fatter, sicker, or they must be requesting C-sections,'" Elliot Main, medical director of the California Maternal Quality Care Collaborative, told the group. "But that's completely bogus. As a doctor I can convince almost any woman in labor to have a C-section."

The reports showed the breadth of variation among hospitals: compare the status quo in Miami to Denver Health Medical Center, a large teaching hospital with an 8 percent (low risk, first birth) cesarean rate; or Crouse Hospital in Syracuse, New York, at 7 percent.[9] If not the patients, what makes these hospitals different? The research suggests that "a large amount of the variation you see in C-section rates, as much as a ten-fold variation, is due to the culture of the obstetric unit and the attitudes of providers," Main told me. Hospitals with a culture of facilitating vaginal birth—those that encourage vaginal birth after cesarean, for example, or where nurse-midwives attend a significant number of births—have far lower rates of C-sections. Denver's chief OB reported to Consumer Reports that one-third of the births at his hospital are attended by midwives, which "helps keep the emphasis on natural birth processes."

Today, there is a robust discussion happening among obstetric leaders and those in the health care "quality improvement" community about the wide variation in cesarean rates, the impact on public health, and what can be done about it. The professional societies of the OB/GYNs, nurse-midwives, neonatologists, and nurses have banded together under the Alliance for Innovation on Maternal Health (AIM) to create "patient safety bundles" and toolkits—like apps for hospitals, though they are old-school checklists and info packets—to better manage complications and bring down cesarean rates. Physician leaders have emerged as voices for change. "A woman's biggest risk factor for the most common surgery on earth is not her personal preferences or her medical risks, but literally which hospital she goes to," says Neel Shah, an OB/GYN at Beth Israel Deaconess Medical Center in Boston who publishes frequently about cesareans. "That's crazy."

In 2015, Shah was offered a position at Harvard's Ariadne Labs, a think tank, and given the challenge: "If you could do one thing to make maternal health better in the U.S., what would you do?" He had three months to figure it out. "Very quickly C-sections were like the ring that ruled the other rings," he told me. This is because a surgical delivery not only has consequences in the short term, but downstream risks as well: for the baby, asthma, allergies, and digestive problems; and for the woman, higher risk of fertility problems, future pregnancy complications, complications of repeat surgery, and higher risk of hysterectomy.

The goal of the toolkit for reducing first-time cesareans is to "build a provider and maternity unit culture that values, promotes, and supports spontaneous onset and progress of labor and vaginal birth."[10] Specifically, women should go into labor on their own; should be free to move, eat, and drink; should be helped to find comfort and relaxation during labor; and should push spontaneously in upright positions—squatting, standing, hands and knees. Basically, the toolkit advises against what happens in most U.S. hospitals.

Surveys of women who recently gave birth paint a picture of women tethered to the hospital beds by various wires and tubes: IV lines with drugs speeding up or inducing contractions, continuous electronic fetal monitoring, epidurals, catheters, maybe a blood pressure cuff and a pulse oximeter, too. They are restricted from food and drink, are left alone for the bulk of the labor, push flat on their backs or leaning back, and suffer trauma to their pelvic floors, if not major abdominal surgery.[11]

Yet the cesarean-lowering initiatives happening in enlightened pockets around the country are backed by statements from physician groups, like one in 2014 from the American College of Obstetricians and Gynecologists and the Society for Maternal-Fetal Medicine on safely preventing primary cesareans.[12] A recent survey of first-time mothers who gave birth in hospitals in California found that among those whose labor was not induced and who did not need epidurals, a mere 1 percent delivered by cesarean section.[13]

"It's really an exciting time," one longtime advocate told me. "The obstetric leadership has made a 180-degree turn. It used to be they wouldn't collaborate with other groups. They told us repeatedly, 'We don't think about the concept of physiologic childbearing, we don't use that language,' and now it is appearing in professional guidance and journal articles!" A decade ago, the obstetric framing wasn't *What can we do to curb C-sections?*

but rather *Maybe C-sections aren't that bad after all.* "Too Posh to Push?" headlines dominated, and the idea that women were driving this trend even seeped into the consciousness of the National Institutes of Health (NIH), which organized a conference on the subject of "Cesarean Delivery on Maternal Request" in 2006.

Several epidemiologists were there to refute the claim that women were seeking elective cesareans—the very premise of the taxpayer-funded meeting. Childbirth Connection had just published its first *Listening to Mothers* report, which found that just *one out of 1,500 women surveyed* had sought out a cesarean. Meanwhile, it found that 57 percent of women who sought a vaginal birth following a previous cesarean, or VBAC, were being denied the option.[14] The International Cesarean Awareness Network documented that around half of hospitals in their sample had outright bans against VBAC. Clearly, the choice to avoid surgery was being systematically denied.

Many physicians were of the mind that an elective cesarean was basically just another way to have a baby, equivalent in risk to a vaginal birth. I spoke to several at the time who were happy to fulfill requests, and some even offered it. The conference concluded that the major surgery "may be a reasonable alternative to planned vaginal delivery."[15] Critics were livid, pointing to reams of data that cesareans carry much more risk. One attendee, a journal editor, quipped that the NIH had effectively "put cesarean section over the counter."[16]

But in the next few years, the ground began to shift. There was more pushback from women, more discussion of other drivers of the trend: fee-for-service medicine, rising malpractice rates and fear of liability, convenience. The media started to tease out these connections, and so did others not historically concerned with the subject, including Hollywood. Ricki Lake and Abby Epstein's documentary *The Business of Being Born* introduced mainstream audiences to the norms of high-tech, modern birth, contrasted to deliveries attended by midwives outside the hospital system (with footage of Lake giving birth in her bathtub), and in the following years the number of home births ticked up. "Doula" became a household word. BBC's *Call the Midwife* drew these providers out of the shadows and onto the screen, as did social media—search "home birth" today on YouTube and the results will be more than 10 million. Several states where certified professional midwives (CPMs) had previously operated illegally passed legislation to license them.

At first, the medical community was defensive. A 2008 statement drafted by ACOG and presented to the American Medical Association calling for legislation against "home deliveries" named Ricki Lake as a dangerous influencer.[17] "Childbirth decisions should not be dictated or influenced by what's fashionable, trendy, or the latest cause célèbre," the final version reads. The group fought (and some state chapters continue to fight) state legislative efforts to license CPMs, who mainly attend home births. Again, the problem was women: "The main goal should be a healthy and safe outcome for both mother and baby. Choosing to deliver a baby at home, however, is to place the process of giving birth over the goal of having a healthy baby."

Then in 2010, Amnesty International dropped a bomb: the report was called *Deadly Delivery*, which sounded like it might detail the plight of women giving birth in a war-torn, resource-poor country but was in fact about the rising rate of pregnancy-related death in the United States. One of its more striking findings was that half such deaths in the United States are preventable. The problem was both too many unnecessary procedures and too little care when truly needed. "Women are not dying from complex, mysterious causes that we don't know how to treat," Nan Strauss, the report's author, told me. "Women are dying because it's a fragmented system, and they are not getting the comprehensive services that they need." In other words, hospitals were failing to ensure the safe births physicians' groups were so vigorously defending.

This uncomfortable revelation came during a broader discussion of the perils of overtreatment and overdiagnosis in health care, and meetings and conferences proliferated during these years to discuss the "perverse incentives" created by fee-for-service medicine, in maternity care and beyond.

Today, even the language around home birth has changed. "Women planning a home birth may do so for a number of reasons, often out of a desire to avoid medical interventions and the hospital atmosphere," ACOG wrote in its 2017 committee opinion.[18] It also urges its members to "maintain a nonjudgmental demeanor" toward home-birth transfers who arrive in labor at the hospital for the next level of care.

"I've been really impressed as far as leadership from the professional organizations that deal with obstetric and neonatal patients, there's been a huge shift," says Jill Arnold. Now the focus is on "the value of labor support, lowering C-section rates safely, and there's been more focus on maternal health overall." Arnold and other birth advocates claim victory in pushing the government's public health initiative, Healthy People 2020, to set the target rate of cesarean section among first-time mothers with single, head-down, full-term babies at 23.9 percent.[19] There's a movement to "put the M back in Maternal Health."[20]

WIDESPREAD FAILURES

It's worth putting this moment into context. For one, we've had this conversation before: in the early 1980s, the NIH appointed a task force on cesareans, and the media called it a "crisis" because the national rate had tripled—to 15 percent. Back then, it was the watchdog group Public Citizen that was shaming hospitals by publishing their C-section rates. We also had physician leaders calling for obstetric reform, and hospitals and HMOs instituting review committees in which obstetricians had to justify every cesarean. These hospitals swiftly reduced their rates of C-sections (counting all births, not just those deemed "low risk") by several points: at one hospital from 25 to 19 percent, at another from 17.5 to 10.2 percent, and at yet another from 28 to 11 percent.[21] Crop tops, high-waisted jeans—the '80s have circled back. But today we are celebrating a national goalpost that matches the worst-performing hospitals of that decade.

Meanwhile, we're not counting maternal deaths systematically—the United States hasn't had an official nationwide estimate in a decade. "Our maternal data is embarrassing," Stacie Geller, a professor of obstetrics and gynecology at the University of Illinois College of Medicine, told ProPublica. "Preventable maternal deaths are not in the basement of our priorities, they are in the sub-basement." Another epidemiologist, who has led studies of maternal mortality, Marian MacDorman, made a direct connection between data and survival: "People are dying because the federal government is not publishing this data."[22] Her 2016 study estimated the number of maternal deaths rose by 25 percent between 2000 and 2014.[23]

Building on the work of Amnesty International, in 2017 Nina Martin of ProPublica and Renée Montagne of NPR revealed in bracing narrative detail—for which they won a Peabody Award—how even women with the most resources (in one case, a neonatal intensive care nurse and wife of a physician, both white, educated, and from a wealthy New Jersey suburb) can be virtually ignored following delivery, even when they report concerning symptoms—even when their physician husband raises hell about concerning symptoms.[24] *USA Today* followed in 2018 with an investigation of dozens of hospitals that revealed "a stunning lack of attention to safety recommendations and widespread failure to protect new mothers." Reporters wrote that "women are left to bleed until their organs shut down. Their high blood pressure goes untreated until they suffer strokes. They die of preventable blood clots and untreated infections. Survivors can be left paralyzed or unable to have more children." They estimated that 50,000 women are injured during birth each year in the United States, making it "the most dangerous place in the developed world to give birth."[25]

According to AIM, the main cause of deadly complications is "denial and delayed response from the healthcare team." But there's more driving this trend. Women who die or nearly die are three to four times more likely to be black. The maternal death rate for black women in Fulton County, Georgia, an area that includes Atlanta, is three times the national average, while the rate for white women there is "too insignificant to report."[26] In New York City, the rate for black women is *12 times* the rate for white women.[27] In New Jersey, pregnant black women are at greater risk of dying than women in Haiti.[28] And these women are not dying because they have more complications or less education.[29] Mills College professor Julia Chinyere Oparah calls it "obstetrical apartheid."

As Linda Villarosa summed it up in the *New York Times Magazine*, "For black women in America, an inescapable atmosphere of societal and systemic racism can create a kind of toxic physiological stress, resulting in conditions—including hypertension and preeclampsia—that lead directly to higher rates of infant and maternal death."[30] That, combined with the "pervasive, longstanding racial bias in health care," explains the epidemic of poor outcomes, "even in the case of black women with the most advantages"—women like Serena Williams, who nearly died of a pulmonary embolism that was ignored by her nurses and physicians following the cesarean birth of her daughter. This world-class athlete spent the first six weeks of motherhood unable to get out of bed.

Villarosa ends her cover story on a pro-doula note. Within two weeks of publication, New York governor Andrew Cuomo pledged a state program to provide more doulas for at-risk women. Premiering two weeks later was the film *Tully*, whose plot centers on a magical postpartum doula who saves an overwhelmed mother from exhaustion. Doulas can indeed be magic—I recommend them without reservation for anyone planning to give birth in a hospital, and they should be accessible to women who can't afford the out-of-pocket costs. There is solid research backing their impact on outcomes. According to the independent researchers at Cochrane, data show they bring down the chance of a C-section by 39 percent. Women with one-on-one, "continuous" support also tend to have healthier babies.[31]

But what seems to be missing from the popular discourse is that *midwives* traditionally provided this one-on-one, continuous support, and they have the clinical skills and expertise to facilitate the birth and intervene in emergencies (as they do in many European countries). A recent five-year study found that the most midwife-friendly states—that is, where they are most integrated into the health system—have the best outcomes for mothers and babies, while the opposite is true for the most midwife-hostile states.[32]

The media focus on the looming "shortage of OB/GYNs," that is, the coming wave of retirements and the number of U.S. counties already without an obstetrician, where women are traveling one or more hours to an equipped hospital and inducing labor or scheduling C-sections so they don't give birth on the highway. This is indeed headline-worthy—the lack of providers endangers people's health and lives. It should be of equal concern that there are so few midwives—the number of births attended by midwives has remained the same for decades: under 10 percent. Midwives achieve births with fewer tears or cuts, fewer C-sections, and fewer mothers who can't hold and nurse their babies because one or both of them are in intensive care. The traditional midwifery model of care is to respect the physiology, not to interrupt or override it as a matter of routine, and to recognize as equally important the social and emotional dimensions of care. Yet rarely are midwives mentioned by the experts or quoted in the media. "Midwife" is thought to be a soft credential.

I don't think this erasure is an accident. Doulas help mitigate the excesses of "institutional birth," but they have no real power in the institution to stop it. They restore a social element of birth that was lost in the twentieth century, but they do not restore the expertise of midwifery. "They're not as threatening as a midwife, because they aren't presenting an alternative to the clinical care that's provided. They're an adjunct to it. And they're perceived as a cheaper option," says medical sociologist Christine Morton, who has studied doulas for more than a decade.

Midwives, on the other hand, do have power and authority where they are autonomous professionals (though in U.S. hospitals certified nurse-midwives often answer to the attending OB). They offer birth spaces removed from the financial pressures of hospitals, where time is money and so are interventions like epidurals and C-sections and neonatal intensive care units. In 2017, ACOG changed its recommendations on postpartum care, urging a routine visit at three weeks rather than the customary six. Home birth midwives typically see their patients twice within the *first* week. If you look closely, the "quality improvement" guidelines are shifting to look more like what midwives have been doing all along: supporting the physiology, intervening when necessary. Yet these providers aren't occupying a key role in reform (or getting enough credit). Why don't we have more autonomous midwives and birth centers? Because they threaten the system, whereas doulas do not.

The new patient safety bundles being adopted by some hospitals also have a demonstrable impact on outcomes. In California, a pilot program led by Elliot Main's group at several hospitals was not only able to lower cesarean rates by several points, but also reduced the number of neonatal complications as well as the number of severe tears in women who gave birth vaginally. Some 160 hospitals across the state have adopted the bundles, and between 2006 and 2013, the state *halved* its maternal death rate.

The bundles address the most common causes of death: hemorrhage, preeclampsia, pulmonary embolism. Sometimes the protocols are simple: compression stockings or blood thinners following surgery can prevent deadly blood clots—precautions that are standard following other major surgeries, but are somehow not standard on maternity wards. It wasn't until *2011* that ACOG recommended them.[33] But Main urges me to separate those bundles from the one on cesareans, which he does not see as a main driver of maternal death. "We're not pushing it as the reason that maternal mortality has risen although it's happened along similar timelines," he tells me. And yet, he concedes the focus on reducing primary cesareans is to prevent the complications they cause in future pregnancies. "The biggest complication of a primary C-section is becoming a prior C-section. Because once you've had scarring of the uterus there are more complications in every subsequent pregnancy."

Shah, on the other hand, makes a more direct connection. "The number one cause of maternal mortality is hemorrhage, and one of the leading causes of hemorrhage is a condition that's caused by C-sections, called placenta accreta," he says. This is when the placenta grows into or through the scar from a previous cesarean, essentially tearing the uterus open when it detaches. This causes a catastrophic hemorrhage that can be uncontrollable. The number of accretas have gone up at least 800 percent in the last 30 years—they were practically unheard of in 1970, and now a hospital will encounter one or two a month, according to Main.[34] "We are facing an epidemic of prior cesarean sections in this country," he says.

While the bundles help direct physicians to make different decisions, the bigger challenge is changing core beliefs. "Some providers have a belief that a cesarean is a safer thing for a mother and a baby," says Main. "I think there is a disconnect because there's an optics problem," says Shah. "If you do a C-section, you don't see the accreta typically because the time from the primary C-section to the really bad consequences of that C-section is on average something like six years." The other problem is a logical fallacy. "If I do a C-section, I'm always right. If the baby is pink and squirming, I think it's a good thing I did the C-section, and if the baby comes out blue, it's a good thing that I did a C-section. It's pretty good to be me," he says.

There may also be some element of choosing what not to see. First C-sections are "very simple surgeries," says Shah. But then they get progressively more complicated, and accretas are now common enough that every OB has encountered one or more. "I've done C-sections where it's like looking at a melted box of crayons," he says. "We're the only surgeons who cut on the same scar tissue over and over again. Think about that. It doesn't magically heal. People don't see what's happening underneath the skin." The immediate postpartum uterus is "a big bag of bleeding blood vessels that's getting 25 percent of what the heart's pumping." When there's an accreta and lots of scar tissue, "you can't tell what's what. That's terrifying."

One way to prevent this life-threatening complication, specific to repeat cesareans, is to prevent the first cesarean from ever happening. This is a stated goal of the Society of Maternal-Fetal Medicine and the American College of OB/GYNs, and of Healthy People 2020. It is also a compromise. "One huge clinical gap nobody will discuss is VBAC. That still is a taboo topic," says Carol Sakala, director of Childbirth Connection Programs at the National Partnership for Women & Families. Among women who've had a vaginal birth, nine out of ten who get pregnant again will have another vaginal birth. The numbers are flipped for C-sections: nine out of ten mothers with previous scars go on to have repeat cesareans. "We're leaving high and dry this generation of women who've had cesarean births and are still getting them."

Sakala's group has surveyed mothers nationwide three times over the past dozen years, and between the second and third surveys something did shift regarding VBAC: "In the second survey a lot of women said my doctor and/or my hospital refused," says Sakala. Then the NIH held a conference on the topic and in 2010 ACOG changed its guidelines to say that most women should be offered VBAC.

By the third survey, just as many women reported undesired repeat cesareans, but fewer women were denied VBAC outright. Instead, during pregnancy they were led to believe a VBAC would be fine, but then toward their due date, or even during labor, they were given reasons for a C-section. The Google search term is "VBAC bait and switch." "The dialogue changed, but the practice did not change," says Sakala. It is extremely difficult to switch obstetric practices in the third trimester, and in many states, including Florida, midwives are restricted from attending VBACs. At that point, women must choose between "showing up pushing" at an unsupportive hospital and hoping for the best, going with another cesarean, or going unassisted at home.

At Magnolia Birth House, women can't VBAC. But Fonte and Taitt know which doctors only do "VBACs on paper" and which do it for real. Their doulas are trained to help women assert their right to refuse a cesarean if they need to. "We're pretty good about getting people information that facilitates their changing providers," Fonte tells me. "The problem is that the pool is pretty shallow." One of those OBs had a VBAC herself, but even she didn't trust her doctors.

THE MIAMI CESAREAN

Dr. Christ-Ann Magloire greets me at 11:30 p.m. at the entrance to the Women's Pavilion at Jackson North hospital wearing teal scrubs and a tropical-patterned surgeon's cap. Before driving over, I had double checked that this wasn't too late for her, but she reassured me a patient was in labor. "She's only 6 or 7 [centimeters], I'm going to be here all night. And anyway, it's for the cause."

The "cause" is the high cesarean rate. The cause is mothers and babies. Up on the labor and delivery floor, Dr. Magloire offers me a seat at the nurse's station in a large postpartum observation area and turns down the volume on the wall-mounted TV—*Real Housewives of Atlanta*. She settles into a swivel chair and drapes a white blanket over her legs, and she is still cold, though it might also be the subject matter that's making her uncomfortable. "It's sick. It's terrible. The statistics are so high, the odds are really in your favor to have a C-section," she says. Three second-year med students are sitting nearby, half studying and half listening to our conversation, which doesn't seem to bother the doctor. "Even me. You know? I kind of got wrapped up in it myself."

Magloire considers herself lucky to have trained in Boston, where the doctors shared the floor with midwives, where "crunchy granola" was a badge of honor, where women who'd had prior cesareans were encouraged to have vaginal births. In Florida, the norms are different. "The number one thing is timing. We don't allow women to go into natural labor. And then we're very quick to intervene, we won't let her progress on her own." For a woman to get into "active labor" in Miami, where her cervix has dilated and contractions are so close together and so strong that the baby descends and she has the urge to push, "she has to be an outlier, where she's so fast they don't have any time to do anything," says the doctor.

Magloire's mother was a midwife in Haiti. As a young girl, she was fascinated by childbirth and used to spend hours staring at encyclopedia pictures of a developing fetus. "I went into OB to become an OB, not a GYN—I never liked the surgical aspect. I really loved maternal and infant health, population health, family planning. I feel like one day I want to work in international health."

As a national health service scholar, Magloire won a scholarship to med school in exchange for several years working in underserved communities. That's how she ended up in Florida. She says the only reason she stayed is that she purchased a home just before the market crashed, and her mortgage is now underwater. "Everything's upside down," she tells me. She describes her own first birth experience not unlike the real estate mess she got caught up in.

The first thing that happened was she went past her due date. Her physician had actually started suggesting a labor induction a week before that, at 39 weeks. "I ignored him," she says. At 40 weeks, she ran her own tests. Her baby was fine, she was fine, so she carried on. "At 41 weeks, he started getting nervous, and he *started* . . ." Magloire says, pausing to let the word sit. She was "overdue." Her baby was "measuring big"—they thought he was 10 pounds. She had too much amniotic fluid.

"That's when I realized I don't really know how anybody else practices," she tells me. She hadn't put much thought into choosing her doctor. "I ended up choosing someone Haitian like myself," she says, someone who didn't work at her hospital, who a couple nurses said was good. "I should have done more research."

She agreed to an induction on a Wednesday. But when the drug they were using, called Cytotec, started causing decelerations in the baby's heart rate, "decels" in obstetric lingo, she signed herself out. "I was about to get on a plane and go back to Boston. I was like, you guys don't know what you're doing." Then she came back on Friday and suggested another method of induction, using a rubber Foley "balloon" catheter, which takes more time but can be a more gentle way to dilate the cervix. The physician and nurses at this hospital were not familiar with the method, so she instructed them.

It also didn't work, and again she signed herself out AMA—against medical advice. But two days later, "I just kind of gave into it. It was Sunday, my mother was leaving Tuesday." A different doctor was on call, and he was "very aggressive." He came into her room, did a vaginal exam, and broke her amniotic sac without asking her or telling her. In Miami, the citywide rule seems to be that once a woman's water is broken, she can no longer get out of bed. They gave her an epidural and Pitocin, but she never dilated past 2 centimeters.

"I cried the whole way from the labor room to the operating room. I felt like, how did I put myself in this situation? I should have just waited. I thought I'd be the exception to the rule," she says.

When she returned to work after her maternity leave, the nurses asked her how the birth went. "I just said, 'Fine. The baby came out.' I didn't tell anybody I had a C-section. I just felt ashamed." Why? I ask. "I should have chosen my provider better, just like most of the women who end up with a C-section. I should have stuck with more pro-vaginal doctors, but back then I wasn't even aware that there was a difference. I didn't know."

Four years later, Magloire was pregnant again, and she was determined not to get "caught up in the same situation." She searched out a doctor willing to attend a VBAC—not an easy quest in this city. She also saw a home birth midwife "on the side." Magloire was one of the few OBs friendly with the local midwives, willing to see their patients for a consult or treat a woman if she transported in labor from an intended home birth. "I was VBAC-y," she tells me. She spoke several times at meetings and conferences organized by Taitt and Fonte. "They're really the ones who brought it to the forefront, who made noise in Miami." They organized women to picket in front of the hospitals that had "banned" VBAC. "Now there's not as much hoopla." Now, the hospitals don't say they ban it. But the rates at hospitals are so low it's tantamount to a ban.

As her second pregnancy went on, Magloire tells me she felt more and more as if she was being "set up" for another cesarean. The last straw was when her doctor told her that she was going out of town. Magloire asked if the backup doctor was pro-VBAC. The answer was no, he's not. "I felt like she was making me go down the same trickery lane," says Magloire. At that moment Plan B became Plan A—or maybe it had really always been Plan A—though she was really not psyched about laboring at home without hospital-grade pain relief. Alas, those were her choices.

She went into labor at 4:30 a.m., spent "all day and night" in her Jacuzzi and shower, and when she wasn't in the water she was wandering from room to room, trying to get comfortable. She gave birth at 7 p.m. standing in her living room, her midwife kneeling on the floor beneath her. She describes it with no love for the labor pains, but giving birth on her own terms "helped close the wound" left by the C-section. She describes all this leaning her elbows on her blanketed knees, looking off into the past. "It's a scar, it's a wound that stays open."

A nurse comes into the room and hesitantly interrupts our conversation. She wants the doctor to come look at the patient in labor—"decels," she says. Magloire rolls her eyes, "You guys are overreading things. She's got Cytotec, Cytotec are decels." Still, she excuses herself, and the med students follow.

On *Real Housewives of Atlanta*, a couple is in a car, discussing some of the darker moments of their relationship, two fellow cast members in the back seat. "Did I ever choke you? I don't remember," the man says to his wife, behind sunglasses. She says he did. "Well, if I did I'm sorry, because maybe I didn't choke you hard enough." The cruel joke sends a wave of shame through the back seat. The wife looks out the window, wiping away tears. The scene cuts to a commercial for Summer's Eve, which no longer calls itself a douche, and speaks millennial: "Because thongs, because yoga, because skinny jeans." I wonder if this TV stays on while recovering mothers tenderly hold their newborns to their breast.

When Magloire returns, I ask her about the Cytotec. Her patient, she explains, needed to be induced for high blood pressure. She doesn't like to induce, but "I know how to do it," she says. It requires certain "dynamics." You're trying to kickstart the body into a process, you can't be too slow about it. The nurses, she complains, don't like to follow orders, and that's why inductions often fail, requiring her to do a C-section.

I ask her how many cesareans she does, generally. "Real ones?" she asks. "Not what these jokers are making me do? One a month." I am not certain I understand—that the nurses are the reason for the C-section? "They're overreading, practicing voodoo instead of medicine," she says. They don't want to turn up the Pitocin every half-hour as is protocol.

As much as Magloire feels she'd been caught up in the system for her own birth, she is telling me that in many ways her own practice is caught as well. I ask her how she'd practice differently if there were no hospital protocols. The first thing she mentions is less electronic fetal monitoring, "because the data shows very well that it hasn't done anything but increase the C-section rate." That would free women up to be more mobile. "Some women want to walk around," herself included. But hospital policy is you have to stay in bed if your water is broken. "When I was home and my water broke I was all over the place." She'd also lift the restriction on eating and drinking, a holdover from the days when C-sections called for general anesthesia. "To me labor is all about passing of time. If munching on a carrot helps you pass the time, then you should have the carrot." Not to mention that eating keeps up your energy.

Her vision is almost identical to the bundle for reducing primary cesareans.

Across town the next day, I meet with Nathan Hirsch, who has been an OB in Miami for 30 years—he also trained up north, at the University of Pennsylvania. I ask him why he thinks Miami's C-section rates are so high. "The primary reason is cultural. There's a high Latin population, it's a herd mentality," he tells me. "When we started practicing 30 years ago, natural childbirth was the main thing—I'm talking about no epidural, water baths, dark lighting, massage therapy. If you didn't do that you were ostracized by families. Today, because the C-section rate is so high, everybody takes it for granted." He adds, "I personally think it's horrible to have your abdomen cut open if you don't need to be." He estimates that 2 to 3 percent of his clients ask for unnecessary cesareans. "We try to talk them out of it," he says, but ultimately it's the patient's choice. Then again, it's not the patient's choice if she wants a VBAC. "We stopped doing it," says Hirsch. "There are not too many private physicians doing it." His practice also doesn't "allow" doulas, "because we've had some who were abusive and interfering with the nurses."

The Latin thing comes up again and again, even though it reveals certain biases, and research has shown that women in Latin American countries like Brazil, who are said to want "vaginal sparing" cesareans, are not necessarily the ones driving the trend. "Wherever you see these skyrocketing C-section rates, they're doctor and hospital driven, they're health-system driven," says Nicholas Rubashkin, an OB/GYN at the University of California, San Francisco, who studies women's autonomy in childbirth globally. "Because when you look at women's values and preferences about C-section prenatally—in Brazil, Argentina, Hungary, and the U.S.—a minority of women would choose electively to deliver by C-section," yet a sizable number deliver that way, "so those women still end up with more C-sections than their preferences indicated."

Still, "if C-sections are being normalized in major Latin American cities, it's impossible for it not to be here in Miami, too," says Taitt. And there may well be a cultural dynamic that has more to do with loyalty than vanity: Latina women often come from large, close-knit families, "all the sisters and cousins had their babies with a particular doctor, and they don't want to rock the boat," says Fonte. "It really is a commentary that we're not pregnant and birthing outside of our social structure."

"I really think it goes back to respect. In our societies, teachers and doctors are the highest," one doula from Haiti points out. You don't question them. Which makes a physician who resists the status quo even more powerful. This doula recalls Magloire speaking at the Gathering Place, not long after her VBAC. "It was the most awesome night of my life. Here's this black doctor with a baby on her lap, from Haiti, my island, talking about how she had a VBAC herself at home, and I'm like what? This is a thing? It was inspirational."

Magloire attributes Miami's cesarean rate to physicians. "I think they don't believe in birth." Men more than women? I ask. "Male or female, especially some of the females. I just think that they see it from an extremely scientific perspective, they don't see it as a natural phenomenon. They feel it's their job to constantly intervene, instead of letting nature take its course."

Still, the previous six deliveries Magloire had attended led to surgery. For this, she blames the nurses, as if they were ultimately in control. The Cytotec, for instance, is really effective, she says. "But it likes to cause drama." In fact, the drug misoprostol (the same drug used in the "abortion pill" regimen) began to be used off-label in the late 1990s to soften the cervix and start contractions, and by the early 2000s several studies showed that it could cause the uterus to rupture. Then it turned out that was mostly the case in women with scars from previous cesareans, which added to the anxiety over VBAC but did not necessarily discourage inducing labor with it. In Miami it's a standby.

"We used to do VBACs all the time," Hirsch tells me. "Then ACOG changed the rules. The rules are if you have a patient who's had prior cesarean, you have to be on the labor floor with her during the entire labor. That's pretty hard for someone who's in private practice." The rules changed again in 2010, when ACOG made it clear that women should still be offered the option even if surgical staff aren't "immediately available," but it hasn't seemed to change hospital policy.[35] The few who are doing VBAC in Miami, including Magloire, charge an extra fee, around $2,500, for the extra time on the labor floor, which patients pay out of pocket.

"To avoid the primary section is the most important thing," says Magloire. "That's why it unnerves me when I have to do a primary C-section. I'm disturbed, because I know the chance of her having a VBAC is low."

PERMISSION TO LABOR

The name "The Gathering Place" evokes in many ways the coalescing of biological and social processes in childbirth—of hormones, of muscles and ligaments, of courage, of support, of supplies—as the boundary between internal and external, spiritual and earthly, dissolves. The physical intensity of that portal opening requires a certain psychic gathering as well, or as one Miami doula told me, "I tell women you have to go in and get your baby." There is enormous power upon the return.

One afternoon, I'm sitting with Taitt and Fonte at their kitchen counter while Taitt chops vegetables for roasting. They are a yin and yang couple: Taitt is black, Fonte is a fair redhead. Taitt's voice booms across a room; Fonte takes a minute to warm up. "This whole way that we birth is the biggest misogynist sexist plot ever," Taitt says theatrically, but she's also serious. "If American women were birthing the way that women are birthing in other countries, we would not be controllable." Fonte adds, "When you have autonomy, when you have agency, when you have information, you feel differently about it, even when you end up with a C-section, even when it isn't the picture-perfect everything that you wanted."

"I felt terrible after my first birth," Fonte tells me over coffee back at Magnolia Birth House. "I had an episiotomy without being told. I had no idea"; she had an epidural and so didn't feel the incision. "The healing from that was worse than the delivery. For sure. It was a year probably before I felt even marginally normal." She also felt terrible because she was furious with herself, "a pretty type A person," for going into it so blind. When the baby was a couple weeks old, she got a form letter from her OB. "I'll never forget this as long as I live, telling me what a great job I did. I was like, *No, I did not. I did not do a good job.*" Part of her anger was in not having the natural birth she had wanted, but "I was also disappointed that I let myself be controlled the way I did."

Taitt and Fonte started the Gathering Place to reach what they call an "underserved" community. And they've gone out of their way to be affordable and accessible and racially diverse—at least half of the mothers and doulas I meet there are women of color. But the women use the word *underserved* more broadly than as a stand-in for low-income.

"I teach a class called Preparing for Hospital Birth, and a lot of times when I'm going through the standard protocols and procedures in the hospital, people are like, 'You can refuse that?'" Fonte tells me. "Um, it's a drug that they're going to put in your veins—you have to consent to that. So yes, you certainly can!" she says. "Grown-ass, lawyer women say these things. So 'underserved' here takes on a new meaning. Lots of people don't have access to information. It isn't just people who don't have a lot of money, or live in a certain area, or don't have transportation to get to their doctor's office. It's also very middle-class, very upper-middle-class women who are lacking the very same information."

Fonte tells me many of her clients are professional, educated powerhouses "who are often very successful, at the top of their game in their field." Still, she says, status quo care in Miami is a great equalizer of disempowerment. "To me this is political work, and it always has been," she says. The hierarchy and patriarchy of the hospital seem to scramble women's gut programming. "Even strong, intelligent, well-educated, successful, powerful women don't act like themselves sometimes in this environment in terms of advocating for themselves and asking questions and getting information." In labor, Fonte will try to gather them back together. She'll often say, "Where'd you go? We need you—the other you? We need *her* here."

Finally, with the birth center up and running, they could offer a place where women were less likely to "lay down," as Fonte and Taitt put it. Where they could hold on to their core selves through the tidal wave of labor and emerge on the other side, power strengthened rather than submerged. But until the spring of 2016, they and their clients needed the same thing: permission.

They wanted to share with me a story that was particularly agonizing. It was an afternoon in March 2015—Fonte got a call from one of the doulas in their network. As head of the doula program, she stays informed about every birth they attend as it is unfolding, and is available for consult. The doula, Esther McCant, had just arrived at South Miami hospital to support a brand-new client. She found her room and walked into a standoff: the woman was not yet in labor, there was no emergency, but the obstetrician wanted to do an immediate cesarean section.

The client was Nathalie Mendoza, a 28-year-old nurse who was having a baby pretty much on her own. She had thought her water might have broken and got mixed messages in triage. At first the nurse had told her it was a false alarm. But then the nurse changed her mind and estimated the baby's weight: 10 pounds. Mendoza was admitted to the labor and delivery ward, where nurses were waiting with IV bags. Now a doctor was telling her natural birth "wasn't an option." Her baby was too big.

Mendoza had only "met" McCant by phone the week before, and had only thought to find a doula at 38 weeks because of the creeping worry that she would end up in this exact situation. The last few months of her pregnancy had been an insurance nightmare that had eroded her trust in the medical system. Mendoza was working as a nurse per diem, and thus had no benefits. Her income was too high for Medicaid, so she had signed up for a basic Obamacare plan through the state exchange. Her first prenatal appointment cost $300 out of pocket.

In her seventh month, she made an emergency appointment because she was ill. "I told the doctor I was super sick, throwing up. I needed IV fluids." He told her she'd need to go to the emergency room. But her deductible was $6,000. "I told the doctor, no, I can't afford the ER." He told her to speak with one of the receptionists about billing. In the waiting room, a woman came out and apologized. It turned out the practice would no longer be delivering at the hospital that her insurance would cover—she would have to change plans or change physicians. Not only could they not care for her that day, they could no longer deliver her baby. Mendoza called her aunt, a nurse, who gave her IV fluids at her home.

Mendoza returned to the practice the next week to plead with them—she was so far along, how could she look for a new provider this late in the game? She tried switching plans. Finally, she stopped working altogether and was approved for Medicaid. She found a new practice through word of mouth, from other women in her childbirth class.

At first, the new practice was worried the baby was too small—Mendoza, young and healthy, naturally thin, had only gained 20 pounds and didn't "look" as pregnant as she was. But then an ultrasound pegged the baby at 8 pounds, which made them worry it was getting too big. They ordered that she have ultrasounds weekly until she gave birth. Mendoza asked the doctor what this meant, what was "too big." "He said I was pretty much borderline." Mendoza was told that at 3,500 grams, just over seven and a half pounds—the average weight for a newborn—she would have a cesarean. Her baby was measuring 3,400 grams. "That's when I started looking for a doula, because I didn't want a C-section."

Mendoza had seen water births on television. They "always seemed more natural, more relaxing," she told me. "Originally I wanted a birth at a birth center. But nobody was supporting me. My family said, 'It's antiquated, it's unsafe. The best thing, the safest thing is to have it in the hospital.'" By that time Mendoza had moved in with her mother.

When she called the Gathering Place to inquire about a doula, she told them about the ultrasounds. Taitt told her if she were at a birth center she would have had just one ultrasound during the entire pregnancy (unless there was a medical indication for more). And furthermore, ultrasounds are notoriously inaccurate for estimating size, off by 10 to 20 percent, so the farther along the pregnancy, the more significant the potential for error—by a whole pound or two. In fact, ACOG has for years recommended against cesareans for size. "She told me a story about a woman at Mt. Sinai [hospital] who they wanted to give a C-section because the baby was too big, and she drove herself while in labor to Jackson [hospital] and was able to have it naturally. So when it happened to me, I always remembered that story—you always have the right to refuse."

In the labor and delivery room, Mendoza told the nurses she wanted to hold off on the IV. She had been asking the triage nurse to reevaluate—she wasn't convinced her water had broken, she had seen fluid on the ultrasound (she'd seen enough ultrasounds to know), she wasn't having any contractions, and "I just knew my baby wasn't 10 pounds."

When the doctor came in, he pronounced the baby too big, her water broken, and a cesarean imperative. "I was crying, I was so nervous," said Mendoza. "I said, 'I know we had talked about this, but I want to have it natural.' He said, 'Well, that's not an option anymore. The baby is too big.' I said, 'OK, I need to think about it.'"

Mendoza met with me on a sunny afternoon almost two years after the ordeal, wearing skinny jeans and a black T-shirt, her chubby toddler with the neighbor next door. She was embarrassed that she still lived with her mother—she had just taken a job as a nurse in a neonatal intensive care unit and expected to be back on her feet soon. When we got to this part in her story, she dialed McCant and put her on speakerphone. McCant remembered the day vividly.

"I always tell my clients, ask for a moment if you need to. Just know that you don't have to make decisions right away," said McCant, who was pregnant with her third baby when Mendoza was due. She named that baby Justice—we could hear his baby talk through the phone. After some time in the hospital room, the doctor came back with two nurses and wanted to know what the decision was. "When she shared her decision that she wanted to do a trial of labor and didn't want a C-section, he went into this whole spiel about Publix," the supermarket chain, said McCant. "He gave this terrible example, that if you knew that in going to the supermarket you were taking a risk you'd get hurt driving, or on the sidewalk, would you do it? He was comparing her decision to not do a C-section to putting her baby in harm's way on purpose, and then it turned into 'I don't know any mom who would want to do that.'"

Mendoza remembered him saying, "It's not about what you want, it's about the baby. What we're concerned about is the baby."

The two women remember the doctor becoming more and more irate, to the point that he started threatening Mendoza. "He said, 'If you try to labor, I'm going to call the department of child services,'" said Mendoza. And with that he left the room. What he was saying didn't make sense to McCant, who had worked as a social worker on child neglect. Furthermore, the baby was fine. The triage nurse had been monitoring him. Nothing about the labor and delivery nurses' body language said there was an emergency—in fact, one of them looked at Mendoza at one point and said, "You're not in labor." "Nathalie asked me, 'Do I have to stay here?'" said McCant, who had Fonte on the phone by that time. "I said, 'No, you don't.' Michelle said, 'No, you don't. And I'd recommend you leave.'"

Mendoza did not leave right away. "I was still in shock. I thought, let me try to negotiate with him," she said. He returned within the hour. "He said, 'No doctor in Miami will let you labor, we have to do the C-section, the baby is too big.'" When he came back the third time, he had a hospital risk manager by his side. "She didn't say much. He was making it seem like it was a hospital issue at this point. He said, 'OK, we'll do an induction, but you have to sign this paper.' It was some kind of waiver. So then I asked him, 'But, Doctor, you just said I could not labor. I'm confused.' He said, 'I don't know what you want,' and he stormed out of the room," said Mendoza. Both women remember him taking off his cap and shoving a table or chair on his way out, startling everyone. "He got really nasty," said Mendoza.

"It was so tense in the room, you could feel the tension, even the nurses weren't really talking to us," said McCant. "So then he came back one more time. The last time he came, he was really calm. He said, 'OK, what is it that you want?' I said, 'No, I don't want to be here anymore,'" said Mendoza. He tried once more to convince her, and when she still wouldn't budge, he called her a "horrible mother for taking this risk." I asked Mendoza: Did he really use the word "horrible"? Yes, she said. She remembered it clearly.

They had been at the hospital for two hours. Fonte, meanwhile, had been working her phone and had found another OB at Jackson Memorial, the county teaching hospital, willing to see Mendoza. McCant encouraged her client to go, but Mendoza was exhausted. "I said I don't want to know anything about hospitals. I want to go home."

And just like that, she got up and left. And she took a nap. And when she woke, she still felt fluid leaking, and her mother coaxed her to go to Jackson, where she was seen by a midwife in triage, who estimated her baby at 9 pounds and said her water had not broken. "I said no, that can't be right." The midwife told her what was "leaking" was her mucus plug. "But the nurse had said the test was 100 percent accurate," Mendoza told her. "Nothing can be 100 percent accurate," said the midwife. "You're not in active labor, and we don't induce for size anymore, and we only do C-sections for babies that are 11 pounds," Mendoza recalled her saying. "So she sent me home."

Mendoza spent the next week not sleeping—she was so upset by what had happened. Her visit with the OB Fonte had suggested went not-so-great—she started talking about inducing if Mendoza went to 41 weeks, which was Tuesday. But Mendoza was already a couple centimeters dilated, and she was having contractions, so it seemed like that wouldn't happen. Still, she called McCant, worried about the encounter, and McCant sent her to the Gathering Place to talk to Fonte. "Michelle really calmed me down," said Mendoza, "so I started focusing more on my breathing." Then McCant arrived, and Fonte said it was OK if they wanted to stay there. Mendoza was in early labor.

"I was looking out the window, looking at the rain, sitting on the birth ball. It was like being in your living room. Calmness. I can't describe it," said Mendoza. "I hadn't slept for a week, I hadn't eaten, I was very irritable. I think Esther came and gave me some soup." McCant added, "And you had honey sticks, trail mix." "I was even able to nap, I got one nap for the whole week," said Mendoza. They played music—Spanish, Latin, reggaeton. The pains got strong and regular.

And then, the thing that laboring women dream will happen happened: the "natural high" kicked in. "I stopped feeling the contractions. I was rocking back and forth. Esther was timing them, she said they're still going on for a minute. I told her I don't feel them." What did you feel? I asked. "It was just breathing. I was so focused on the breathing, the pain wasn't there anymore. Before it was like a level 10, now it was like at a 2." McCant saw that the contractions were getting close together and told her it was time to go. "I did not want to go back to the hospital. I was holding off as much as I could," said Mendoza. "She was sipping on raspberry leaf tea, she was taking her time. You drank one cup for hours!" said McCant. "That's how much she wanted to avoid the hospital. She was like, 'Why can't I just have the baby here?'"

Mendoza was so calm when she got to the hospital, the midwife in triage asked why she was there. But when she checked her, she said, "Your doula was right." Mendoza had dilated to 6 centimeters, the benchmark clinicians use for when "active labor" is usually in full swing.

Mendoza didn't have her baby for another 14 hours. From triage, she went to the labor floor. "They strapped me to the monitor, I could no longer eat any food, they strapped me to an IV. My labor stalled completely." After pleading with one of the doctors, she was allowed to get up and sit on her birth ball, right next to the fetal monitor.

How did you feel? I asked. "I felt like I wanted to go back to that little safe space at the birth center. I was trying to visualize that and go back to that." When they broke her water, the pain came back, and she got an epidural.

"I was anxious. I was very nervous again. I didn't want any interventions but I caved in to them. I said do whatever you have to do, I just don't want a C-section." By around noon, it had been 24 hours since they'd begun at the Gathering Place, and McCant needed a nap. She went to a nearby Panera and laid her head down on a table.

The doctor mentioned a C-section if there was no baby by 2 p.m. Mendoza negotiated for Pitocin and more time. Serendipitously, the nurses and doctor were busy for the next few hours with another birth. In that time, Mendoza dilated. All of a sudden it was happening. McCant and the doctor returned, nurses broke down the lower third of the bed, turned down the epidural, raised the stirrups, and Mendoza started pushing. She wanted to change positions and squatted for a few contractions. "Other doctors wouldn't have let me do that," said Mendoza. "I had seen birthing videos, being vertical, being upright, that's what really works." While she was squatting, she says, she felt the baby descend. She heard the nurses say "We can see the head!" But she couldn't hold herself up for much longer and, exhausted, lay back flat on the bed. Mendoza pushed for another few minutes, and the baby was born, and weighed 9 pounds, 3 ounces.

OBSTETRIC VIOLENCE

In the canon of women's stories of being bullied, threatened, or abused in labor, Mendoza's had a happy ending. In New Jersey, Lindsay Switzer was at Shore Medical Center, 9 (out of 10) centimeters dilated, on hands and knees with her midwife, feeling the urge to push, when the OB on call, Natalia Rezvina, walked in, asked if Switzer wanted a spinal block (Switzer said, "No, thank you"), and then asked about her first child's delivery (vaginal). "It was at that time she said I needed a C-section—*without examining me, without reviewing my son's heart tones, and without any further discussion as to other options*," Switzer later wrote. When Switzer tried to ask questions, the doctor threatened to call "legal people" if she didn't sign a consent form for surgery.[36]

Her midwife told her, "Lindsay, you're being bullied." "But I didn't know what to do with that information. I was naked and in pain and scared, and believing there was something wrong with my baby and with me," Switzer later wrote.[37] She signed the papers and went into surgery, which was over by 6 p.m. "I thought I was okay for a couple of months—you say, well, I had a healthy baby. But I was having panic attacks. I couldn't lie on my back in bed because it reminded me of being in the operating room. I was diagnosed with PTSD and an anxiety disorder, and I'd never had any problems before." In a written apology, Rezvina responded that that she was focused on the baby's "non-reassuring fetal heart tracing." The doctor's employer, Regional Women's Health Group, LLC, apologized for her "bedside manner" and assured Switzer that it was enrolling Rezvina in a behavior modification course. The baby was born with no signs of having been in distress.

In Alabama, Caroline Malatesta's baby was crowning—about to be born—when nurses *held the baby back* because the doctor was not yet there. Malatesta was having her fourth baby. She'd had her first three at a different hospital, but chose Brookwood Baptist Medical Center based on its marketing campaign for a new Women's Center, which was "all about supporting and empowering women." "Before then, I didn't know there were options. I was hearing of friends being allowed to move around during labor, use the restroom, drink water, avoid stirrups, and birth in different positions. I always had been confined to the bed with a bedpan or catheter, only allowed to eat ice chips, and on my back in stirrups for delivery. I always was prepped from the waist down with surgical cloths and washed with antiseptic prior to delivery. I just figured that's how childbirth was done everywhere," she later wrote.

During a prenatal appointment, her new doctor told her all of that was backward and unnecessary and promised she'd be able to move around and labor in any position. But when that day came the nurse who greeted her at Brookwood told her to stay in the bed. Once admitted, Malatesta's water broke and the baby crowned. She could not bear to stay on her back and flipped to hands and knees and began "breathing the baby out." When the nurse came in, she pulled Malatesta's wrist out from under her and pinned Malatesta on her back. More nurses joined. "I desperately tried to flip back to my hands and knees, struggling against the nurses to do so. The nurses held me down and pressed my baby's head into my vagina to delay delivery as he was trying to come out," wrote Malatesta. This went on for six minutes, and caused her lifelong nerve damage, "the worst birth injury" her doctor had ever seen in his decades-long career. "I've been left with a debilitating medical condition, my sex life is gone, I see a therapist, and I'm on medications both for pain and to ward off panic attacks," Malatesta told Yahoo in 2015.[38] When questioned by attorneys, the nurses and the on-call doctor could recall little about Malatesta's birth. But a notation in her medical chart indicates that she'd been instructed not to push. Malatesta's primary nurse, Melissa Graham, responded in a deposition that the nurses believed that if Malatesta pushed, the baby would be born before the doctor arrived.[39]

In California, 27-year-old Kimberly Turbin was having her first baby at Providence Tarzana Medical Center, pushing on her back, in stirrups, when the doctor, Alex Abbassi, took out scissors and murmured to the nurse he was about to cut an episiotomy. Turbin noticed the sharp metal near her vagina and asked what was up. "I'm going to do the episiotomy now," he said. Turbin, who had previously explained to the nurses that she was a rape survivor and asked them to proceed with her gently, protested, "Why, why can't I try?" There was arguing, the nurse tried to convince her it was OK, she had an epidural and wouldn't feel anything. Her mother scolded her in Spanish to not argue with the doctor, to let the doctor do his job. "No, don't cut me!" Turbin said clear as day. The mother told the doctor to go ahead. Then the physician made one cut, then another, and another, and another, and more. Twelve cuts in all. You can hear each snip audibly in the video, available online (major trigger warning).[40] When the baby was wrested out, everybody (except Turbin) cheered.

These are just some of the cases we know about because lawyers and advocates got involved. Switzer won an undisclosed settlement; Malatesta won an unprecedented $16 million after the case went to trial. Turbin called 80 lawyers before she found one willing to represent her, and won a settlement, prior to which Abbassi surrendered his medical license with a claim of "age-related cognitive defects."[41] When the advocacy group Improving Birth launched the #breakthesilence campaign, hundreds of women submitted pictures and stories: "After refusing an episiotomy, my OB ripped me open with his bare hands." "I was pushed down and held to the bed when I resisted a cervical exam." "I was forced into an unnecessary cesarean WITHOUT ANESTHESIA." Other stories have trickled up to the media, like this one, which was heard first on the podcast Birth Allowed and made it into a Vice story on the "Hidden Epidemic of Doctors Abusing Women in Labor": a woman is laboring in her Alabama hospital room, standing up and leaning over the bed, when the doctor enters and wants to do an exam. She declines. He straddles her from behind. "'So, this is how we're going to do this,' he says, before pulling up her skirt and forcing his hand roughly into her vagina."[42]

These stories point to a problem underpinning the U.S. maternity crisis that I think cuts deeper than cesarean section, that is vaster than maternal death and injury—a dark force lording over the ring ruling all other rings: entitlement to women's bodies—the denial of a person's right to determine who and what enters their body, to respect, to give and refuse consent, because they happen to be pregnant. At the extreme end are women who have been court-ordered to have cesareans and other interventions, and on the flip side, women criminalized for the outcomes of their pregnancies—charged with murder for miscarriage or stillbirth. This isn't just a problem in medicine—the state and courts are complicit. Attorney Lynn Paltrow attributes this to decades of anti-abortion legislation that gives fertilized eggs, embryos, and fetuses more rights than the people who carry them, and to courts that have "no coherent understanding of what it means to fully include human beings with the capacity for pregnancy as fully protected and fully included in the U.S. Constitution." The organization she founded, the National Advocates for Pregnant Women, has documented around 1,200 such cases in the last 30 years. A majority of the convictions and incarcerations are of women of color.

These outliers exist in a culture of everyday breaches that are considered routine maternity care: women told they "have to" be induced, or have "mandatory" vaginal exams; women told they "must" have continuous fetal monitoring, or an IV (also shown to have no benefit), or no food—per "hospital rules"; women told they are not "allowed" to get out of bed, or go past their due date, or push how they want to push.

Mark Spence is an OB/GYN and the medical director of Magnolia Birth House (the law requires that an OB fill this role), and he meets me there one morning. If clients need to transport to the hospital during a birth, he's the midwives' first choice. Otherwise he has his own busy practice. "I had a fight with a nurse this morning," Spence tells me. "She says, 'The patient wants to eat. But we have a no-eating policy.' First of all, there's no documented study about why a patient can't have oral intake." He points out that women come into the ER having just eaten McDonald's and end up having cesareans. "The difference is we would have taken on that liability" if the ER patient had eaten while admitted. The morning patient insisted on eating, and the nurse was furious. "It comes down to a power struggle," he says, but it shouldn't be. "Hand the patient a form for refusal" so that it's documented, which should protect the hospital in case of any future litigation. "I don't understand what the problem is."

There were no shortage of stories among several doulas who gathered one night at Magnolia to tell me about what they witnessed in Miami hospitals: laboring women spoken to as if they're children, told inaccurate information about their progress, sexual asides to male partners, coercion, and worse. "They're preparing you for a C-section as soon as you walk through the door," said a labor and delivery nurse who moonlights as a doula. Many recalled obstetricians saying variations of "I was all set to cut you" after a baby is born vaginally. And they pointed to the city's episiotomy rates as evidence that many doctors cut anyway—at some hospitals, 30 percent of women delivering vaginally receive episiotomies.

"I've seen doctors make sexual jokes in the room while the mom is pushing. They'll nudge the dad, 'I'll make sure it's all good for you after,'" said a doula of many years. "In any other setting those would be grounds for sexual harassment." Another recalled a birth she attended, in which the woman had brought her mother and father, both doctors. She had been laboring for hours when she asked for an epidural, but by the time the anesthesiologist arrived she had changed her mind—she felt ready to push. But her father and the doctor wouldn't take "I changed my mind" for an answer. "They literally held her down and said she needed the epidural. I was standing there thinking, how can I save her from these people she invited to her birth?" said the doula. "It was like watching someone get raped."

One doula tells her clients to have a man on their birth team who will be willing to stand up for them. "We know where we are—if you're talking about a space where patriarchy is present, it's the hospital," she said.

Christine Morton, the medical sociologist, led a survey of nearly 3,000 doulas and labor and delivery nurses in the United States and Canada over the course of 2012 and 2013. Two-thirds said that they had witnessed providers "occasionally or often" performing procedures without giving the patient a chance to agree to them. Nearly one in five witnessed providers doing things "explicitly against the patient's wishes." One in three reported providers threatening women "that her baby might die" when a patient resisted. One in ten said they witnessed racially or sexually demeaning language. Morton and her coauthors needed to raise funds on Indiegogo to analyze the data—"It's a research topic that isn't high on the list for funding organizations," she told me. And yet doulas are important sources. "Clinicians often work in isolation [from] their colleagues," but doulas are witnessing it all. "You'd hear these horrible stories that doulas had witnessed or their clients had experienced, and I wanted a way to roughly assess the frequency with which those occurred." The next step is examining how "an interaction that leaves someone feeling that they aren't considered human by the person taking care of them" might impact the health outcome. "That's the piece that I think needs to be measured."

From the perspective of advocates sitting at stakeholder meetings, crafting quality measures and bundles and toolkits, things are getting better. At least we're moving in the right direction, says Neel Shah. But even those same advocates question how much evolution is trickling down to "rank-and-file" clinicians, and the doulas and midwives on the ground tell me it's getting worse. Kimm Sun, a home birth midwife in New York, tells me women (who often seek her out for their second pregnancy) aren't telling her their birth stories, "these are trauma stories." Amy Willen, a nurse-midwife in Chicago, writes that she's attended hundreds of hospital births but "can't think of one in which I did not have to struggle, fight with, or otherwise protect the mother-baby dyad from some amount of dehumanization and disrespect for the sacred."

Adult patients have the right to refuse *any* medical intervention, for any reason, period—the legal concept is autonomy. ACOG is clear on this: "Pregnancy is not an exception to the principle that a decisionally capable patient has the right to refuse treatment, even treatment needed to maintain life," reads its ethics guidelines.[43] Yet in the egregious cases that have bubbled up, the clinicians involved clearly never got the memo.

In Switzer's case, the doctor emphasized that she wanted "to help ensure the health of the child and to try to avoid brain damage due to lack of oxygen," but she also believed she had the right to compel surgery. "I have two patients. I don't have just one patient . . . that is why I disagree with the statement of your, of the American, whatever, ACOG, that the desire of the mother has to supersede the desire of the fetus," Rezvina said in a sworn deposition (her native language is Russian).[44] In Turbin's case, the doctor can be heard saying, "What do you mean, 'Why?' That's my reason. Listen: I am the expert here." In Malatesta's attending physician William Huggins's deposition, an attorney asked whether it was true in general that doctors could "override the momma's choice about how she labors and delivers," and he concurred: "The doctor is the one who ultimately has the choice of how things are going to happen."[45]

The courts are part of the problem, too. Hermine Hayes-Klein, an attorney who founded the organization Human Rights in Childbirth, tells me, "This is something I really puzzled over when I was first doing this work—how do you tell women they have a right when the right is so routinely violated? Can you say they have the right to refuse C-sections when there are judgments for court orders for C-sections? The answer is yes, you can," she says, because the right to bodily autonomy—the right to not be touched if you don't want to be touched—is a universal human right. "The duty of the government and the law is to reflect and protect those rights, and when it doesn't, it's illegitimate, it's acting wrongly."

In practice, clinicians feel ownership over the outcome of a birth, and thus ownership over the body giving birth. They fear legal liability for a bad outcome—that they will be sued if the baby dies or suffers damage, and they will lose (there is little fear of a bad maternal outcome). But is this fear justified? "It's a false God," says Stuart Fischbein, an obstetrician in Los Angeles. "I think they use that as a canard to justify what they do. Yes, it's horrible when you get sued. It's life changing. And I understand that, but ultimately our obligation is not to avoid being sued, our obligation is to take care of women who need us."

Part of the problem is that the culture of obstetrics remains especially paternalistic, or as doula and author Elisa Albert puts it, "obstetric violence is the last culturally acceptable form of violence against women."[46] Cristen Pascucci, who led ImprovingBirth and founded Birth Monopoly, told me she had never identified as a feminist until her first birth experience. "All of a sudden I was like, Oh, this is the kind of infantalizing, insulting, degrading treatment that feminists have been bitching about." The real tragedy is that many women submit to it, have come to expect it, and accept it.

A majority of the women surveyed in the *Listening to Mothers* surveys reported old-school, non-evidence-based, unethical practices—68 percent of those birthing vaginally, for instance, pushed lying flat on their backs. Of the women who had episiotomies, only 41 percent had a say in it. Yet they consistently rated their care as "good" or "excellent"—84 percent in 2013.[47] "Women don't inherently believe that they have a human right to high-quality access to health care," says Loretta Ross, the activist and scholar who had a large role in developing the "reproductive justice" framework. We were talking big picture, not just maternity care. "So even if we were to address the macro issues of changing the way health care is delivered, and changing the way health care is researched, we would still have the problem at the more micro level of changing what women demand from the health care system."

In her first letter to Somers Manor OB/Gyn, Lindsay Switzer, who is an attorney, called her treatment "borderline abusive." It was only through therapy that she felt more strongly about what happened. Malatesta initially felt "betrayed" by the hospital and only confided in her husband. "I was worried people would think I was being dramatic, because it's not socially acceptable to complain about your birth if you have a healthy baby," she wrote. The dawning recognition of "birth trauma" and "obstetric violence" and "birth rape" is "women naming their experiences," naming something previously unnamed, says Hayes-Klein, just as "sexual harassment" used to be "just something that happened when men and women worked together."

And these women are swimming against a strong cultural current in which women don't have agency in childbirth, the "narrative that women don't birth babies, babies are delivered by white coats," says Hayes-Klein. "Cultures that want to keep women under reproductive control do so in large part through keeping them literally ignorant about how their reproductive systems work, and we are about birth. You have to be lucky to chance upon information," she says. "Because *What to Expect* isn't going to tell you. It's going to tell you to listen to the white coat."

The impassioned organizing of a handful of individuals and groups—the blogs, books, and films—have not flipped this paradigm. Birth activists are waiting for their #metoo moment. "That's one of the ways in which birth is this forgotten area of feminism," says Hayes-Klein. "Childbirth is based on a prefeminist model of women, in which they're sort of obedient and passive and pretty ignorant about their bodies and do what they're told."

BREECH LIABILITY

Hayes-Klein wanted to tell me about a case that was on her mind—she was trying to help this person get legal representation in her state. This woman had planned a home birth, but when her midwife examined her in labor, she felt the baby's buttocks descending rather than its head—the baby was breech. This midwife had previously delivered breeches and had the skills to attend her client as planned, but the state had recently restricted licensed midwives' scope of practice—they could no longer attend breech births. She told her client they'd have to go to the hospital.

When they arrived, a nurse told the woman she'd have a C-section. The doctor arrived and confirmed, but the patient refused. When she kept refusing, the doctor asked her partner to step outside the room and asked *him* to sign the consent form. He refused. The nurses kept trying to get the woman to consent to surgery while she was quietly contracting, the baby pressing down.

Finally, a new person entered the room, likely the hospital's risk manager, saying they couldn't be liable for a death. She asked the woman to sign papers stating that she was refusing surgery "against medical advice," which she did. At that point, the hospital essentially kicked her out. Nurses pulled out the IV lines and monitors they had urgently attached, and refused her admittance to a room. She was almost fully dilated and feeling the urge to push. A sympathetic nurse directed them to a different hospital, an hour's drive away.

The woman fought the urge to push during the entire car ride. When she arrived, the baby already emerging, the doctor on call told her she'd need a C-section. Again she refused and continued pushing. Nobody touched her except her midwife, still by her side though her hands were tied by a licensing rule change. She helped her patient to lean forward into a semi-squat as the baby was caught by nobody and emerged onto the hospital bed, perfectly healthy.

Several minutes later, she was able to hold her baby, but the moment was spoiled by a nurse who had taken hold of the new mother's free hand and used it to slap her own face while the nurse scolded her, saying "Bad girl! Bad girl!"

"What they were slapping her for was that a breech baby had come out of her vagina, and that wasn't allowed at this hospital," says Hayes-Klein. The first hospital violated federal law, she says, referring to the Emergency Medical Treatment and Active Labor Act, which prohibits hospitals from turning pregnant patients away when they are having contractions. The staff at both hospitals acted unethically and illegally. "Bullying her is illegal, bullying him is illegal. Kicking her out of the hospital is illegal. It's all illegal but they're assuming she won't get access to accountability and to justice," says Hayes-Klein.

And there was more to the story. The hospital called the state's department of children and family services, which attorneys say is not uncommon when a delivery room situation escalates, particularly for women of color. The family spent the next 24 hours unable to leave the hospital so that mother and baby could be tested for drugs—a plastic baggie tied around the infant's genitals to capture his pee. The social worker was sympathetic and ultimately closed the case.

Hayes-Klein wanted me to hear this story for two reasons: First, as yet another example of abuse and dereliction of duty. And second, as an example of how restrictions on care providers and classifications of "high risk" encroach on women's autonomy. "The change of rules meant that midwives couldn't support her with a baby coming out of her vagina, but then she goes to the hospital and they say sorry, breech babies aren't allowed to come out of vaginas here, either," says Hayes-Klein, and then she's punished when she attempts to exercise her constitutional right to refuse surgery.

Midwives' scope of practice is frequently where advocates compromise: in several states, they are prohibited from attending breech, VBAC, and twin births—the dominant discourse on home birth is that it's only acceptable and appropriate for "low-risk" births. On its face, this is a reasonable argument: breech and twin births require specific skills, VBAC carries an extra risk of the cesarean scar rupturing. A woman planning a VBAC, for example, might decide it prudent to be in a hospital with ready access to an operating room. But what if that hospital is going to deny her labor support? If a midwife can't attend her but the hospital won't either, what are her options? There is solid evidence that these births are still "low risk" in the hands of skilled providers. But advocates like Hayes-Klein point out that the evidence is beside the point. "They're withdrawing support for physiological birth in or out of hospital," and that's a monopoly, she says. "A hospital has a different set of incentives and market pressures if it knows the woman can walk out and give birth with a midwife than if it knows she has nowhere else to turn."

Stuart Fischbein, the obstetrician in LA, had for many years been the go-to for twins, breeches, and VBACs; he was also happy to take transports from home birth midwives, and none of it was popular with the administration at Cedars-Sinai Medical Center—nor was a consensual relationship he had with a patient—all of which, he says, led to his resignation from the hospital in 2007. The midwives he knew suggested he start attending home births. "My first comment was to laugh, but then they invited me to come to a couple births, and those were unbelievably beautiful," he says. So he began taking on home birth clients—almost all of them clients his midwife colleagues were restricted from attending. "I found it completely liberating, because now I can do what I'm trained to do."

Rixa Freeze, a historian who studies breech birth, says ours is "a culture in which litigation and worries about malpractice often subsume a woman's ability to choose what happens to her body . . . If you don't offer vaginal breech you're forcing a woman to have a C-section, which is both unethical and illegal. But it happens every day." Fischbein argues this ethics violation begins a step earlier, in residency, where OBs are no longer learning the skills required to be able to offer a vaginal breech or twin delivery. (VBAC, he says, "is nothing special.") "The skills that make my profession unique are the ability to do things like put on forceps, do a breech delivery, do a breech extraction on a second twin, turn a baby [in utero so it's facing head down]," he says. These skills aren't being taught anymore. "We're not even trained for the 85 percent of women who are normal."

If the system granted pregnant patients their bodily integrity—in other words, granted them agency and responsibility for their choices—physicians would be "liberated" to use their skills (and restricting midwives would be anathema). Instead, the OB profession has given those skills up. "There's been enough evidence since 2002 to suggest that breech birth is a reasonable option," yet hardly any physicians or residency programs will offer it, says Fischbein. "Why is that? Well, it's because it doesn't fit the model by which they want to practice." He points out that restoring women's access to skilled providers for breech alone could lower the national cesarean rate by 2 to 3 points, yet vaginal breeches and twins and VBACs never come up in the national policy conversations—the Healthy People 2020 goal excludes them—instead, surgery is assumed. "The root is that women are not at the center of care," says Nicholas Rubashkin. "It's very hard for a woman to go to an individual hospital and say 'This is my right'" if there aren't skilled providers and a supportive system. "We see women pushing for their rights and getting really abused."

Even if it would be in physicians' interests to relearn these skills and center care around patients' rights, the courts haven't encouraged it. Most malpractice cases aren't about violations of bodily autonomy; there is no professional risk in denying labor support. Lynn Paltrow's sober assessment is that in practice, women don't have the protections we think we have. "Is there a point in pregnancy when women lose their civil rights?" she asks rhetorically, intimately familiar with hundreds of cases in which judges failed to recognize them. The courts "will apply principles of equality" when the question is over whether a woman has the same rights as a man, "but if we need to account for the fact that half of the people who are supposedly protected by the Constitution can get pregnant and need health care that's different from men then we're completely confused and unable to guarantee equality," she says. The remedy may need to be sweeping and radical, perhaps in the form of an Equal Rights Amendment. Says Hayes-Klein: "How much would change in the birth room if it's really clear to everybody there that the woman has the right to make all the decisions about her care on the basis of accurate information and support for her decisions?"

Is there a bundle for that?

6: WOMEN'S HEALTH, INC.

SEX SHOPS USUALLY declare themselves, but A Woman's Touch in Madison, Wisconsin, is more of a destination, the kind of place people find by word of mouth. It's on a low-traffic industrial side street, next to the railroad tracks and a bike path. GPS guides me to an unremarkable office building. I enter through a heavy glass door and walk down a fluorescent-lit, linoleum hallway with a stainless steel water fountain. The windowless shop is also stadium bright, with industrial gray carpet and corporate ceiling tiles. The vulva-shaped chocolate lollipops and wall of vibrators tell me that I'm in the right place, but it feels more like I'm walking into a health clinic than a sex shop. And in many ways, I am.

The store was founded in 1996 by Ellen Barnard, a social worker, and Myrtle Wilhite, an internist. They began seeing the usual clientele—couples looking for creative suggestions, women, young and old, who had never had an orgasm. Wilhite had recently left medicine and thought she'd just do the bookkeeping. But then people started coming in who were medical refugees: those who had lost function after starting a medication; women with pelvic pain, vaginal dryness, intimate skin problems that prescription creams weren't helping; men with erectile dysfunction; cancer survivors whose sexual lives had vanished.

People with medical problems quickly comprised about half their clientele—often they were expressly referred to the shop by their physician, even for issues like recurring urinary tract infections. "When the health care community heard that there was a doctor here, they started sending people to us with any question about sex or sexuality that they couldn't answer," Barnard tells me when I visit the shop, "which was just about everything."

"That's how we started broadening out, and realizing that there was this huge need." For the most common questions, they produced more than a dozen text-heavy brochures, which they give away gratis. So many women came in complaining about vaginal dryness and pain with sex during menopause—most of whom wouldn't consider even topical estrogen because of personal or family history of breast cancer—that Wilhite, a scientist at heart, spent "hours, days, months" hovering over medical and scientific journal articles to research "what do we know about healing skin, what do we know about vaginal moisture, how do I put it all together to help women?"

The shop owners developed a program, which they trademarked Vaginal Renewal—a regimen that combines Wilhite-approved moisturizers and low-frequency vibrators. The idea is to stimulate the tissue, which restores blood flow, which promotes healing. "We can increase blood flow without mucking around with estrogen at all," Wilhite explains. For a time they had a line of vibrators manufactured solely for Renewal. The University of Wisconsin began testing the protocol with gynecological cancer patients and found that it helped preserve function better than standard dilator therapy.

Barnard and Wilhite even recommend Renewal for recurring UTIs, to rehab the skin around the urethra, which buffers it from bacteria, and for trans women who've had bottom surgery to create a vagina. They get grateful calls and emails from around the world. "I can talk for hours about all the things we've learned that the medical establishment doesn't understand," says Barnard. Very few gynecologists specialize in sexual health issues. Wilhite, who trained in internal medicine and epidemiology, says she and most doctors she's encountered—even gynecologists—had minimal training in vulvar, clitoral, and pelvic anatomy. And forget about sexual response. "Did I learn what I know now in medical school? No, I did not," she says.

Luckily, the medical community has embraced them. "Because they don't have solutions," says Barnard. The few FDA-approved drugs for "female sexual dysfunction" have been disappointments. And the jury is still out on the latest trend: vaginal infrared laser therapy. In addition to running the shop, the women go out into the community to teach health care providers. "In that way we've really become one of the major sexual health resources for the medical and therapeutic community."

A lot of the problems they encounter are side effects of something medical: psych meds, antihistamines, cancer treatments, hysterectomies, genital surgeries, and hormonal contraceptives can all affect one's libido, arousal, and orgasm. "I can't tell you how many times a day we have young women who are taking" hormonal contraceptives, including IUDs, says Wilhite. "They come in with symptoms of severe vaginal atrophy. They are so dry, they are so uncomfortable." She and Barnard emphasize that sexual response is also a marker of health in general. "Because to get all those systems to fire off, all those nerves, all that blood, all the structures, the mind-body connection—that's a great test of health, how well is this organism doing?" says Wilhite. And while they do see healthy people just browsing for lingerie or a toy, they also see a lot of chronic illness, even among people in their 20s and 30s. "We're seeing tons and tons of people affected by the obesity epidemic: younger men who are struggling with erectile dysfunction and their partners who are struggling with dryness and diabetes-induced changes in arousal and orgasm," says Barnard. "I think half the people I talked to yesterday had type 2 diabetes."

Diabetes and heart disease are "direct links" to sexual dysfunction, she says. "The bottom line is, sexual function is completely dependent upon good, healthy blood flow to all the little bitty blood vessels, so we call erectile dysfunction the canary in the coal mine, because men generally have ED four or five years before they have their first heart attack." For women, too, metabolic disorders affect blood flow and nerve function. "If you don't have neural function, you don't have sexual arousal," says Wilhite.

Occasionally someone has a problem that needs a medical solution, "but more often than not when we're talking about sexual wellness, other than the basic physiology stuff that has to be addressed, it's much more complicated than any medication or any medical treatment can solve," says Barnard. It's more head-to-toe wellness—especially the head, and Wilhite attributes problems there to 25 years of abstinence-only education. "When we opened the store in '96, I thought we were going to raise women up to the sexual comfort that young men had with their own bodies," she tells me. Instead, men have just regressed. "They're less sexual than any generation before them. These young people don't know how to pleasure themselves. We had to write a brochure, *Masturbation for Men.* I mean, are you kidding me?" she says. "Meanwhile, they're getting unprecedented rates of sexually transmitted diseases, because we're treating [young women] with IUDs, so nobody's using condoms." She mentions a recent "cluster" outbreak of syphilis and HIV in a Milwaukee high school.[1]

The shop owners have a triage system in place: they've trained their staff to talk customers through common issues, and they'll step in for more complex cases. They recommend a "good sex diet" (modified Mediterranean) and review potential lifestyle changes, from the cut of one's jeans to flossing (it decreases inflammation) to exercise. Sometimes they encourage switching to a different birth control pill or to a nonhormonal method. Other clients need help talking through what sexual capabilities survive cancer.

I found my way to A Woman's Touch because a professor suggested it was an example of feminist health in action. It is, and also happens to be one of the last surviving independent, women-owned sex shops. Here's a thriving corner of Main Street, not Wall Street. And at A Woman's Touch, the sex toy business pays the overhead for what is essentially a community clinic.

It is also a living tie to the lineage of feminist health centers that emerged following *Roe*, aided by Medicaid reimbursement for abortion. These clinics were "vanguard organizations that were fertile soil for many of the movement's innovations," wrote anthropologist Sandra Morgen. They forged a new model of basic GYN care at a time when women had to go through humiliating pelvic exams just to get birth control. "Feminist health clinics sought to restore the partnership between consumers and health care providers."[2]

These places thrived during the brief window before the Hyde amendment ended public funds for abortion, in 1977, and before abortion clinics became punitively regulated—with Targeted Regulation of Abortion Providers laws mandating the width of the hallways and such. Meanwhile, women (not MDs) were able to do counseling, Paps, even blood draws—everything but the abortions themselves. They were passionate about changing the standard of care. They had a strong patient-centered philosophy, closer to what today we'd call a reproductive justice framework (though the term did not yet exist). Today, the patient-doctor relationship is ideally more or less a shared decision-making process. Back then, "there was no range of styles," says Cindy Pearson, executive director of the National Women's Health Network, who entered the movement through a San Diego clinic in the late '70s. "You were either compliant or a bad patient."

The medical establishment took the women's centers as a direct challenge and in some cases tried to put these competitors out of business. The founders of the Feminist Health Center in Tallahassee filed and won an antitrust suit against their local hospital after they caught administrators on tape conspiring to deny them backup care.[3] In LA, Carol Downer was famously charged with "practicing medicine without a license" for recommending yogurt for vaginal yeast—police raided the LA center's fridge, confiscating workers' lunches. For the most part, however, these non-professionals were challenging the way care was being delivered, not necessarily the care itself.

"The feminist women's health centers could have been great laboratories for preventative strategies, but they ended up being more like the health care system—just for women," says Barnard. She and Wilhite are trying to expand that paradigm. "What is it women really need to know when they want to stay healthy and age gracefully and go through menopause without horrible symptoms and be sexual beings?"

The other thing that sets A Woman's Touch apart from the zeitgeist is that the "treatment" for sexual dysfunction, while innovative, is low tech. They offer no simple "pill fix." Rather than medicalizing sexual health, the shop owners often call out someone's dysfunction as a side effect of medicine itself. And they are in a unique position to do so.

Ever since the little blue Viagra pill became a blockbuster, the pharmaceutical industry has been racing to develop a pink one—and funding professional conferences and "public education" campaigns to establish "female sexual dysfunction" as an epidemic in need of a cure. Manufacturers have tested testosterone gels and nasal sprays, antidepressants as libido enhancers, even estrogen mimickers similar to those used in cancer treatment. But in the nearly 20 years that they've been trying, only three drugs have won FDA approval. They aren't very effective and cause fun side effects like yeast infections and fainting. While the sexual medicine community has brought more needed attention to conditions like vulvar pain, it has very close ties to the pharmaceutical industry. In several instances, industry has also established close ties with the women's health advocacy community.

PHARMA'S LITTLE HELPERS

In October 2014, the FDA held a "patient-focused drug development" meeting, to which 50 female patients arrived from across the country. These meetings were new for the agency. The rationale was to bring patient perspectives to bear on the pharmaceutical pipeline, before a drug gets to market—part of legislation that promised a speedier drug approval process in exchange for more funding provided by pharmaceutical companies.[4] The meetings thus far had focused on chronic illnesses like sickle cell disease, fibromyalgia, chronic fatigue syndrome, hemophilia, and HIV. They could get emotional: sufferers (or the parents of afflicted children) speak for the record about debilitating symptoms; the toll on work, relationships, family, dreams; and their desperation for better treatments.

The meeting in October was about "female sexual dysfunction."

The talk was raw and real, ranging from lack of interest to lack of sensation to outright pain. Some women acknowledged having "duty sex" for their relationships: "I might not even want to have sex but if he wants sex then and I give it to him then, yes, I was a good wife today," said one woman. As the FDA summarized, "Several participants attributed the onset of their condition (either sudden or gradual) to specific life events, including childbirth, hysterectomy or mastectomy, intrauterine device complications, early-onset menopause, discontinuing hormone therapy, and adverse reactions to medications."[5]

The meeting was also about equality—how men have two dozen FDA-approved erectile enhancers, while women have zip (this wasn't totally accurate—at the time there were three FDA-approved treatments for vaginal pain and female-arousal problems, and not one libido enhancer for men). Equality was a recurring theme among the speakers. But they also talked about a specific drug, then called flibanserin, which targeted low libido—the formal diagnosis at the time was hypoactive sexual desire disorder. Several of the women had in fact been enrolled in clinical trials for flibanserin and reported that it had salvaged their libidos, saved their relationships, and changed their lives. "We need approval," one said plainly, voicing the urgency in the room. "Just say yes," said another. Most of the patients who spoke disclosed that the drug's maker, Sprout Pharmaceuticals, had paid their way to Bethesda.[6]

By early 2015, possible "gender bias" at the FDA thwarting approval of a promising "pink Viagra" was a major media story. The *New York Times*, *Washington Post*, *Los Angeles Times*, and other outlets ran stories quoting leaders of a campaign called Even the Score, which was agitating for parity in sexual medicine.

The campaign won the support of several well-respected organizations that don't usually take a stand on a particular drug's approval: the National Organization for Women, the American College of Nurse-Midwives, the National Association of Nurse Practitioners in Women's Health, Black Women's Health Imperative, CHANGE—Center for Health and Gender Equity. NOW president Terry O'Neill appeared in two videos on the campaign's web site. The campaign worked the media so well that *Time* magazine listed Sprout's drug, by then renamed Addyi, as "the number one inanimate object that drove the news in 2015."

An approval hearing for Addyi was scheduled for June of that year. It became a referendum on women's sexual equality. "It's time to start believing what women say about their sex lives," Jan Erickson, government-relations director for NOW, told the advisory panel. The crowd, packed with Even the Score members who had arrived on buses wearing matching teal scarves, cheered. There was just one problem: the drug, which had *twice* before been rejected by the FDA (once as an antidepressant), could barely show that it had any effect over a placebo, and it caused some troubling side effects, like dizziness, low blood pressure, and fainting.

This didn't seem to bother its boosters. As experts and health advocates presented their concerns about the drug's safety record and lackluster performance, the crowd *hissed.* They applauded speakers like Lori Weinstein, who spoke "on behalf of the 75,000 members of Jewish Women International who share our belief that FSD [female sexual dysfunction] has been overlooked for far too long . . . We believe the science is there for the approval of the drug."[7]

In August, the FDA announced its historic approval, overturning its own internal reviewers' recommendations. The campaign had won. So had Sprout CEO Cindy Whitehead. In under 48 hours, she flipped Sprout and Addyi (its only product) to pharmaceutical company Valeant for a dazzling $1 billion.

It was one of the most successful pharmaceutical public relations stunts in the history of the FDA. It also revealed a serious vulnerability within women's interest groups.[8] Even the Score's leaders said the campaign "evolved from discussion among the women's groups," as the *New York Times* reported.[9] The documentary filmmaker Liz Canner, who directed *Orgasm Inc.*, about the high-stakes race for a female counterpart to Viagra and who had attended the June hearing, told me she suspected otherwise. Canner and I collaborated on some investigative reporting and learned that Even the Score hardly grew from the grassroots—rather, it was *Sprouted.* Several organizations we called said the idea had been presented to them by two insiders. One of those people was Audrey Sheppard, the former head of the Office of Women's Health at the FDA. Sheppard was a card-carrying women's health advocate, but in this case she was working for Sprout.

Following her tenure at the FDA, Sheppard began consulting with industry, acting as an intermediary between device and drug manufacturers and women-focused advocacy groups in DC. By the time Sprout was priming the market for its libido drug, this had become her full-time gig. Her web site describes "a boutique firm specializing in unmet needs in women's health."

Sheppard began organizing luncheons, conference calls, and private meetings with leaders to introduce them to flibanserin in 2013. At first, those meetings were focused on the drug's ostensibly promising new data. But by early 2014, advocates told us she was back knocking on their doors with Whitehead by her side, this time with a different sales pitch. Now there was talk of the need to fight gender bias at the FDA.

"They raised the argument that led to Even the Score," said Susan Wood, a former head of the FDA's Office of Women's Health and now director of the Jacobs Institute of Women's Health at George Washington University. Wood and others doubted that premise. "This wasn't about the FDA being sexist, it was about the data," she told us. The data was poor. "Awful, just awful," Cindy Pearson had said.[10] It showed that women who took Addyi had on average eight-tenths of one additional "sexually satisfying event" per month over women who took placebo—a negligible benefit.

Canner and I called other groups that sponsored Even the Score. Board members at the American College of Nurse-Midwives, Jewish Women International, and Black Women's Health Imperative told us they were surprised to learn of their organization's involvement in the pro-Addyi campaign—some said they thought they were supporting a "sexual health equity" campaign, not a particular drug, and following our inquiries the midwives' college rescinded its support. "To me, it really looks like we and probably some of those other organizations were tricked into being part of something that we were never intending to endorse," one board member told us. Sheppard declined to comment. In 2017, Even the Score disappeared from the Internet.

These groups may have been "uninformed but well intentioned," as one advocate told the FDA, but if you scrolled down the About Us page of Even the Score's web site, past the logos of the two dozen societies, associations, and organizations, it was clear that Sprout was a sponsor. And the campaign was slick, expensive, and well connected: it included well-placed parodies of Viagra ads, a petition drive that garnered 55,000 signatures, and a joint letter from 11 members of Congress, spearheaded by Debbie Wasserman Schultz, to the FDA urging the agency to approve the drug. Behind this machine was Blue Engine Media, a PR firm with ties to both of Barack Obama's presidential campaigns. Some of the groups, like the Center for Health and Gender Equity, the National Consumers League, and the Society for Women's Health Research, took contributions from Even the Score or Sprout directly.

One bioethicist and a social psychologist later wrote in the *Journal of Medical Ethics* (part of the *British Medical Journal*) that Even the Score was "cleverly disguised as a campaign to empower women" based on "deceitful and inaccurate information" that employed an "unethical use of moral arguments."[11]

The other interesting thing about Even the Score was if you wandered among the list of two dozen sponsor organizations, you started slipping on a lot of Astroturf—that is, groups meant to look like grassroots patient-advocacy efforts but were actually crafted by industry. Professional societies like the American Society for Reproductive Medicine and the International Society for the Study of Women's Sexual Health (ISSWSH) don't hide their corporate partnerships—Sprout Pharmaceuticals was the "platinum" sponsor of ISSWSH's 2016 annual meeting.

Other outfits that signed on to Even the Score, like Red Hot Mamas, EmpowHER, Blue Thong Society, and His and Her Health aren't even non-profits. Red Hot Mamas runs menopause education meet-ups in hospitals around the country, and it also produces industry-influenced content—since 2015 in partnership with the Hormone Health Network—"to bring fresh, new resources to women, including educational materials and patient guides for menopausal women, as well as information for endocrinologists." The Network (www.hormone.com) is an arm of the Endocrine Society, which has industry partnerships with just about everyone: Pfizer, Merck, Lilly, Abbott, Amgen, AbbVie, Medtronic, Boehringer Ingelheim.[12]

EmpowHER's site is also full of pharma-sponsored content. Hisandherhealth.com seems to be written by bots ("Viagra is a protected and compelling oral treatment for men with the erectile brokenness and incontinence of physical, mental or blended reason").[13] The Blue Thong Society is a social club for "fun, fabulous, smart, and sassy" women who choose blue thongs over blue hair. Their corporate sponsors are Enterprise Rent-a-Car and Blue Ice Vodka.

Many of the groups appeared to have more credibility—they were real advocacy organizations founded by real people with boards of directors and mission statements. The executive director of the National Consumers League, Sally Greenberg, told the FDA her organization was "the oldest consumer organization in the U.S., founded in 1899 by pioneering women during the progressive era" who "fought passionately for women's equality and fair treatment." The league accepted a contribution from Sprout, according to the *New York Times*—Greenberg was one of Even the Score's most vocal media sources. "This is the biggest breakthrough for women's sexual health since the pill," she told the *Times*. She also insisted that Even the Score would carry on after Addyi: "It's never been about one treatment."[14]

The Society for Women's Health Research was founded in 1990 by physicians Florence Haseltine and Susan Blumenthal. Both were working for the NIH and pushing for women to be included in studies and clinical trials (the joke remains that even the lab rats are male) and for more federal funding for research on women. They succeeded, founded the *Journal of Women's Health*, and helped draft the 1991 Women's Health Equity Act and the 1993 NIH Revitalization Act, mandating the inclusion of women and minorities in clinical research.

But over the next decade, the society's "sole mission . . . to improve the health of women through research" expanded as lobbyist Phyllis Greenberger took on more operations. By 2002, Blumenthal and Haseltine had handed over the reins entirely. During Greenberger's tenure, the organization became a high-bandwidth conduit for pharma-funded "public education" campaigns, like "Know My Bones," about postmenopausal osoteoporosis, underwritten by Amgen, maker of Prolia (which has been shown to *increase* risk of fractures with long-term use). In 2002, it teamed up with Novartis on "The ABCs of IBS" (irritable bowel syndrome) as part of the drugmaker's rollout of Zelnorm, which was taken off the market in 2007 because of cardiovascular risks.[15] The society took money from Eli Lilly to help rebrand Prozac to treat "premenstrual dysphoric disorder."[16] And in 2010 there was "Sex Brain Body," designed by PR giant Ogilvy, sponsored by Boehringer Ingleheim, maker of none other than pink Viagra hopeful, flibanserin. For Greenberger, the partnerships help fulfill the organization's mission. "Back in the day, women's health meant contraceptives and hormones," she told a pharmaceutical marketing magazine in 2015. "We've finally convinced the world that women's health encompasses all products, whether for depression or bone health."[17]

These are examples of "disease awareness" campaigns or what the industry calls "condition branding"—drug companies can't legally market a drug until it's approved, so instead they market a disease. They know a drug manufacturer won't be perceived as the most credible source of information, so often they'll create what looks like a patient advocacy group to spread the word. Or they'll use an existing non-profit, Pearson explains. This has complicated the women's health movement's goal for more informed consumers. "We wanted more information. We got more information—and a lot of marketing that masquerades as information," she told me, even from sources that women would assume they can trust. Groups like the Society for Women's Health Research "have always been comfortable taking industry money, and often their positions are in line with industry." Pearson says she and her staff use the society's campaigns to forecast what drugs are coming down the pipeline.

The National Organization for Women was a different story—it doesn't usually get involved with drug campaigns. According to the insiders I talked to, the leadership knew Even the Score was a pharma job. They had been warned about the data. But the sexism argument was too compelling. It made sense—the FDA had held the morning-after pill political hostage for years (Susan Wood left her post over this). And the structure of NOW is such that a small handful of national staffers decide which campaigns get stamped with the iconic NOW logo. This one was discussed at a 2014 board meeting with chapter leaders from across the country, for about 30 minutes, but it was not put up for a vote; the decision to sign on was left up to staffers. To some, it fell to one side of the infamous generational divide threatening the group's relevance. The women in charge identified with the cause; others were skeptical.

Where did this leave real women's health advocacy? Even the Score revealed the reach of industry's tentacles, as well as the depleted reservoir of true watchdogs. A small band of dissenters wrote letters to the FDA and op-eds arguing that drug approvals should be based on science, not politics. But they were no match for the Blue Engine PR machine, and those in opposition admitted they were slow to respond because of their relationship with Sheppard. "A lot of us who know and respect Audrey through the years, even though we disagreed with her on flibanserin, we were reluctant to actively work against her," said Diana Zuckerman, executive director of the National Center for Health Research, one of a handful of DC health watchdog groups that do not accept industry funding. "By the time the campaign was created, we were too late," Wood said. "The groups had already signed on."

For all the bluster about women needing this drug, Addyi turned out to be a sales dud and a liability for Valeant. Many insurers refused coverage. It was supposed to achieve $1 billion in sales by mid-2017 but barely cleared one percent of that. One condition of its approval was a black-box warning of risks including dizziness, drowsiness, fainting, nausea, and, when mixed with alcohol, unconsciousness (kind of like a date rape drug). The norepinephrine–dopamine disinhibitor would need to be taken every day, not just when someone was in the mood to get in the mood. A 2016 meta-analysis in *JAMA Internal Medicine* looked at previously unpublished clinical trials, along with those reviewed by the FDA, and concluded that "the benefits of Flibanserin treatment are marginal."[18] But hey, sexual equity.

Another group on the Even the Score roster was HealthyWomen, which boasts a Dr. Oz endorsement and calls itself "the nation's leading independent, nonprofit health information source for women." Yet you can trace almost all of the web site's content back to one drug manufacturer or another: Amgen is mentioned in stories on migraines; content for doctors about endometriosis is sponsored by AbbVie (it has a drug in development); Allergan (and its drug Restasis MultiDose) is mentioned again and again in an article about dry eye. Radius Health is behind a 2017 poll finding that "82 Percent of Postmenopausal Women Miss Critical Connection Between Osteoporosis and Bone Fractures."[19] (Its new drug Tymlos, for osteoporosis, had just been approved by the FDA, with an estimated cost of $19,500 per year.)

The "marketing juggernaut" of osteoporosis screenings, as one reporter called it, is its own illustrative example of industry capture of both the media and the nonprofit sector. Back in the mid-1990s, Merck was facing lackluster sales of its debut bone drug, Fosamax. Even if women could be convinced to request a screening, their physicians had no easy way to test for bone density. So Merck pushed manufacturers to make portable testing machines. Then it created the Bone Measurement Institute, a nonprofit subsidiary. According to a Columbia University Business School study of the company, "The goal wasn't only to sell the drug to the elderly who had osteoporosis. Merck officials said they were aiming for the 40 million postmenopausal women in America."[20] The *Seattle Times* reported that in 1995, there were 750 bone-measuring devices in the United States. Four years later, Merck reported 8,000 to 10,000.

Zuckerman recalled attending meetings of yet another women's group, the National Council of Women's Organizations (a lead sponsor of Even the Score), where the agenda seemed to be bigger than women's concerns. In the beginning, "it was a nice coalition," she told me—primarily a way for DC feminists to network. For a time, her group was a member. "Then [the National Council] got involved in women's health issues . . . and started doing things that were very questionable," for example, a luncheon in the late '90s, sponsored by which company she couldn't recall, where guests were given bone density tests—this was before anyone had heard of osteopenia. The point was, now these leaders had heard of it.

By 1998, Merck had successfully lobbied Congress to pass the Bone Mass Measurement Act so that Medicare would cover the testing, and then came out with a new version of Fosamax to treat a new condition, "osteopenia." At last, the drug achieved blockbuster status, as middle-aged women across the country worried over whether they too had osteopenia. And they almost certainly did, because osteopenia merely puts a label on the normal decline in bone density as women age. As Alan Cassels and Ray Moynihan put it in their 2005 book *Selling Sickness: How Drug Companies Are Turning Us All into Patients*, "Using a raft of sophisticated public relations techniques, this informal alliance has tried to convince a generation of healthy women that they are at risk of breaking a bone at any moment and that their very lives are in peril."[21] Women's groups like HealthyWomen continue to be part of that alliance.

HealthyWomen was also host to a flibanserin campaign, "Sex and a Healthier You," sponsored by its original developer, Boehringer Ingelheim. It also promoted the discontinued sterilization device Essure through a stealthy site called "Family Size Matters," whose mission was to "help raise awareness on family planning for women who are done having children" and which was sponsored by Bayer. Clicking on the site prompted a quiz, and depending on how you answered it would lead you to the site for either Essure or the Mirena IUD. If HealthyWomen's content doesn't make the group's industry connections clear, the dozen-plus companies that have appeared on the list of corporate advisors over the years do: among them are Bayer, Eli Lilly, Ethicon (Johnson & Johnson), Merck, Novartis, and Pfizer.[22]

HealthyWomen isn't all marketing—it ran a pro bono "Keep the Care" campaign in 2017 in support of the Affordable Care Act and its mandates for women's preventative care. It has a due date calculator. But it also "welcomes partnerships with industry leaders, including pharmaceutical companies, consumer product companies, managed care companies, hospitals and health systems and media establishments." The real giveaway is its board: at last glance it had zero medical professionals. Most members are pharmaceutical marketing executives, with names like GlaxoSmithKline, Johnson & Johnson, Merck, and elite PR agencies peppering their bios. It offers no financial information on its web site—considered poor form for a legit nonprofit. Federal tax filings show it has taken in around a million dollars in grants each year. In an email, a spokesperson acknowledged that some funding comes from "industry supported educational programs," but the group's goal is "to educate consumers and health care professionals through objective, research-based health information reviewed by medical experts to ensure its accuracy."

Like the Society for Women's Health Research and the National Consumers League, HealthyWomen wasn't always like this. It began as the National Women's Health Resource Center, founded in 1988 by Violet Bowen-Hugh, an OB/GYN who was one of only six women to enter George Washington School of Medicine in 1957, and who was "dismayed by the lack of credible, scientifically based data on women's health."[23] The HealthyWomen site launched in 2005 and current CEO, Beth Battaglino, took over in 2006.

In 2014, Battaglino showed up at the FDA's patient-focused hearing on female sexual dysfunction. She told the room about one of HealthyWomen's recent surveys—of 1,000 women, 61 percent said their sexual relationships or lack thereof were "distressful." This word choice was specific—low libido isn't a diagnosis per se unless it causes the person "personal distress." Battaglino did not mention that the survey had been paid for by Palatin Technologies, another pharmaceutical sponsor of Even the Score.[24]

Even patient community groups can be co-opted by industry. For

20 years now, HysterSisters is where many women land when they start Googling about whether they should have a hysterectomy. That's what Jennifer Nelson of St. Paul, Minnesota, did in 2017 after her physician recommended a robotic hysterectomy for a large fibroid that was causing her misery. "Everything I read on the site was 'real' patients raving about the robot. I thought it must be great," she told Health News Review (a media watchdog that announced in 2018 it would cease publication by year's end for lack of funding). She had horrible complications following that surgery, requiring several more to repair her bowels, a colostomy bag, treatment for severe sepsis, and more. Studies suggest that robotic hysterectomy offers little surgical benefit and increases costs.[25] But when she returned to HysterSisters to share her harrowing experience, her post was removed by the web site.[26]

Founded by a schoolteacher in 1998 after her own hysterectomy, HysterSisters grew so large it needed more servers. To keep the cost free to members, "we manage our financial obligations with the help of our sponsors, advertisers," and member donations, the site explains. One of those sponsors is Intuitive Surgical, manufacturer of the robotic da Vinci Surgical System.

ESTROGEN FOREVER

For more than half a century, one of pharma's biggest target markets for "disease awareness" has been older women—in the beginning, the marketing message was that the end of a woman's fertile years was a public scourge as dire as smallpox. The 1966 industry-funded book *Feminine Forever* declared menopause "a tragedy," that in the absence of estrogen a woman would "be condemned to witness the death of her own womanhood." Drugmakers like Wyeth, Upjohn, and Searle effectively rebranded menopause a disorder of "estrogen deficiency" and set about selling women and their doctors "replacement therapy." The ads for Premarin in particular laid on thick social pressure to medicate: on one side of a two-page spread is a bus driver with the caption, "He is suffering from estrogen deficiency"; on the next page is an angry passenger: "She is the reason why." Another ad shows a father shielding his two children from their raging mother: "Almost any tranquilizer might calm her down," reads the copy, "but at her age estrogen might be what she really needs."

At the market's height in 2001, menopausal hormones were the inflation-adjusted equivalent of a $5 billion industry.[27]

Pharma's successful run in defining menopause, however, was heading toward a roadblock. In the early 1990s, thanks to efforts of feminists and the first female NIH director, Bernadine Healy, the National Institutes of Health launched the Women's Health Initiative (WHI) study, the first to look at large-scale prevention efforts to address threats to women's health like heart disease and breast cancer. One arm of the study tested whether estrogen protected women from heart disease, as drug companies had long claimed. The hormone trials study enrolled 27,000 women between 1993 and 1998 and was supposed to follow them for eight and a half years, but by 2002 the results were clear enough that the NIH had to call it off.[28] Hormone "therapy" led to an increased risk not only for heart attack, but also breast cancer and stroke. At a press conference, Jacques Rossouw, the director of the WHI, said that based on the findings, women should not start hormone replacement therapy, and should quit if they had.

Overnight, it seemed, physicians scrapped prescriptions and women flushed their pills down the toilet. In the 2012 documentary film *Hot Flash Havoc*, the visual for this is the A-bomb mushroom cloud. That image could have represented women's anger at being guinea pigs for decades, but the film points its outrage at the NIH, arguing that as a result of its scientific inquiry, women's menopause symptoms returned with a fury, and hot flashes were the least of it: osteoporosis, depression, joint pain, insomnia, muscle atrophy, dry eyes, dry vaginas, sex drives out the window, relationships destroyed—cue the mushroom cloud. "It's truly a tragedy, they have wrecked people's lives," says one doctor. "It was morally irresponsible," says another.

Pharmaceutical companies like Wyeth (which has since merged with Pfizer) saw their profits plummet in the years following the NIH bombshell. But the data didn't deter them from promoting estrogen. Instead, Wyeth in particular waged a public relations campaign in the pages of medical journals and in the halls of medical conferences, tweaking its message to promote hormone use for younger women—under the age of 60 and within ten years of menopause. The women in the WHI study, the argument goes, were just too old.[29]

That campaign also found its way to the Society for Women's Health Research, whose 2002 annual charity ball was sponsored by Wyeth and themed "Coming of Age." "It was like they were doing an ad for Wyeth," one participant told Alicia Mundy, who wrote an investigative piece about it in the *Washington Monthly*. The week after the gala, Wyeth presented the society with a $250,000 check at a sixtieth anniversary event for Premarin.[30]

"Hormone therapy is definitely being reframed," Adriane Fugh-Berman, professor of pharmacology and director of the Georgetown University–based watchdog organization PharmedOut, told me in 2012. She coauthored a 2011 study that analyzed some 50 opinion articles following the WHI and found that more than half were "promotional in tone," attacking the WHI, downplaying the risks of estrogen, exaggerating its benefits, and implying new ones. It also found that eight out of ten authors studied had declared payment from menopausal hormone manufacturers. This made historical sense, she said. "First it was sold to keep you 'feminine forever,' then it was sold as disease prevention, now it's being recast as safe in the low-dose formulation."

Hot Flash Havoc seemed to fit right in with this history of industry PR. Except "there is not a penny of pharmaceutical money in this movie," Alan Altman, an OB/GYN and the film's medical advisor, asserted. "We have every major menopause expert in the country interviewed in the film and they all say the same basic thing"—that the WHI got it wrong. I had met Altman at a conference of the International Society for the Study of Women's Sexual Health, where he mentioned the film whenever he had an audience. He was also ending his term as president of the society, and he was particularly vocal about menopause as a disease of "estrogen withdrawal," which sounded very much like an updated version of estrogen deficiency. When I pressed him on the point, he made clear he wasn't saying that *all* women need to take estrogen. Yet at one point he joked with the audience, "Who is this asymptomatic postmenopausal woman and where can I find her? I'll take her out to dinner."

Like most of the experts in the film, Altman had extensive relationships with drug companies: he was a speaker for Novogyne, Ther-Rx,

Warner Chilcott, and Solvay and was on the advisory board for Upsher-Smith, Novogyne, QuatRx, and Wyeth.[31] When I followed up with him by phone, he was in Atlanta giving a sponsored talk. "But I do that because I believe in what estrogen does. They haven't bought me," he said.

While the film had been produced without industry funds, the experts had numerous conflicts of interest. Sheryl Kingsberg, a psychologist at the Cleveland Medical Center, has a long history of financial relationships with pharmaceutical companies: Boehringer Ingelheim, Wyeth, Johnson & Johnson, Trimel, BioSante, Procter & Gamble.[32] In the film, she offers this metaphor: "Consider a grape. Without estrogen, it shrivels up into a raisin." Wulf Utian, who cofounded the North American Menopause Society and was an outspoken critic of the WHI, had taken large sums from Wyeth.[33] Anita Clayton is a psychiatrist and frequently called upon media sexpert (including on Even the Score) with rare mention of her connections to companies including Palatin, Pfizer, Trimel, and Sprout.[34] Nor did the film make any of these disclosures. Also in the film: Phyllis Greenberger, then CEO of the Society for Women's Health Research, which held a private screening and reception in DC in 2010. In 2016, the film was updated and revised, with Goldie Hawn narrating, and aired on PBS with underwriting from the society.

When I brought up the question of industry influence on the movie with Altman, he denied any whatsoever. "This movie was not made because of a pharmaceutical company or to sell anything, it was to get the truth out about the misrepresentation of the WHI study." He found it "extremely annoying" to have to defend the film's or his own credibility. "That's ridiculous. But that's the way the culture is now. You know, pharma is a bad thing, and if you receive 20 cents from a pharmaceutical company that means you're totally influenced," he said. (According to ProPublica's Dollars for Docs database, which compiles financial disclosures compelled by the Sunshine Act, Altman took in nearly $45,000 between 2013 and 2015 in speaking fees and associated travel. There's no data prior to 2013, before the act went into effect.) The WHI looked at the wrong women, he reiterated—too old. "Estrogen is a preserver of good function. It doesn't repair bad function 20 years down the road," he told me. "You should be angry as a woman."

Anger, it turned out, had funded the film. Heidi Houston, the executive producer, and other female investors did not merely have a rough ride with "the change." They were thrust into early menopause by surgery or drugs and left to manage the fallout on their own, with no warning or treatment from their doctors. And they were pissed. When Houston was 44, her doctor asked if she was done having kids and offered to stop her period with progestin, as a matter of convenience. "I had no idea he was going to put me into early menopause," Houston told me, and he gave her no warning of the symptoms. "I had joint pain so bad I could barely walk in the mornings," she said. "The next thing was headaches. Then the next thing, I am having these mood swings." She had heart palpitations, then her cholesterol started going up. "I had no idea that it was related to menopause at all for two years, that's why I said somebody needs to make a movie to figure this out."

Michelle King Robson, another investor who is also the creator of EmpowHER.com, jumped on board because of her own hysterectomy. Her doctor suggested removing her uterus because of her digestive problems—they seemed worse when she had her period. The doctor also recommended removing her ovaries, because they might become cancerous. She was never asked her about her cervix, but that was removed, too. "I thought I was sick before," Robson told me, sitting in her palatial home in Scottsdale, Arizona. "Then I really tanked." She had trouble getting out of bed. She began having suicidal thoughts. She went to nine doctors in search of relief.

Another woman in the film is Karen Giblin, who founded Red Hot Mamas, the menopause support group, in 1991. She was just 40 years old when she had a hysterectomy for endometriosis and heavy bleeding, which threw her into surgical menopause. "My surgeon was excellent, but he didn't really prepare me for the menopause that followed," she told me. She went to the bookstore and found one book on the subject, which she felt compelled to hide under a magazine while in line to pay. An elected representative in Ridgefield, Connecticut, at the time, she founded Red Hot Mamas to break the silence and taboo around menopause. The meet-ups are festive, with music and red boas for all attendees. Women commiserate about symptoms and hear local MDs speak. They also go home with pamphlets underwritten by the major industry players. (Giblin says she met her second husband at a dinner sponsored by Solvay Pharmaceuticals.) Today the taboo has lifted, but she worries many women are "hormonally challenged," because they're fearful, since the WHI, of taking hormone therapy.

What's ironic is that for all the medical community's focus on hormones for otherwise healthy women who've entered the menopausal years, the WHI showed that women who've had their uteruses and/or ovaries removed *do* benefit from replacing lost estrogen. "Surgical menopause" *is* more like a disease than a normal facet of aging—an abrupt ovary shutdown can cause severe fatigue, depression, and sexual dysfunction for which the mushroom cloud is no hyperbole. And people whose ovaries are gone or no longer functional are in fact at a higher risk for many life-shortening conditions if they are not taking hormones. This nuance was lost in the media coverage that followed the WHI bomb.

Meanwhile, anyone who is taking hormone therapy and quits cold turkey will likely suffer withdrawal symptoms, and this abrupt break was basically what the NIH advised when it released the WHI findings. So it's entirely possible that women who'd had hysterectomies and were wrongly taken off their hormone regimens were unnecessarily harmed, while other women taking hormone replacement therapy were thrust into the havoc of withdrawal—a perfect chaos for pharma to swoop in and promise order.

Just as Even the Score had tapped into a real need and valid skepticism among a certain demographic, so had the film. It didn't need industry backing, at least not directly. "The industry creates an atmosphere. If you get to enough key opinion leaders, then marketing messages become conventional wisdom. People who don't have conflicts of interest begin repeating them as well," Fugh-Berman explains. "I've been yelled at by entire rooms of doctors, I've been told that denying women hormones was genocide." Indeed, surveys of OB/GYNs in the years since the WHI have found that about half don't believe the results of the government study, which included more than 16,000 women.[35]

Several times a week, a woman will walk into A Woman's Touch in Madison for help negotiating vaginal dryness and pain with penetration—what Wilhite and the medical community call vulvovaginal atrophy.

For those women, it is distressing. They no longer have access to a reliable source of pleasure and intimacy.

Women's circulating estrogen decreases in menopause, though their ovaries don't shut down altogether. And like the rest of our skin and muscle, the vulva and vagina experience some thinning and drying. But that doesn't necessarily predict dysfunction. Loren Wissner Greene, an OB/GYN and bioethicist at New York University, recommends lube or estrogen cream, which has far fewer downsides than taking pills systemically. Greene and other physicians point out that women who stay sexually active through menopause tend to do better than women who don't. "Use it or lose it," they say. Sex, it turns out, is a preserver of good function.

Perimenopause—the years before the menstrual cycle ceases—is actually the period we associate with the worst symptoms: hot flashes, bleeding, sleep and mood disturbances. According to Greene and other experts, around 10 percent of otherwise healthy women have symptoms that are severe enough to warrant treatment. That's far less than the 70 percent claimed by experts in *Hot Flash Havoc*, but it's a sizable minority.

Meanwhile, there is a lack of clear understanding and consensus around the hormonal physiology of the transition to menopause. It's not as simple as a decline in estrogen. In fact, irregular periods and spotty ovulation indicate that what declines during perimenopause is progesterone, while estrogen levels fluctuate. Endocrinologist Jerilynn Prior has studied treating hot flashes with progesterone and found that, surprisingly, it is as effective as estrogen. "Even though their own estrogen levels are high and progesterone low, the standard of care is birth control pills or [estrogen-progestin] hormone therapy, neither of which have been shown to work," Prior told me.

Prior is the author of *The Estrogen Errors*, and one of those errors, she argues, is confusion over perimenopause and menopause. Menopause *follows* the "havoc"—by that time estrogen levels have tapered, and the classic symptoms have usually subsided. "If people in their general discourse confuse phases of women's lives that are totally hormonally and experientially different, then how can their treatment be very appropriate?" she asks.

Greene is skeptical of what she calls the "propagandizing" of female sexual dysfunction. Our bodies change as we age, and sexual function depends on everything from how hot we are for our partner to whether we're obese, stressed out, breastfeeding, on antidepressants, getting cancer treatment, or have had a hysterectomy. Wilhite blames our sugar-loaded Western diets for bad symptoms (she counsels women to eat more vegetables and lay off the bread and wine). This may explain why women in Mexico, Japan, and Southeast Asia report fewer or none of the symptoms we do.[36]

Hormones have their place as treatment. But as preventive medicine? Even if women start earlier? At lower doses? There's no evidence. Older women are not suffering from "estrogen deficiency" any more than everyone over 40 is suffering from youth deficiency.

One of the most unfortunate outcomes of the estrogen myth is that it masks the impact hysterectomies have on some women. In *Hot Flash Havoc*, these stories are presented in the context of normal aging. "Hormone therapy" becomes the savior of a man-made catastrophe. And as a result of the producers' own health challenges and dependence on pharmaceuticals, the industry has dependable allies in them. Robson has traveled to DC several times to speak on behalf of various drugs, including flibanserin/Addyi. "Generations of women have suffered in silence for far too long, far too long," she said at the patient-focused hearing. "It is time for the FDA to act."

THE GARDASIL GIRLS

The history of medicine is marked by several drugs that have captured the energy and passion of women's groups. In 2007, the It drug was the newly approved vaccine against human papillomavirus (HPV), Gardasil, which manufacturer Merck claimed would prevent cervical cancer.

In January of that year, Christine Baze, a singer-songwriter from Boston, flew to Marco Island, Florida, for a meeting of a group called Women in Government (WIG). She was there to talk (and sing) to about 60 state legislators about the invasive cervical cancer she had discovered at age 31 and barely survived, and the "Pop Smear" concert and tour she started to raise awareness of Pap screening and to share her excitement about the new vaccine.

Baze didn't fly on her own dime to Florida. Nobody at the conference did. WIG had picked up the airfare and hotel tab for all the attendees. How could this group of public servants throw around that kind of cash? Among its donors was Merck, which paid Baze $7,500 to speak at three other events.[37] Baze was inspired to "jump on the HPV vaccine bandwagon on the biggest level," she told me. Part of that bandwagon was lobbying state governments to mandate the vaccine for girls in public school—this was the true purpose of the WIG meeting in Florida. The vaccine was designed to prevent two high-risk strains of HPV that had been estimated to be responsible for some 70 percent of cervical cancers. But clinical trials showed the vaccine was only effective before exposure to HPV, thus the CDC recommended it target girls aged 11 to 12. WIG members were the perfect audience: in a position to sponsor bills in state legislatures mandating the vaccine, as nearly two dozen states would attempt to do, or push governors to issue executive orders, as Rick Perry of Texas would try to do.

But some public health experts raised concerns about mandates. For one, the clinical trials hadn't shown that the vaccine had any impact on cancer—they couldn't with only a handful of years of data. They only showed a reduction in abnormal cervical cells, most of which resolve on their own. There was the question of public value. We already had a highly effective method of cervical cancer prevention: the Pap test.

Long before the vaccine was in the pipeline, cervical cancer was considered an almost entirely preventable disease. It grows very slowly, over 10 to 20 years, so testing every three years catches cellular changes that can be watched and treated if necessary. HPV infections are mostly transient and benign—the body's immune system clears the vast majority, even the high-risk strains. The virus is so common that some 80 percent of sexually active people have had it by the time they are 40. So while it's true that HPV is present in most cervical cancer, most HPV is harmless. One potential benefit of a vaccine is that if women have fewer abnormal Pap results, they would have fewer harmful biopsies and procedures to remove abnormal cells—procedures that cause scarring and contribute to childbirth complications. Then again, if everyone followed the guidelines to do Pap screenings no more frequently than every three years, that would also reduce the harms.

Another problem was that the vaccine would afford only limited protection from HPV infections, waning at about five years—if a girl got the vaccine when she was 11, would it wear off just in time for her to start hooking up? Merck specified in its labeling for Gardasil that girls and women who received it would still need to get regular Pap screening. But there was danger in people believing they had been vaccinated against cervical cancer. What if they stopped getting Pap tests? "There is a real risk that cervical cancer will increase in the U.S.," Diane Harper, a Dartmouth researcher who helped design and implement clinical trials for both Merck's Gardasil and GlaxoSmithKline's Cervarix, later told *Discover* magazine.[38]

In the 1920s, cervical cancer was the number one cancer killer of women; as Pap testing became routine, in the 1950s, cervical cancer deaths in the United States began to fall. Today, cervical cancer represents just .8 percent of cancer cases in the United States. The National Cancer Institute estimated there would be roughly 13,000 cases and 4,000 deaths in the United States in 2018.[39] (Worldwide, the number of deaths is much higher, around 250,000.) They occur mostly in women over age 50 with concurrent infections like HIV, and poor women and women of color are disproportionately represented, pointing to disparities in access to care, not a lack of awareness. Still, Baze didn't want anyone to go through what she did, so she rocked in order to, as she put it, "save the hooch" (her version of "cooch," or slang for vagina).

WIG had in fact put cervical cancer on its agenda as early as 2004, which was also when Merck began its "public education" campaign. As Judith Siers-Poisson reported in a four-part investigation for *PR Watch*, "Merck used their deep pockets to make sure that even before the FDA had approved Gardasil, there was a growing awareness of and concern about—one might even say fear of—HPV among U.S. women. The marketing juggernaut was multifaceted and meticulously planned."[40] WIG had at that point a roster of some 20 pharmaceutical or medical funders: in addition to Merck and GlaxoSmithKline (which had Gardasil competitor Cervarix in the pipeline), there was Digene (which manufactures an HPV test), Novartis, Eli Lilly, AstraZeneca, Bayer HealthCare, Pfizer, Bristol-Myers Squibb, and Pharmaceutical Research and Manufacturers of America, the lobbying group for the industry. "It appears that word has gotten around that WIG is ready, willing and able to cooperate with those invested heavily in health care policy," wrote Siers-Poisson.[41]

By 2006, WIG's web site featured a legislative policy toolkit with sample legislation for state mandates, fact sheets on HPV and cervical cancer, and maps showing pending HPV vaccine bills. At its peak in June 2007, that map showed that 23 states and the District of Columbia had introduced HPV mandate bills, with Virginia the first state to pass a law. Merck's hand in this was not necessarily obvious to representatives. Health Policy Monitor reported that California Democratic assemblywoman Sally Lieber, who introduced a bill in late 2006 to require girls entering sixth grade to be vaccinated, had declined a meeting with Merck and was sponsoring the legislation "because of the unique opportunity it presented to prevent cancer with a vaccine—something that has never before been possible." Lieber did, however, meet with WIG, according to Health Policy Monitor, without knowledge of its ties to Merck.[42]

One high-level public health expert I talked to expressed concern about the backlash mandate bills would cause. Among the vaccine's other problems, it had landed on rocky political turf: the religious right objected to it on grounds that in preventing a sexually transmitted virus, it would give teens license for sexual promiscuity. The expert recalled a conversation with a state legislator who had introduced a bill to mandate the vaccine among school-aged girls. "I'm a vaccine advocate, and I was trying desperately to keep them from introducing a bill to mandate this. I said no, you don't want to do this," this person told me. "Where do you think she got the idea? A woman's health conference sponsored by Merck."

Former president of WIG Susan Crosby insisted to *PR Watch* that WIG is "a totally unbiased, unprejudiced group." And perhaps it was just sincerely persuaded by the cancer prevention argument. Andrea Boland, a Democratic senator from Maine, told CorpWatch that at the Florida meeting there was a "pull to get on board" in promoting HPV vaccination, "and when I raised questions, the response was 'Do you want your daughter to die of cancer?'"[43]

In 2009, Columbia researchers Sheila and David Rothman documented in the *Journal of the American Medical Association* how Merck had also pushed its award-winning marketing plan through three professional medical organizations, which gave their physician members industry-crafted language to promote Gardasil to their patients as the first-ever "cancer vaccine." At least one group, the American Society of Colposcopy and Cervical Pathology, also encouraged doctors to lobby for state mandates. "They seem to be repeating the marketing message of Merck," wrote the Rothmans.[44]

Then there were the direct-to-consumer ads. If you were on a large college campus in the late 2000s, they were everywhere. Full-page ads in the school newspaper. Foam drink warmers at the student health center. Billboards. And of course prime-time TV spots. The "One Less" campaign featured teen girls mostly on their own doing middle-class teenage things: horseback riding, playing soccer, knitting, skateboarding, step dancing. The girls say they want to be "one less" cancer diagnosis, "one less" death. "Ask your doctor about getting vaccinated with the only cervical cancer vaccine: Gardasil." The girls in the ad enthusiastically take up the message, chanting "O-N-E L-E-S-S" while skipping double dutch; one even labels herself by stitching "one less" on her hoodie.[45]

By 2008, Gardasil sales had surpassed blockbuster status, at $1.4 billion. As the Rothmans put it, "to achieve this penetration, the marketing of this vaccine broke with traditional practices." "I'll give Merck credit—there is absolutely nothing factually incorrect in Merck's advertisements," Diane Harper told *PR Watch*. "But the interpretation of the rock stars, and the media, and of everyone else is that this vaccine will completely eliminate cervical cancer. I've worked with ABC, with NBC, and even on their nightly news, their headline is 'HPV vaccine prevents cervical cancer.' It's true, that is a true headline, but it is not accurate."[46]

It was true in theory, but now, more than a decade later, there's still no indication that the vaccine prevents cancer—the data still doesn't exist to support that claim, and won't for many more years if it's true. Meanwhile, journalists and researchers who've looked back at the clinical trial data have found it less impressive than initially reported. Jeanne Lenzer, now a contributing editor of the *BMJ*, broke down the numbers for *Discover* in 2011: According to Merck's own data, vaccinated girls and women saw an overall 17 percent decline in abnormal cervical cells. Most of those abnormal cells resolve on their own, so a 17 percent decline isn't necessarily a predictor of a significant reduction in cancer. "Whether Gardasil will reduce cervical cancer deaths in real-world conditions has simply never been answered. It might—but that would take a long-term study, and one that should be done *before* it's widely promoted," she wrote.[47]

And there are lingering questions about safety. Tom Jefferson, a physician and research fellow with the Centre for Evidence-Based Medicine in Oxford who is reviewing 206 studies of HPV vaccines, many unpublished, tells me, "There are some apparent benefits, intermediate benefits. It looks as if [the vaccine] may be preventing precursors of cancer." But he points out that since most of these abnormalities regress on their own, the benefit is not clear. Fewer abnormal Pap results does mean that women don't need as many follow-up visits and procedures. "That's the good news. Then on the other side, you've got these harms—real, perceived, we're not sure yet," he says.

Physicians in the United States, Denmark, Japan, Mexico, and Italy have documented case reports of people developing what are broadly called autonomic disorders following HPV vaccination. In Denmark, neurologists opened special "syncope" clinics to evaluate girls and women with these symptoms, which generally include fatigue, headache, chronic pain, cognitive dysfunction, and difficulty standing, and fall under different names: postural orthostatic tachycardia syndrome (POTS); dysautonomia, small fiber neuropathy, and symptomatic dysfunction. Doctors may also diagnose these symptoms as chronic fatigue syndrome, fibromyalgia, or chronic regional pain syndrome.

Louise Brinth is a Copenhagen neurologist who evaluated more than 300 cases of girls and women who developed such symptoms after HPV vaccination. She and other specialists brought dozens of case reports to the attention of the European Medicines Agency (EMA), urging further research to determine if the association with the vaccine is causal or coincidental. So far both the EMA and Cochrane, which conducts systematic reviews to guide evidence-based practice, conclude, based on published studies, that there's no relationship between HPV vaccination and long-term neurological problems.

Brinth wrote a 60-page response to the EMA, noting that HPV vaccines "have not been shown to have yet prevented a single case of cervical cancer death . . . We have evidence demonstrating that the vaccine prevents precursor states and that is as good an indication as it gets. I believe that the HPV-vaccines have the potential to counter both mortality and morbidity—both death and suffering—in the long run. However, we are dealing with a preventive measure and this calls for a very high focus on safety."

Tom Jefferson at Oxford is one of several researchers challenging both the EMA and Cochrane on the conflicts of interest of their HPV vaccine reviewers and the inadequacy of the clinical trials, none of which, he says, compared vaccine recipients to a control group that got a true placebo.[48] Another recent analysis published in *BMJ Evidence-Based Medicine* concluded, "Cochrane's conclusions on HPV vaccines are based on poor science and thus not relevant."[49] Jefferson has been a vaccine researcher for 25 years, generating systematic reviews for Cochrane, the World Health Organization, pharmaceutical companies, and government entities. He tells me, "No vaccine is 100 percent safe. It's a question of a trade-off between benefits and harms." One thing that makes the calculation a bit different for the HPV vaccine than others is that "if there are harms, they're here now, whereas the benefits are far in the future. And historically harms have been understudied, underreported, underinvestigated, and ignored."

A recent eight-month investigation by Slate looked back at the original clinical trials' ability to determine safety and concluded, based on interviews and thousands of pages of documents, that they were "flawed from the outset," wrote author Frederik Joelving. "To track the safety of its product, the drugmaker used a convoluted method that made objective evaluation and reporting of potential side effects impossible during all but a few weeks of its yearslong trials."[50]

Sorting this out will require untangling deep conflicts of interest and transcending the highly charged discourse on vaccines in general. In Buffalo, New York, neurologist Svetlana Blitshteyn has evaluated patients from around the United States with symptoms identical to those Brinth has documented. "In neurology we have been trained to ask patients who present with certain neurologic symptoms whether they've been vaccinated. Because sometimes in certain patients that's a trigger for certain neurological adverse events," she tells me. "In some cases in my opinion, POTS can also occur after vaccination, just like Guillain-Barré syndrome," which is an accepted adverse event in adults following the flu vaccine, for instance. Patients often come to her after being dismissed by several other physicians, often after being referred to a psychiatrist for anxiety or even admitted to a psych unit. "We have to be the patients' advocates rather than tell them it's all in their head and they're crazy and it's not real," she says.

Like Brinth, Blitshteyn also questions the reviews that have concluded there is no increased risk with vaccination, because POTS and other autonomic disorders go by so many different names and are largely unknown to primary care doctors, so they are underdiagnosed in general. But a complicating factor is that teen girls are the population most likely to get POTS. "There has to be a special study done, where prospectively a large number of patients are followed closely: those who were vaccinated with Gardasil and those who weren't, to see which arm develops those disorders and then compare numbers. Anything else is going to be full of flaws," she says.

"I have been in this highly explosive field for four years now," wrote Brinth. "I want to voice my ever increasing feeling of our considerable inability to be nuanced and balanced when discussing vaccines—both their efficacy and side effects . . . We are in desperate need of a shift in paradigm, a groundbreaking one, or the future of public confidence in vaccines will be lost."

Back when Merck's award-winning marketing campaign was in full swing, some journalists and researchers were asking tough questions and shedding light on the vaccine's potential drawbacks. But U.S. politics precluded any reasoned debate. Right-leaning groups attacked Gardasil as the "promiscuity vaccine" and opposed mandates on moral grounds. Women's groups had prepared a defense, and feminist journalists followed their lead. Leading up to the FDA approval, the National Organization for Women ran a "women's health project effort involved in public education activities concerning FDA review of a new vaccine," according to its 2005 annual report, and its legal defense fund supported legislative mandates.[51] In *Ms.* magazine, Cindy Wright wrote breathlessly in 2007, "Even if I had to pay full price, how could I say no to the first-ever cancer vaccine? How could anyone? Who would consider not giving our daughters the best chance of avoiding a deadly disease?"[52] The venerable *Boston Globe* columnist Ellen Goodman called Gardasil "extraordinarily safe and effective against a lethal disease" and warned parents: "Caution: Too much suspicion can be bad for your daughters' health."[53]

Canadian women's health activists, however, had begun sounding alarms about the vaccine's dubious benefits when it was first approved, wary of a new product and the marketing juggernaut behind it. They reached out to their American colleagues but notably could not persuade watchdog groups like Our Bodies, Ourselves and the National Women's Health Network to sign on. "They couldn't get buy-in from their boards for such a critical message," Anne Rochon-Ford of the Canadian Women's Health Network told me. Our Bodies, Ourselves blogger Rachel Walden initially supported state mandates but expressed some regret after Merck's marketing tactics became apparent. As Siers-Poisson put it in *PR Watch*, the political climate had "produced a knee-jerk reaction. Instead of carefully examining the issue, the response from some has been to endorse the vaccine simply on the grounds that if the Right is against it, they should be for it."

Furthermore, Merck's ad campaign had a certain postfeminist appeal, conveying "that vaccination is empowering," wrote scholar Tasha Dubriwny in *The Vulnerable Empowered Woman.* "The Gardasil girl's ability to choose to vaccinate and her role as an adolescent who is 'free'—that is one who has a certain degree of independence from her mother and other family members—are linked by an overarching theme of postfeminist girl power."

In 2009, the CDC's Advisory Committee on Immunization Practices recommended the vaccine for boys, and in 2014, the FDA approved Merck's new formulation, Gardasil 9, which protects against seven high-risk HPV strains, along with two that cause genital warts (also thrown into the original Gardasil as a bonus). But to this day the cancer benefits are theoretical.

Recent medical studies touting the vaccine's effectiveness are either funded by Merck or the authors report conflicts of interest, some of which are disclosed in medical journals but rarely make it into mainstream media coverage, which has almost exclusively been positive. In December 2017, a ten-year study, published by the journal *Pediatrics*, made headlines that the vaccine showed long-term safety and efficacy.[54] "HPV Vaccination Immunity Remains Strong 10 Years Later, Especially for Preteens," was *Forbes*'s. "The vaccine was virtually 100 percent effective in preventing disease in these young individuals," Daron G. Ferris, an OB/GYN and lead author of the study, stated in a press release put out by the Medical College of Georgia at Augusta University, where he is a professor. "Now we need to push for more young people to get vaccinated."[55] This study was funded by Merck, and Ferris had accepted $60,000 in consulting and speaking fees for Gardasil specifically in 2014 and 2015.

Another study, published in September 2017 in the *Lancet*, looked at the newer Gardasil 9 and reported on the absence of high-grade cervical abnormalities in women followed for six years.[56] "There is no question that the vaccine works," said lead author Warner Huh, who helped develop the vaccine (echoing Ferris's promotional tone). "The challenge is to get the new vaccine into widespread use among young women."[57] Huh even suggested that the vaccine could replace Pap screening: "Looking forward, with widespread vaccination, it is highly likely that cervical cancer will evolve into historical interest only, and screening, like Pap smears, might go away altogether."[58] This study was also funded by Merck, and Huh received $30,000 in consulting fees for Gardasil in 2014 and 2015.

Even a recent Consumer Reports headline was unequivocal: "Why Your Daughters (and Sons) Need the HPV Vaccine."[59] Researchers have found an association between HPV and a range of other cancers, including penile, anal, and throat cancers, so now the rationale is that vaccination will prevent those, too, though it is still theoretical.

When the FDA approved Gardasil 9, a fresh marketing push followed. But now it's not only Merck promoting the "cancer vaccine" message; the CDC is also using that language. Since 2014, the pharmaceutical giant and taxpayer-funded agency have been connected through the National HPV Vaccination Roundtable. At a meeting in February 2018, which took place in Atlanta, the director of communication unveiled the "We're In" campaign for member organizations and providers to show their solidarity with the mission. "What does 'We're In' mean? It means you and your organization: Understand that the HPV vaccine is a cancer prevention vaccine and want to spread the word," the PowerPoint slide explained.

Baze attended that meeting and is featured in the 2014 film *Someone You Love*, which Roundtable members and public health departments all over the country utilize "to educate and help others emotionally connect what HPV can do to you, or someone you love," she explains. The conversation has shifted away from the controversies of ten years ago. (Baze tells me that looking back, she feels the focus on state mandates was the wrong approach.) In the intervening years she has given HPV talks to college, high school, and even middle school students—and has attracted several sponsors: Merck, GlaxoSmithKline, Qiagen/Digene, Roche, Gen-Probe, and Hologic/Cytyc. "I do feel we're on the cusp of something beautiful and something great," says Baze, "and I want to be able to say I was part of that."

THE MORE OPTIONS, THE BETTER

By now it should come as no surprise that when safety concerns arise about certain already approved pharmaceuticals, establishment women's groups haven't exactly been on the front lines raising red flags. This is true for contraceptive drugs and devices, and especially true of one long-established organization in particular—one that millions of Americans have put on donation speed dial during the Trump years: Planned Parenthood.

Picture another FDA meeting, this one on December 8, 2011—a joint meeting of two advisory committees, one for Reproductive Health Drugs and one for Drug Safety and Risk Management. The large group met to discuss a "fourth-generation" progestin, drospirenone, featured in then-popular oral contraceptives Yaz and Yasmin, made by Bayer, as well as several other less prominent generics. By then, several published studies were suggesting that the drug caused roughly twice the number of blood clots as previous-generation Pills, which can lead to permanent injury, stroke, heart attack, even death. The FDA had received thousands of adverse event reports, including some 200 deaths. The meeting would determine if the fourth-generation pills should remain on the market.

Cindy Pearson of the National Women's Health Network spoke during the public hearing and, for historical context, evoked the activists who had disrupted a hearing on the Pill four decades prior—the founders of her organization. They were "upset that what was in many ways an enormous advance was also dangerous." As a result of her feminist health forebears speaking up, Congress required drug labeling, and manufacturers created lower-dose pills. "It appears as clear as epidemiological evidence can make it be clear that drospirenone containing pills are taking the arc of history and progress backwards. They are more dangerous than earlier combinations of pills, and they have no well-established, unique benefit," she said.[60]

What was also becoming clear was that Yasmin's (precursor to Yaz) original manufacturer, Berlex Laboratories, had evidence of the increased risk years earlier—even during clinical trials—and failed to report it to the FDA. Former FDA commissioner David Kessler detailed all of this in a 196-page report that he generated for the ongoing litigation against Bayer, which acquired Berlex in 2006—the company would ultimately settle thousands of claims, paying out some $2 billion to women who suffered blood clots and another $80 million to others who had strokes or gall bladder injuries. Kessler accused the drugmaker of omitting data showing the increased risk from the original drug application, and quoted internal corporate documents from 2004 in which scientists reported a "several-fold increase" of blood clots for Yasmin compared to three other oral contraceptives, and a "10-fold higher" rate of total serious adverse events.[61] Bayer executive Leo Plouffe Jr. defended the company's integrity to NPR: "We've always had a very open communication with the FDA. We've responded openly to all requests for information from the FDA."[62] Kessler's report was under seal until December 6—two days before the FDA meeting. It was not given to the advisory panel members or discussed at the meeting on a technicality: because it hadn't been submitted in the requisite 30 to 60 days prior.[63]

Yaz and Yasmin were blockbuster hits in the world of contraceptives—and another bang-up marketing job. Ads promised clear skin—an adolescent dream come true—and relief for "premenstrual dysphoric disorder (PMDD)," or severe PMS. "Now there's a pill that goes beyond the rest," said a 2008 TV ad. What was true was that Yaz went beyond birth control for FDA approval: it was the first pill to request additional indications in conjunction with preventing pregnancy—treating acne and PMDD. But Adriane Fugh-Berman of PharmedOut told the FDA that while this was a "very clever" move by the manufacturer, "there are dozens of randomized, controlled trials showing that other oral contraceptives are effective for treating acne . . . Yaz has never been shown to be superior." As for PMDD, "a condition invented previously by another drug manufacturer," there was also no "reliable evidence" that Yaz alleviated period symptoms any more than any other pill.[64] Ads implied even more benefits, like weight loss, and extended the claims to Yasmin, though that formulation didn't have the additional approvals. Kessler concluded that "Bayer's economic success was achieved, in part, by marketing and promoting Yasmin and Yaz for off-label indications in violation of the law and its duty of care."

By 2008, these two products captured nearly one-third of the oral contraceptive market.[65] The acne and PMDD indications shouldn't have given doctors license to prescribe them for those symptoms exclusively—regulators calculate whether a contraceptive's benefits outweigh its risks compared to the risks of pregnancy, thus acne and PMS (and irregular periods) don't stand up. In 2009, the FDA required Bayer to run a $20 million corrective ad campaign making clear that people shouldn't take Yaz because they think it will cure pimples or PMS.[66] But the Pill in general has become standard treatment for a panoply of ailments brought to GYN appointments.

At the hearing, one woman recalled her doctor suggesting the Pill for "irregular cycles" when she was 16. The patient had seen the ads for Yaz and heard that they would help with PMS and acne, so she asked for that brand. "What teenage girl wouldn't want to take a pill that promises all that?" Another woman's doctor suggested Yaz specifically for pelvic pain, even though she was overweight, over 35, and had problems taking hormonal contraceptives previously (all known risk factors). "It's a low dose," the woman recalled her doctor saying. "The benefits will outweigh those risks." Both women developed life-threatening, permanently disabling blood clots. There were more tragic examples, like a Maryland law school grad, an athlete, who was prescribed Yaz for irregular periods. Her mother and father spoke—she had died of a heart attack. Another mother recalled giving her terrified 20-year-old daughter CPR on Christmas Eve, unable to save her from pulmonary embolisms in both lungs.

When Dr. Vanessa Cullins, then vice president for medical affairs at Planned Parenthood Federation of America, spoke, she didn't address these grief-stricken speakers. Instead, she acknowledged—several times—that drospirenone doubles the risk of such tragedies, but said this is "an acceptable risk and has been deemed an acceptable risk in the past. All of these products should remain on the market without FDA-imposed restriction because a twofold risk is still extremely rare, and it is dwarfed by the [blood clot] risk that is seen in pregnancy and during the postpartum period."

Four years later, Planned Parenthood's chief medical officer, Dr. Raegan McDonald-Mosley, spoke at another emotional FDA hearing on safety questions surrounding another Bayer product, the permanent contraceptive implant Essure, which the company has since taken off the market. "Planned Parenthood has always recognized the importance of a wide array of contraceptive options, and our role as a provider is to inform a woman about her options, with the inherent risks, benefits, and alternatives of each," said McDonald-Mosley. Yet when the FDA issued a black-box warning and ordered Bayer to create a patient booklet detailing risks (like migration of the device and perforation of other organs, pain, bleeding, and systemic allergic reactions) to be read and signed by both patient and physician, Planned Parenthood declined to use it.[67] When I asked the organization to provide the "consent" materials it was using, it declined to share them. Yet McDonald-Mosley told the FDA at the hearing that in 2014, adverse events "such as recurrent or constant pain" affected up to 7 percent of those who got the device through one of their affiliate clinics.

The committee meeting on drospirenone ultimately voted 15 to 11 that the "benefits outweighed the risks," and thus the products should remain on the market. An investigation by the *Washington Monthly* and

British Medical Journal later found that four of the panelists who voted yes had financial ties to Bayer—ties that elided the FDA's policy against conflicts of interest.[68] Meanwhile, another panel member, Dr. Sidney Wolfe, director of the consumer advocacy organization Public Citizen, which had raised concerns about drospirenone's safety, was barred from voting due to "intellectual conflicts of interest."[69]

The rationale for a yes vote was summed up by Anne Burke, a physician and committee member (one of the four who had a financial relationship with Bayer): "I acknowledge that there does seem to be a moderate increased risk, it's still lower than the risks of pregnancy."

This is the uber-rationale for all contraceptives, and one that feminist watchdogs have questioned repeatedly. "All birth control pills are approved on the basis that they are less risky than pregnancy. So no matter how many blood clots they might cause or even how many deaths they might cause, it's less than if the woman were pregnant," Diana Zuckerman explains. "But our point is that when there are 90 different pills on the market, why are you still comparing it to pregnancy? Why aren't you comparing it to other pills?" Or other methods? "No contraceptive should be compared to the risk of getting pregnant; they should be compared to the risk of the most similar other contraceptive!" says Pearson. "It's just ridiculous."

Furthermore, as Betsy Hartmann points out in her critical history of birth control *Reproductive Rights and Wrongs*, "Why should the measure of risk center solely on women?" Women can't help but bear the risks of pregnancy alone, but the risks of contraception could be shared.[70]

At both FDA hearings, Planned Parenthood's reps stated they had no conflict of interest to report, but the relationships were a little more complicated. As Planned Parenthood disclosed, Essure was the only female sterilization method that its clinics could offer. The other dynamic at work was more ideological than financial. As Cindy Pearson explains, "We know from past research that the more options that are available for women, the higher the percent of women who want to be contracepting will. So any new method is an advance."

The "more options, the better" philosophy permeates the world of family planning, which tends to remain agnostic on risky products, from Essure to Yaz to Depo-Provera. But at what point is an option so risky that it is not worthy of being one? Historically, the bar has been pretty low. A product like the Dalkon Shield, or Norplant, or Essure is made available to the masses and only deemed unacceptable (almost always by the court or by public opinion—hardly ever by the FDA) once tens or hundreds of thousands are exposed. In countries where the United States provides aid, the threat of maternal mortality is used to justify free and low-cost distribution of a product like Depo-Provera, now in a self-injectable form called Sayana Press, which studies suggest makes women more susceptible to HIV.[71]

The emphasis is on effectiveness. And uptake. More options means more uptake, and funders of service providers may even expect certain deliverables—a target number of IUD insertions or prescriptions written, for example—to justify their continued support. One funder in particular was behind a strategic campaign that began more than a decade ago to remake the IUD's image and get more women on what are now called long-acting reversible contraceptives, or LARCs. "In December 2006, I got a call from an anonymous foundation, and they said they would like to help women use the most effective methods of contraception," Jeffrey Peipert, an OB/GYN at Washington University in St. Louis, told Bloomberg News. "They said, 'You come up with a program to promote and encourage the use of the most effective methods.'"[72]

Peipert suggested piloting a program where everything from condoms to IUDs would be free, removing cost barriers. The anonymous foundation put up $20 million for the program, called the Contraceptive CHOICE Project, which recruited nearly ten thousand local women and teens, and generated a widely cited 2010 study finding that when given the choice, three-quarters of patients will choose the "most effective" method: an IUD or implant like Nexplanon, in which hormone-releasing capsules are inserted under the skin of one's arm (a descendant of Norplant that is supposed to be easier to remove).

But advocates quickly raised questions about what the program itself called the "LARC First" model of care, in which clinicians present the contraceptive options in the order of most effective to least effective. So no matter the patient or their situation, the provider's preference for them is a LARC, and that goal is embedded into the encounter. Or as Cindy Pearson put it, "You walk in, you have two kids, you want to wait a couple years before your third, LARC first. You're 16, you haven't had sex yet, just feeling kind of happy, like you might want to—LARC first. You've been on oral contraceptives for years, life is happy, LARC first!" Under that model, it's not surprising that the study would find women overwhelmingly "chose" LARCs—patients tend to go where doctors steer them. In the years following the St. Louis study, both the American College of Obstetricians and Gynecologists and the American Academy of Pediatrics cited it in new guidelines recommending that LARCs be the "first-line recommendation," even to adolescents.[73] The program was replicated in places like Iowa and Colorado, the latter in particular generating headlines proclaiming it a "startling success," attributing it to halving the teen pregnancy rate as well as slashing the number of abortions, while saving the state $65 million over eight years.[74]

In the tradition of John D. Rockefeller III, the anonymous donor behind this project turned out to be Warren Buffett. He also gave seed money to the nonprofit Medicines360 to develop the lower-cost IUD Liletta. "For Warren, it's economic. He thinks that unless women can control their fertility—and that it's basically their right to control their fertility—that you are sort of wasting more than half of the brainpower in the United States," said Judith DeSarno, the longtime family planning advocate Buffett hired to lead the CHOICE initiative. But, as advocates soon pointed out, if women's rights were the primary concern, why the agenda to push one method over another? In particular, a method over which the user has little control once it's initiated? "While we strongly believe . . . LARC methods are an integral part of a comprehensive method mix, we also are concerned that unchecked enthusiasm for them can lead to the adoption of programs that, paradoxically, undermine women's reproductive autonomy," wrote Anu Manchikanti Gomez, Liza Fuentes, and Amy Allina in a 2014 commentary titled "Women or LARC First?"[75]

It did not escape these and other advocates that programs targeting "high-risk" populations were "especially worrisome given the long-standing devaluation of the fertility and childbearing of young women, low-income women and women of color in the United States, and the perception that these women have too many children." Meanwhile, advocates began hearing complaints that clinicians weren't being trained to remove the devices; that no thought had been given to how a woman who got an implant for free would be able to get it removed years later when it expired (or when they were ready to get pregnant); and worse, that some LARC First–trained clinicians were refusing to remove devices from unsatisfied customers.

Ashleigh Oxford in Atascadero, California, "went from a happy, go lucky 31-year-old to a depressed walking zombie in just 3 weeks" after getting a Kyleena IUD. At that point she went back to the clinic in nearby Paso Robles to have it removed. The clinician put her in stirrups, inserted a speculum, removed the speculum, and then told her it looked fine. Oxford was confused—"It's still in? You didn't take it out?" she said. Then began the argument. Oxford asked her again to remove it, the clinician said she didn't think that was a good idea, give it six months and then come back. Oxford insisted. "But what will you do for contraception?" the clinician asked. "What happens when you have an abortion?" This went on for several minutes until Oxford, shaking with anger, demanded she "get the fucking thing out now." Finally, the clinician obliged. Oxford wrote this up in a public post on Facebook that garnered more than 600 comments and was shared 8,200 times.[76]

"I felt like as a woman she would have been more understanding. I'm on Medi-Cal [Medicaid] . . . maybe she thought I was irresponsible because I'm a single mom," Oxford told me. "It was like my power as a woman and as an individual went out the door."

Such anecdotal reports have since been borne out by research, and in some states, Medicaid will cover removal only if it is deemed "medically necessary." South Dakota Medicaid's 2016 billing manual stated it "will not reimburse for the removal of the implant if the intent is for the recipient to become pregnant."[77] (This does not appear in the 2018 manual.)[78]

In 2017, SisterSong Women of Color Reproductive Justice Collective and the National Women's Health Network published a white paper outlining a "LARC Statement of Principles," which was signed by dozens of organization, including, to its credit, Planned Parenthood. Jessica Gonzalez-Rojas of the National Latina Institute for Reproductive Health, another cosigner, emphasized that her group is not "anti-LARC." "What's problematic is when there are programs that solely look at

LARCs as a panacea," she told me, for teen pregnancy in particular. "A lot of these programs do this because they see young women giving birth as a problem, because they see black women giving birth as a problem, because they see immigrant women giving birth as a problem. A lot of this is really fueled by eugenic principles that still exist."

The media narrative has for the most part ignored the reproductive justice critique. The week the AAP announced its policy change, Slate's headline was "Parents, Get Your Teenage Daughters the IUD." "While a lot of parents might be nervous about their teen daughters getting IUDs, it's actually a really great idea. Even if your daughter isn't having sex yet, odds are that she will be soon enough," wrote Amanda Marcotte. In Jezebel, Adele Oliveira began her piece in the same vein: "It's hard to think of a segment of the American population that could benefit more from long-acting contraceptives than the teenager." Oliveira quotes a Santa Fe public school nurse who works with a group of teen moms: "I pushed IUDs quite a bit . . . My students weren't very good at taking their birth control pills or getting their Depo-Provera shots on time."[79] A 2018 headline on the site Rewire (which also receives funding from Buffett) exclaimed: "DIY Birth Control Shot Can Help Advance Reproductive Justice."[80]

This is not to say that individual clinicians have conscious biases. In the world of public health, unplanned pregnancy is a diagnosis. In the clinical setting, it's seen as a failure of care. In some places, a woman who walks out the door without a LARC or a shot of Depo is seen as that failure personified. A recent paper in the *Journal of the American Medical Association* concludes that LARCs are "underutilized," representing 14 percent of contraceptive use.[81] "Each year, 43 million women, nearly 70 percent of all reproductive-aged females in the United States, are *at risk* for unplanned pregnancy," wrote the authors (emphasis mine). They conclude that the "majority of patients are medically eligible" for IUDs and implants, and point to barriers of "expense, misunderstanding about safety, and inadequate counseling." Nowhere in the paper do the authors mention side effects. "We've really pushed IUDs to the point where there are underserved women who can't get them out," says North Carolina OB/GYN and researcher Rachel Peragallo Urrutia. "I think sometimes we're blinded by the desire to prevent unplanned pregnancies."

The problem with a laser focus on effectiveness is that it ignores a person's values and desires, not to mention the complexity of the human condition. As Loretta Ross likes to point out, "Not every unplanned pregnancy is unwanted, and not every planned pregnancy is kept . . . You just can't make those kinds of generalizations and speak to the reality of how women make decisions," she says. Maybe for a mother wanting to space her children, an unplanned pregnancy isn't going to be the end of the world. Maybe a single 20-something would rather protect herself against STIs and deal with the occasional mishap. Maybe a teen exploring her sexuality would rather not risk altering mood or libido. It's not like a woman wanting to manage her fertility is the same as a person with a bad toe infection, says Pearson. For that, hell yes, you want the most effective treatment. "But when you come in for contraception, it's about sexuality, it's about your period, it's about are you in school, are you spacing kids," she says. "Contraception is life. It's not a medical problem."

And yet, contraception has fallen under medical purview thanks to history. The U.S. birth control movement's first hurdle was getting out from under obscenity laws. Margaret Sanger led that charge by courting professionals—researchers and physicians. And she helped win physicians the sole legal right to distribute contraceptives, even though she herself—a nurse—had fit diaphragms in the Netherlands, where midwives were the main providers. "So completely has birth control become identified with the medical profession that it is sometimes difficult for us today to imagine how it could have been otherwise," wrote historian Linda Gordon.[82]

While the birth control movement had roots in the radical leftist and feminist movements of the late nineteenth and early twentieth centuries, it soon came into alliance with environmental conservationists (who blamed overpopulation—that is, women—for world conflict) and eugenicists (who blamed the "unfit" for social ills). The founding of Planned Parenthood in particular was the product of this evolution. Sanger herself said "more children from the fit and less from the unfit—that is the chief issue of birth control."[83] Planned Parenthood's original name was the American Birth Control League, which advocated "racial progress." These forces found synergy in the well-endowed "population control" movement, which for a time had its own office in the executive branch and flooded universities with funding.[84]

From the beginning, population control had a close relationship with the medical industry. John D. Rockefeller's Population Council would go on to develop Norplant and had a hand in promoting many "easily abuseable contraceptive technologies into already abusive population control programs," wrote Hartmann. The feminist movement pushed back against this reproductive imperialism in the 1970s, arguing that women would be better served by aid money spent on clean water and food security, and by securing their basic rights. "Development is the best contraceptive" became the new slogan, and Rockefeller himself announced at a conference that "women increasingly must have greater choice in determining their roles in society."[85]

Then came the '80s. By the time Depo-Provera was approved by the FDA for contraception in 1992, the drug had been given to tens of millions of women worldwide. (The National Women's Health Network tried and failed to block the approval; a 1982 FDA public board of inquiry had warned, "Never has a drug whose target population is entirely healthy people been shown to be so pervasively carcinogenic in animals as Depo-Provera." Upjohn, the manufacturer at the time, responded that the adverse effects observed in animal studies were not directly relevant to potential side effects in humans.[86]) In 2012, the Gates Foundation contributed to a $4.3 billion campaign to bring contraceptives to millions of the world's poorest women, many in Africa. The Family Planning 2020 initiative, a consortium of NGOs and governments, pledged to expand access to multiple forms of contraceptives. In 2014, Gates negotiated with Pfizer to make the self-injectible form of Depo. An article in the *Lancet* called all this activity "the rebirth of family planning."[87]

This commitment to long-acting methods is succeeding in bringing women more long-acting methods. But as Hartmann wrote, "technological innovations are not 'neutral'; instead, they embody the values of their creators." She questioned why less risky barrier methods haven't been valued by the powers that be. "The contraceptive revolution of the second half of [the last] century has been influenced more by the pursuit of population control, prestige, and profit than by people's need for safe birth control. Millions of dollars have flowed into the development, production, and promotion of technically sophisticated contraceptives such as the pill, injectables, and implants, despite their health risks, while the improvement of safer and simpler barrier methods has been virtually neglected."[88]

While forces greater than women's needs and desires have shaped the birth control landscape, and coercive population control practices and ideologies persist, many women have also welcomed even the riskier products with open arms. In the early 1980s, Ross wrote several articles critical of Depo-Provera, which in addition to being distributed internationally was being used off-label in the United States, primarily on poor young women of color.[89] She realized that many of the young women around her were taking it by choice. "Hell, half my staff was on Depo-Provera," she told me.

Once a product is on the market, it has achieved the status of a "choice." If it isn't yet on the market, it can be presented as a "choice" women should have. Within a skewed framework of "risks versus benefits," it's a tough road for reproductive justice activists, especially when the most vocal critics of the more harmful products often have an anti-abortion, anti-contraception agenda. This is the case for Depo: in a 2011 report, the Rebecca Project raised flags about DMPA's potential connection to HIV infection and the ethics of international distribution, and called for congressional hearings into the matter. But the small, respected organization was experiencing a coup—the report's author, it turned out, was tight with right-wing extremist groups, and he effectively shut out the organization's feminist founders.[90] "That's part of the tragedy of the problem," says Ross. "Because how do you offer a legitimate and sustained critique of Depo without getting in bed with the dog that has the most fleas?

"That's what complicates our work."

7: THE CASE FOR HOME ABORTION

THE SOLA VARIETY of papaya resembles a pregnant uterus, so much so that humans use the fruit to learn one method of modern reproductive health care: manual vacuum aspiration, or MVA, a low-risk, low-tech method of first-trimester abortion that requires little or no anesthesia.[1] As one doctor remarked at a conference in 1973, where the technology was introduced to physicians from around the world, "it's something we will be able to bring practically into the rice paddy."[2]

This, too, is the fruit I have been given to practice on. I've placed it on a table across from me, and I'm focused on the neck, where its stem grew, which evokes the cervical os. The tool I'm using is a large plastic syringe with a bendable plastic straw-like thing, called a cannula, where the needle would be. At the top of the syringe is a bivalve, to create one-way suction.

I carefully peel the remnant of the papaya's stem, then set the bivalve by pressing two plastic tabs, then pull the plunger on the syringe. For learning purposes, my cannula is 8 millimeters wide—larger than necessary for a very early procedure—roughly the size of a drinking straw. I press it gently into the brown dot on the fruit. The skin gives, and the instrument slides in.

I'm with a small group of learners in a living room—I have agreed not to say where or with whom—cannulas and vinyl gloves scattered about the coffee table, the smell of tropical fruit in the air. That morning, we had been guided through gentle speculum insertion by willing volunteers—a quasi-GTA model. Now with our papaya wombs, our teacher explains that on a real cervix, a provider might need to start with smaller-diameter cannulas to gradually open the sphincter. Gentle pressure and patience can achieve this, she says, without the anesthetic or sedation typical in modern clinics.

Very slowly, I push further into the round fruit until I feel resistance—what would be the uterine fundus, then I retract a bit. By flipping the bivalve, the suction I created in the syringe pulls from the cannula, and some bright orange pulp and gray seeds travel through the straw, which prompts me to shout out, "It's working!"

The MVA with a handheld syringe and plastic cannula is now the standard of care around the world for any "pregnancy loss," including miscarriage, which allows it to exist in countries where abortion is outlawed. Originally distributed by USAID, in 1973 the government handed the job to the North Carolina–based group Ipas, which has introduced it to more than 100 countries.[3] A 2015 Ipas publication cites several studies that found no significant difference in outcomes of women who were treated by physicians and those treated by "mid-level providers," and notes how that term wrongly implies a lower level of care. "Multiple studies have shown that the safety and effectiveness of care provided by these cadres is equivalent and sometimes better than that provided by their professional counterparts."[4] A 2012 World Health Organization report concludes, "Abortion care can be safely provided by any properly trained healthcare provider, . . . e.g. midwives, nurse practitioners, clinical officers, physician assistants, family welfare visitors, and others."[5]

"I would feel comfortable with you doing an MVA on me," says my teacher later that day, while just she and I are debriefing over tea. I am flattered, but stunned by the fact that I could theoretically do this for someone, were it to come to that.

Maybe it has already? Ninety percent of counties in the United States have zero abortion clinics. Mississippi and six other states have just one for the whole state. Several more have fewer than five. As I write there is a bill in the Iowa state legislature to ban abortions at six weeks; another in Ohio to ban them altogether; another signed into law in Idaho that mandates that clinics offer abortion "reversals." According to the Guttmacher Institute, just 1 percent of procedures happen in physicians' offices. "Keep Abortion Legal" is an iconic NOW protest sign. It was the bare minimum ask, and the Supreme Court is poised to shut it down.

Underground abortion is a thing again.[6] I found my instructor—who is equally fearful of law enforcement and anti-abortion vigilantes and thus doesn't want to be identified—because others have found her. Over the past five years, a decentralized group of providers has multiplied to a few hundred. They are trading in herbs and pills, reviving the practice of menstrual extraction, and even learning to do clandestine MVAs. They're offering this mostly at low cost or no cost, completely outside the medical system.

Many of these providers are already familiar with vaginal exams and accessing the cervix: they are midwives, though no matter their license, abortion at home is outside their scope of practice. Others have no license to lose: they are students or doulas, or they are just fed up with the waiting periods, enforced ultrasounds, and fictitious scripts clinic patients must hear; or perhaps they've had enough of the overpriced, gruff clinic that has a monopoly on access in their community; or they feel compelled by the absence of any clinic at all. Still, it's all happening on a spectrum of illegal to probably illegal. Thirteen states have criminal abortion laws on the books that could be used against such providers. And abortion seekers themselves could be charged—six states have laws specifically making self-abortion a crime. In any state, a person could be charged with practicing medicine without a license or unlawful dispensation of a drug. "I would say they face substantial risks in providing care to people if they're not an abortion provider under the imprimatur of the law," says Farah Diaz-Tello, senior counsel for the SIA Legal Team, which is working to decriminalize abortion wherever it happens.

Even as access is spotty and legality hangs in peril, the people seeking out these providers "are not desperate in the way we think," one provider tells me. "They're desperate for someone to provide them with care that's compassionate, for someone who cares about their story, for someone who wants to know how they're feeling months after. They want someone who gives a shit about them. And they want to do it on their own terms, in a place that's comfortable, with people around them who care about them."

Typically, these providers start by helping their friends or family, often because they are asked to. Most are dispensing misoprostol, one of the drugs in the two-drug RU-486 "medical abortion" regimen, aka the abortion pill. "Miso," as it is known colloquially, causes the uterus to contract. Because it has several other uses, it is cheap and easily accessible throughout the world. Midwives carry it legally to treat postpartum hemorrhage. Even your local vet has it to control canine stomach acid. Miso is very effective in causing an abortion on its own, 75 to 85 percent effective up until 12 weeks. If the abortion is incomplete, a person could present to a clinic or emergency room as if they were simply having a miscarriage. No blood test will detect the drug, and there is no clinical benefit to disclosing that one took it. Advocates have called it a "game changer."[7]

But this American-grown grassroots provider community is offering more than miso. They know the herbs that disrupt progesterone (the hormone that sustains the pregnancy), others that contract the uterus, and others that soften the cervix. They're recommending herbs on their own or in the place of mifepristone, the first drug in RU-486, which is expensive and harder to get. Some providers have sterile cannulas of increasing diameter and boxes of vinyl exam gloves and three sizes of plastic specula on hand. And they have security protocols: encrypted emails and apps, pseudonyms, and a healthy mistrust of reporters.

Yet they also want to be known. They want women to know to look for them. They want genderqueer and trans folks to know they're a nonjudgmental resource. They want women of color, young women, indigenous women, poor women, undocumented women—anyone who for whatever reason can't or would rather not walk into a clinic—to know they're there. They have a vision for a different paradigm of care, one that harkens back to an era before abortion was "between a woman and her doctor," when pregnancy, childbirth, and pregnancy *loss* were managed by women in the community—midwives. They want more providers to start offering this to their communities.

"You could totally do this," my teacher tells me.

I just look at her. That's crazy, I say. I admit my greatest fear would be causing someone an infection. What was that movie? The one where the old lady sweetly administers to several London women with the same rubber catheter? (*Vera Drake.*) I admit to other worries: hemorrhage, puncturing the uterus, or worse, other organs. We run through the scenarios: the cannulas are sterile in their paper and plastic packaging, and so long as they touch nothing else, the risk of an infection developing is extremely low. Plus, we have antibiotics now.

In terms of perforation, the cannula is rounded and closed at the top (there are two openings on either side). It's soft and flexible, not sharp. If one goes slowly and gently, it would be extremely difficult to injure the uterus. The illegal-era tragedies happened with razor-sharp curettes, which are looped, spoon-like metal instruments, or knitting needles, hairpins, the infamous coat hanger—whatever women could get their hands on, if their own hands were all that they had.

Think about the "Janes," she tells me. Between 1969 and 1973, this underground network of housewives and college students in Chicago learned how to do D&Cs—that is, they dilated cervices and scraped out uteruses with those sharp curettes, which they were responsible for sterilizing. And they did this with just local anesthetic (for safety reasons, in case everyone needed to leave a location quickly), at a time when physicians would put women under general anesthesia in the operating room for the same procedure. The Janes performed some 11,000 D&C abortions without a single death. "What we're doing is way less risky than what the Janes were doing," she says.

Hemorrhage is very rare. It has happened twice in the 2,000 or so abortions recorded by the current underground network, and both were managed in the emergency room.[8] It's also a risk of medical abortion the way it is administered by clinics: women swallow the mifepristone in the clinic and take the miso with them to bleed at home. The instruction given to women in case of severe bleeding is to go to the ER. But it can be hard to know what's OK and what's not—miso cramps can be intensely painful—and the whole thing is scarier if you're alone. Part of the home-provision philosophy is that the provider stays with the woman during the loss, just as a midwife would be present for a labor.

Alison Ojanen-Goldsmith is a researcher at the University of Minnesota who has taken on the task of quantifying this off-the-grid provider network and their outcomes. There are of course limitations to this kind of study, but "we hypothesize that the majority of care is incredibly safe," she told me. Several studies in countries with less reliable emergency services have shown that MVA is safe in the hands of non-physicians. One study out of Nepal showed that women were about as accurate in dating their pregnancies as technicians with ultrasounds. And Ojanen-Goldsmith points out that those who seek out community care often have a more expansive notion of "safety." "For marginalized populations who've experienced medical trauma, maybe the clinic isn't the safest."

When I tell the New York physician assistant Virginia Reath about this new underground, part of her is clearly proud—she was part of the '70s movement to spread speculum epiphanies and remembers seeing the plastic cannula and handheld syringe for the first time at a conference and being awestruck by its simplicity. As a physician assistant, she started a program to train doctors how to do MVAs, even though legally she couldn't provide them. In 1995, she worked with the ACLU to successfully challenge New York's law, which defined physicians as abortion providers but did not explicitly prohibit other licensed professionals, such as physician assistants and licensed midwives.

"Ultimately I support people doing them," she says. "The only thing I would say is you have to make sure the patient recognizes what the risks are"—and that they take responsibility for it. "Because if you don't know how to control a hemorrhage—I've had patients start bleeding out on the table. Even with a simple MVA," she says. The patient could have an undiagnosed clotting disorder or an oddly shaped uterus. "If that happens to an inexperienced person, that's a scary thing," she says. There will be a sea of blood, and you have to use brute strength to massage and "wake the uterus up." Any "serious" training should include basic protocol for managing a hemorrhage, she says, and anyone doing an MVA should be prepared.

When I was around 12, my friends and I watched *Dirty Dancing* on VHS at every sleepover. The image of Penny sweating and shaking on a bed after her back-alley abortion became for me the nightmare scenario of what a reversal of *Roe* might create. It's no coincidence that Penny is saved by a legit doctor with clean instruments and an IV bolus.

It turns out the screenwriter was very intentional about this plotline. "When it came time to shoot it, I made it very clear that we would leave in what is, for me, very purple language: references to dirty knives, a folding table, hearing Penny screaming in the hallway," screenwriter Eleanor Bergstein told Broadly on the film's thirtieth anniversary. "The reason I put that language in there was because I felt that—even with it being a coat hanger abortion—a whole generation of young people, and women especially . . . wouldn't understand what [the illegal abortion] was."[9]

In her definitive history *When Abortion Was a Crime*, published in 1997, Leslie Reagan wrote in the epilogue: "If *Roe v. Wade* were to be overturned and abortion made illegal again, the history of when abortion was a crime suggests that the results would be dire indeed . . . some women will die; many more will be injured. The old abortion wards will have to be reopened, a public health disaster recreated."[10] This has been the pro-choice narrative for two generations.

Illegal abortion looks very different now. "Handmaid's Tale IRL: What if *Roe* were to go?" asked a 2018 panel at South by Southwest. The three panelists all spoke of how women are getting their hands on misoprostol and calling on friends or doulas (or friends who are doulas) to hold their hand. Groups are forming to support the self-inducers, they said, collecting and dispensing pills. One of the panelists, Judith Arcana, was an original Chicago Jane. "What's going to happen when *Roe* is overturned is that a lot of people are going to use a variety of methods, and it's going to be the task of people who mean to do good and right and be righteous folks in the world to learn about all the kinds of things in addition to pills," she said. "There will be such people. There are such people now."

My instructor is confident (or cocky, some would say) that most people, with minimal training, could offer various methods safely. "Pills?" she laughs. "Anybody can do pills." A quick Google search will turn up the proper dosage of misoprostol depending on the week of gestation. The World Health Organization spells it out. The European NGO Women on Web, led by Dutch gynecologist Rebecca Gomperts, has been sending pills to women all over the world, though not to the United States, for a dozen years. (In 2018, Gomperts changed her mind about the United States and began prescribing the pills remotely, which are fulfilled by a pharmacy in India and sent by mail. The reason, she told CNN, was that the organization was being flooded with thousands of emails from U.S. women desperate for help. "I realized it was time," she said.[11]) But even MVA with a sterile cannula is low risk—minimally trained providers around the world have proved it so.

"This is not your grandmother's illegal abortion," she says.

THE CLINIC COMPROMISE

On April 10, 1970, the New York state legislature passed what was called the Cook-Leichter bill, which effectively legalized abortion throughout the state. This influenced the *Roe v. Wade* decision three years later and turned New York into a destination for thousands of desperate women who had the means to get there. It was the beginning of the end of the dark days of back-alley butchers. Yet in the realm of forgotten history is the fact that this was not cause for celebration among New York's radical feminists. In fact, the movement's most ardent leaders were devastated.

When the bill was originally introduced, it called for the wholesale deletion of the laws on abortion from the New York criminal code, or "repeal." This would have meant that abortion reverted to the same status as any other medical procedure: broadly governed by the Department of Health, but not specifically regulated. To communicate this concept clearly, New York feminists had distributed copies of a "model abortion law": a blank piece of paper.[12]

Up until it passed the state Senate, Cook-Leichter was effectively a blank piece of paper. But anticipating challenge in the assembly, its authors added restrictions, including that the procedure could only be performed by a physician and prior to 24 weeks gestation.[13] Confusingly, the media called the rewritten bill a "repeal bill," and it is still referred to as such.[14]

As author Ninia Baehr later put it, "Because our radical history has been hidden from us, most of us . . . do not realize that the legality we seek to defend was in fact a compromise of the original demand for repeal. If you repeal something from the law, you take it out of the law entirely. If you legalize something, you grant control to the state."[15] The radical feminists did not want to grant control of abortion to the state. They wanted women to control it themselves.

Lucinda Cisler was a 32-year-old architect and city planner turned radical feminist when the bill was wending its way to the governor's desk. She and her partner, James Clapp, a math teacher, had quit their jobs the previous year and founded the local NOW chapter's offshoot New

Yorkers for Abortion Law Repeal, "because it was in the air that things were about to change," she told a historian.[16]

If Cisler was able to envision cityscapes decades into the future, she also had a knack for predicting the failing infrastructure of our twenty-first-century reproductive justice edifice. In early spring 1970, Cisler penned what is now considered a classic missive to her sister activists, titled "Abortion Law Repeal (Sort of): A Warning to Women." In it, she advocates with crystal clarity (and prescience) why feminists needed to dig deep and find their grounding on abortion distinct from the broader abortion rights movement. That broad movement included physicians and public health advocates, whose main goal was to deal with the crisis of botched procedures.

Feminists, Cisler argued, had to be vigilant about their reasons: not to liberate doctors, whose hands were tied by the criminal code; or hospitals, whose septic abortion wards were overflowing; and not even to protect women from unscrupulous providers. "Such reasons are peripheral to the central rationale for making abortion available: justice for women."[17] At the core of why women needed abortion law *repeal* was their right to self-determination and bodily integrity. "Without the full capacity to limit her own reproduction, a woman's other 'freedoms' are tantalizing mockeries that cannot be exercised," she said.[18]

Cisler saw what would happen if the movement settled for less. "In our disgust with the extreme oppression women experience under the present abortion laws, many of us are understandably tempted to accept insulting token changes" and other "seductive fake-repeal bills and court decisions" cropping up around the country. These laws would not "legalize" abortion in the way many people believed they would, she warned. Women would not suddenly have the "right" to an abortion. The state would retain control, deciding which abortions were OK and who could perform them, and that would likely be just physicians, which would keep the price artificially high. Women would still be in the position of appealing to the patriarchal medical system for their freedom.

Cisler predicted that poor women would lose out, which they did in a big way when the Hyde amendment prohibited federal funds from paying for abortions in 1977. She also predicted gestational limits, parental consent laws (because at the time, some states required a husband's consent), and even criminalization of women themselves should new technologies allow them to take matters into their own hands: "In looking not so far into the future, this restriction would also deny women themselves the right to use self-abortifacients when they are developed—and who is to say they will not be developed soon?"

She also predicted how activism would founder. "The possibility of fake repeal—if it becomes reality—is the most dangerous: it will divide women from each other. It can buy off most middle class women and make them believe things have really changed, while it leaves poor women to suffer and keeps us all saddled with abortion laws for many more years to come."

Cisler's warning notwithstanding, NOW and NARAL (originally the National Association for the Repeal of Abortion Laws) maintained support for the New York bill in spite of its new substance. New Yorkers for Repeal made the difficult decision to actively oppose it. "We were considered horrible people who just wanted women to die," Cisler later told a historian.[19] In 2018 I reached her by phone at a rehab facility in Manhattan, where she was reluctantly living. "All we were saying was leave the door open for what developed, not to monopolize it with doctors. The doctors didn't want to do it much anyway," she said.

In protest pictures Cisler stands out in gingham dresses with her hair tied neatly back or under a handkerchief. A California native who goes by Cindy, she had won the 1955 Betty Crocker Homemaker of Tomorrow Award for her high school, then graduated from Vassar College and the Yale Architecture School. For her thesis she designed a new dorm building. "Built-in closets frequently occur just where we want to put something else," she wrote in an alumni magazine article coincidentally titled "A Room of One's Own: The Architecture of Choice." "I have revived the old idea of a wardrobe, moving on hidden casters to become a maker of spaces rather than a large immobile obstacle to one's ideas."[20] If the feminist idea—and ideal—was the total repeal of abortion laws, the built-in closet of the collective imagination was internalized paternalism and what we'd now call a lack of intersectionality. "Most middle-class women have indeed been bought off by New York's law," Cisler wrote in a postscript:

> Compromises once enacted are almost impossible to budge. Why then have we behaved so differently when it comes to so basic and personal a right as the legal capacity to decide what is to happen inside our very bodies? Why do we refuse to see that "justifiable" abortion granted to some is not a right but a most tenuous privilege, and that as long as any woman belongs to the state every woman is a chattel? Can it be that we really like being property after all?[21]

Part of what made Cisler so confident was that she knew abortion technology was changing—even in 1969. That year, she and Clapp hosted a five-part series on New York City's community radio station WBAI. In the second part, titled "Abortion Inside and Outside the Hospital," they interviewed Dr. Bernard Nathanson, a Cornell-affiliated OB/GYN. After he described the D&C in graphic detail, Cisler asked about vacuum aspiration, which she said was being used to treat some botched procedures. He only knew it was being used in Europe, and reported that it required less skill, and no anesthesia. "Some of these techniques are suitable for outpatient use, I understand, particularly the vacuum aspirator method," she said. The doctor wasn't sure. Clapp pressed on, "How about a sort of compromise—not on your kitchen table, not in a hospital, but in a nice sterile clinic."[22] The law was being written for physicians, but Cisler saw that innovation would enable those with less training to provide the service. And she knew of the women doing so already in Chicago.

In 1971, Cisler met some of the radical "self-helpers" from the Los Angeles Feminist Health Center but had mixed feelings about them. "I don't care how many abortions you did yourself with your own hands, that's not to me ultimately as good a use of your time as changing the damn law," she told me. But those women had commandeered the speculum, which led to the development of menstrual extraction. This was the truly radical centerpiece of the self-help health movement. Once women could insert a speculum, they had uncovered the entrance to the womb, into which they learned how to thread the newly invented sterile plastic cannula and use suction to extract its contents. They also contributed to the innovation of the manual vacuum aspiration technique, which would make it more available to non-physician providers.

When Carol Downer, a newly radicalized mother of six, saw a cervix for the first time, "It just clicked!" she said. For decades this anatomy had been shrouded in white-coat mystery; physicians were the gatekeepers. "I was like, 'Well, of course!' The only way they can keep abortion illegal is to keep us in total ignorance of our bodies. Because once you see it you realize that abortion is so simple . . . We realized we could do this," she told an interviewer in the 1980s.[23] The story of how this group developed menstrual extraction is also the story of how the modern clinical abortion procedure evolved to be less invasive, less risky, and more accessible throughout the world. For a century, the medical approach to removing tissue from the uterus had been dilation and curettage (D&C), which required anesthesia in the operating theater. After dilating the cervix, the physician would insert a sharp curette into the uterus and scrape its contents out. There was a real risk of perforating the uterus and introducing infection.

Soon after her cervical epiphany, Downer and fellow activist Lorraine Rothman visited a local illegal abortion clinic run by a man named Harvey Karman (who went by "Dr.," though his credential was a dubious PhD) to follow their hunch that it wasn't rocket science. Karman had begun his involvement in abortion as a kind of underground travel agent, arranging trips for women to doctors in Tijuana. But when some came back having been harassed or worse, he began performing D&Cs on his own. He recalled in 1973 that these "convinced me that it didn't have to be emotionally or physically traumatic."[24]

One of Karman's early patients contracted an infection and died, for which he served two years in prison. After this, according to some sources, he began reading the medical literature out of Eastern Europe, where abortion was legal and physicians were using electric suction in lieu of surgical instruments. At first, physicians were using suction curettes, metal cannulas, and later hard plastic cannulas. Inspired by this, he cut the end off a plastic syringe and attached some plastic tubing to it, thereby creating manual vacuum suction.[25] This tubing would later evolve into what would be known throughout the world as the Karman cannula (though he never patented it), which would become one of the most revolutionary innovations in reproductive history.

The feminists were divided on Karman. He had swagger, openly defying the law and even training women, whom he called "paramedics," to perform the procedure. He also had James Bond looks and drove a Jaguar, yet charged just $25 for a less-than-9-weeks procedure and $40 between 9 and 12 weeks. "We didn't like him, but we did take advantage," says Downer. "We were just the 'dumb' local women, Harvey's fan club. We were just hanging around. We wouldn't have an appointment, we'd just go in. Nobody said anything to anybody."

Rothman observed Karman's cannula method and envisioned even more improvements: his device had no safeguard against pumping air back into the uterus, which could cause an embolism. Also, what if the contents being extracted were greater than the syringe's volume? That would require a clumsy transfer. She "took the apparatus home and spent the next week haunting hardware stores, grocery stores, chemistry labs and aquarium shops," Downer and Rebecca Chalker wrote in their *Book of Women's Choices*, and she fashioned a homespun version with a mason jar, rubber stopper, and two sections of plastic tubing, one that attached to Karman's cannula, another that attached to the syringe. She called it the "Del-Em," which Downer shied from explaining when I met her. "It's just a nonsense thing that we dreamed up," she told me. "It's not to be shared."

The Del-Em did two important things: it created a bypass so that air could go only one way, and it allowed the woman desiring the extraction to pull the syringe herself, which theoretically would protect anyone else in the room from culpability. Karman's original device was a standard syringe modified with "side-arm catchers . . . which need to be made specifically." These popped out once the plunger was fully retracted, locking it in place—"vitally important because of the danger of air embolism," Karman and Berkeley physician Malcom Potts wrote in a 1972 *Lancet* article describing the device.[26] The modern manual vacuum aspirator used today, patented by Ipas, features a bivalve, which not only creates a stronger suction than the original concept, but prevents the user from accidentally pushing air into the uterus during retraction. Based on Downer and Chalker's account, this innovation was Rothman's idea. If the modern MVA features a "Karman cannula," perhaps it should also acknowledge the "Rothman bivalve."

Rothman and Downer went on a 23-city tour, boxes of plastic specula and Del-Ems labeled "TOYS" in case they got pulled over. The workshop began with a slideshow: "Happiness is knowing your own cervix," stated one slide. But maybe happiness was really *accessing* your own cervix. One activist told reporter Elizabeth Fishel coyly that "interest in menstrual extraction often develops naturally out of the" self-help clinic. That was the women's goal all along, to "get as many women as we could interested in the self exam, learning ME, and taking over women's health," Downer told me.

Interest developed at the movement level as well. There were underground periodicals like *The Monthly Extract* and *The Witch's Os*. "Friendship circles" formed—groups of women who would regularly do menstrual extraction on each other, using the Del-Em, perhaps as a way to skip periods, perhaps also as a way to keep up skills, in case a friend (or friend of a friend) needed to extract more than a period. "It was wink-wink," says Virginia Reath. "Because once you knew how to use a speculum, once you saw what a cervix was, once you started getting familiar with that part of the body, you knew you could help somebody."

Word got around, and as Fishel reported in 1973, 100 self-help "clinics" were functioning around the country, offering what is essentially a very early abortion for less than $50. Looking at this history, one can see the faint outlines of an alternative reality, had abortion been decriminalized on terms different than *Roe v. Wade,* had Cisler's dream of repeal been realized. But history went on its path, and self-help effectively ended with the *Roe* decision.

In the early 1970s, some American hospitals were experimenting with electric suction with a sharp metal cannula, under the guise of treating incomplete miscarriages.[27] This still required a fair amount of dilation and ran the risk of perforation (and the suction was difficult to control—it could be too strong). Manual vacuum aspiration with a plastic cannula allowed for a more controlled, more discreet, "non-traumatic" extraction. When Karman wrote up his innovation with Potts, who was head of the International Planned Parenthood Federation at the time, it drew the interest of USAID, and the agency negotiated a contract with the Battelle Corporation to manufacture thousands of "menstrual regulation" kits, which were sent around the world.[28] So manual vacuum aspiration—the kinder, gentler abortion—became a major export, while it remained largely unused in the United States. "Doctors had been trained to think that abortion was difficult and dangerous, and it took them a decade to adjust to the fact that it is a simple, straightforward procedure, often completed in four or five minutes," said Potts. "The epidemiological evidence since the 1960s has shown that this is the safest way of terminating a pregnancy."[29]

In 1973, in anticipation of the Supreme Court decision, 100 professors of OB/GYN signed a famous letter, published in the *American Journal of Obstetrics and Gynecology*, calling on their colleagues to learn the electric vacuum aspiration technique and fulfill the need that would arise: they accurately estimated about one million procedures each year. But they still did not see abortion as simple or straightforward: "The practice of abortions in doctors' private offices is to be condemned," they wrote.[30]

Forty years later, another 100 signed a new statement detailing the phalanx of restrictions on women's access and physicians' practice, including the way politicians have interfered with resident training. (It took 23 years for the accrediting organization of OB/GYN residency programs to require training in abortion, but a federal amendment introduced by Republican senator Dan Coats allowed programs to bypass it and still maintain their federal funding.[31]) In several states medical students by law can't learn "abortion," which denies the reality that the safest way to end a pregnancy is also the safest way to treat a miscarriage. So physicians who aren't trained in "abortion" will have less experience treating miscarriage. But the physician authors of the recent letter stop short of criticizing their colleagues, the vast majority of whom don't offer abortion as part of their practice, leaving women to navigate the phalanx—or pushing them to avoid it entirely.

Today, abortion must be accessed through the health system yet is something apart from the health system. This was not what the feminist health movement envisioned. Clinics emerged after *Roe* for several reasons: abortion still carried too much stigma for physicians to openly offer it in their practices, and feminist activists didn't trust them to provide it anyway. Feminists wanted to ensure the care was respectful, the patients informed, and the decision theirs alone.

Thus began an uneasy "mutual dependency" between feminist activists and (mostly) male physicians. "Activists needed the doctors, in most fundamental terms, because *Roe v. Wade* and subsequent decisions had made clear that abortions could not be performed by anyone other than a physician. But the doctors needed the feminists as well because the medical community as a whole had no idea what it meant to deliver abortion legally, in outpatient settings, to a large group of healthy women," wrote UC Berkeley sociologist Carole Joffe and others.[32] The abortion clinic as we know it, in other words, was a compromise.

"The freestanding clinic is and was a very good idea. However, it accentuated the separation of abortion from the rest of medicine," Joffe tells me. That's one of the downsides. The other is that the anti-abortion movement has largely shaped the clinic experience. "Part of the reason women don't like going to clinics is because they're not very welcoming places. When you go to the dentist you don't go through metal detectors. This is not how people want to give abortion care, this is the result of the violent anti-abortion movement."

Had history gone a different way, had another case or a wave of abortion repeal legislation remade the landscape, what would it look like now? The clinic system has rendered abortion visible and vulnerable—clinics are brick-and-mortar targets—while the act of obtaining an abortion is a public spectacle, from the walk past the picketers to the group recovery rooms. The entire experience, even the words that come out of a provider's mouth, has been proscribed by the state. And more importantly, as Joffe and colleagues put it, "abortion care has become further marginalised from mainstream medicine. The existence of the clinics arguably helped relieve many abortion-sympathetic physicians from the perceived burden of becoming an abortion provider themselves."

Even physicians who get training in medical school, who want to provide in-office abortion to their patients, often join practices that will not let them, or practice at hospitals that will not let them, either for insurance reasons or because the other partners don't want "the taint" of abortion, says Joffe. "It has become so politicized that if you do abortions you know you'll be picketed, you know you'll lose patients," she says. Even if they try to do it quietly, word will get around. So practices often require partner physicians to sign contracts that they will not offer terminations. "They have to sign contracts that they won't even work one day a month at a Planned Parenthood," says Joffe.

When mifepristone was approved by the FDA in 2000, Joffe was among the observers who thought "this is going to change everything."

That was also the gist of a *New York Times Magazine* story on the drug, titled "The Little White Bombshell." Optimists predicted the number of providers would double. "Well, it didn't really work out that way," Joffe admits. Medication abortion is just as regulated as the surgical procedure—the FDA mandates two provider visits (down from three) to obtain the two-drug regimen, while 18 states have preempted telemedicine from enabling a workaround, and still other states ban non-MDs from dispensing it. It is by far easier for someone to just order miso online. Or call a doula.

THE LUNCH HOUR ABORTION

Several years ago, life slammed into me from two directions at once: first, a painful breakup; then, a positive pregnancy test arising like a phoenix from its ashes. Breakups I had gone through, but somehow I had never needed an abortion. As I entered my 30s, I became aware that the calculus of an oops would be different than it had been in my 20s, when my ovaries would have spirited me to a clinic. But now I was staring at 35, uncertain of my future fertility, future relationships, future, period.

After a week of agonizing Skype and cell calls (we weren't even living in the same city), ending it seemed the only reasonable thing to do. But my instinct was no longer the clinic. My instinct was to avoid the clinic. First, I tried to find a group doing menstrual extraction. When that didn't work, I called a midwife friend to ask about herbs. She suggested a regimen, though she warned me it was not a sure thing. She also made clear that once I started the herbs there was no turning back. They would absolutely affect the development of the embryo. I should investigate other options should they not work within a couple of weeks.

I swallowed the "lodging" dose of bitter tinctures at 2 a.m. one night after another excruciating conversation (I don't recommend this). I took the herbs dutifully for a week, discreetly squeezing dropperfuls into glasses of water wherever I happened to be. I began to feel what I can only describe as a pelvic queasiness, like I needed to purge, but nothing was coming.

I needed to line up a plan B, and there were several within reach by subway. But I was clinic-averse. Too public, too assembly line, too medicalized, too impersonal. I knew of a couple providers in private practice who did abortions in-office—indeed, I had seen one for Pap tests, but just the month before I had received a letter that she was closing up shop. I was in a privileged position, surrounded by safe options. But I wanted more than safe.

A recent conversation came back to me. It was with a doula and activist who had fresh opinions that resonated with me about the way we do abortion—why did it have to happen in clinics, why couldn't it happen at home as well? She'd given birth to her first child in the comfort of her own home, under the care of a gentle, skilled midwife, and it had been empowering. When, a few years later, as a single mother working and studying full time, she needed an abortion, she wanted the same kind of experience. But her midwife didn't offer this, and neither did other midwives in the community.

She learned of a group of women in Chicago, about four hours' drive from her home, who had revived the practice of menstrual extraction. My contact reached out to them but they couldn't make the trip to her, nor she to them. She could find nobody else offering the home abortion she wanted. So she resigned herself to the clinic, where she negotiated a manual vacuum aspiration without sedation.

Still, she found the experience humiliating and traumatic, from the waiting room where nobody wants to make eye contact to the stranger who did the procedure to the recovery room, where "they sit you in a chair and give you Coca-Cola, there's just a woman in the room filling out paperwork. There's no, How are you doing? How are you feeling?" she said. "I thought to myself, they could do a lot better than this. There could be so much more for women here." Was there a movement for abortion reform? I asked her. "To humanize the experience? That's not a term that would go over really well in the pro-choice community."

What about me—why did I really not want to go to the clinic? An emergency room is public, medical, impersonal, but I wouldn't hesitate to go there if I had a broken limb or needed stitches. Thinking through it now, it's clear my aversion was about shame. The shame of not feeling I had my life together enough to have a baby. The shame of staying in a relationship that would end in such spectacular failure. The prospect of sitting in that waiting room felt like a public shaming, like punishment, and the grief I was going through was punishment enough.

It turns out the lockdown atmosphere is the reason many people give for disliking the abortion clinic.[33] Ojanen-Goldsmith interviewed 25 people who had either received or provided alternative abortions and found a common motivator was a "prior in-clinic abortion," as well as "the desire for privacy, control and active participation" and "gaining bodily knowledge and autonomy."[34]

A heightened experience of medical care in general, the abortion clinic is also a headache of redundant tests and paperwork and protocol. In one locale, a provider tells me that "women are signing up for a six- to eight-hour process. There's blood testing, a urine sample, vaginal exam, and vaginal ultrasound. Then mandated counseling. Then they're in the queue for the one doctor working there, which means more time in the waiting room. Then mandatory post-procedure monitoring." And that's in a state without a mandatory 24- to 72-hour waiting period.

The procedure itself is also unnecessarily medicalized. Many providers use electric vacuum aspiration, which requires a special machine that makes an unforgettable sound, though according to a 2015 survey, 80 percent of clinicians reported having used manual vacuum aspiration, up from 49 percent in 2002.[35] The vast majority of women elect for sedation—called "general" frequently, though it is not (general requires a breathing apparatus).

One doctor who sometimes performed abortions at Planned Parenthood told me that while anesthesia slightly increases the risk of complications, "They can make the assembly line faster this way, and charge more." An unconscious patient also obviates bedside manner. Sedation is overkill, this doctor and others told me, but it fits into a system that rewards intervention and speed, and it fits with the social stigma involved with clinic care that women would rather check out.

This was not what activist doctors envisioned the post-*Roe* era would look like. Malcolm Potts, the former director of the International Federation of Planned Parenthood, told a reporter in 1973 that when used in the early first trimester, the new suction method with plastic cannula would require little to no dilation, causing minimal pain and reducing the need for anesthesia. The reporter paraphrased: "The vast majority of patients are able to go about their normal activities within minutes of the procedure, a fact that has given it the nickname of the lunch hour abortion."[36]

Back in my predicament, I searched harder for a group doing menstrual extraction, to no avail. I probably could have found misoprostol if I'd looked, but I really didn't want my uterus to feel worse than it already did. I wanted the now-damaged pregnancy out. I called around to clinics in New York but found it difficult to find one that would do manual vacuum aspiration—most said they did electric—let alone one without sedation, with one exception: Early Options, which still prides itself on its trademarked SofTouch (it's a simple MVA) in an environment "just like a doctor's office." At the time, the procedure cost a cool $950—nearly three times as much as Planned Parenthood.[37] The "lunch hour abortion" had become a luxury item, out of my budget.

My next-to-last resort was the practitioner who was about to close her practice. I had her private email. She called me back right away. She'd make an exception for me. "This is why I do what I do," she said. A week later I was in her exam room, surrounded by moving boxes with my feet in stirrups while she rested an ultrasound wand on my cervix. "There's the sac," she told me, pointing to the tiny white circle on the screen. "There's not much embryonic activity."

She had used herbs successfully herself, she revealed, and it looked like they'd had an effect in my case. My body just hadn't let go yet. Maybe it would still, but this was my chance for it to be over, and I took it. She injected a local anesthetic into my cervix—the most painful part of the procedure—and put a cool washcloth on my forehead while she did the aspiration. It was over in five minutes. I felt 15 pounds lighter, and relief. The grieving was hardly over, but at least now I could begin moving on. A friend was reading a magazine in the waiting room, and we went and had lunch.

As an experiment, I decided to call around to see what my options would be if I needed an abortion and was still clinic-averse in early 2018. With one phone call I found a doula who said she'd do a menstrual extraction for me "as an act of friendship." And if I needed miso, someone she knew had a stash handy. I had to laugh at how easy (and free!) this would have been just five years later. The doula had only been doing this for about a year—after the 2016 election, a midwife had called her with urgency. "She was like, I want to teach you this stuff and I want to teach it to you soon."

The election of Donald Trump is a major touchstone for several off-grid providers I talked to, but this community had been building during Obama's second term, during which time hundreds of restrictions were passed and abortion declined to its lowest level since 1972.[38] Out of the robust birth doula movement grew a more political group of "full spectrum" doulas, who connected their work with the reproductive justice movement: they would support any pregnant person no matter the outcome—abortion, miscarriage, birth, stillbirth.

For some doulas who were accompanying women to clinics and seeing them through medical procedures or hanging with them at home while they took the pills, it wasn't a huge leap to begin offering options that would save their friends the time, expense, hassle, and indignities of the system. And they had a historical basis for this evolution.

YOU WERE ONCE THIS PROVIDER

In early 2013, Molly Dutton-Kenny submitted a several-thousand-word essay called "The Midwife as Abortion Provider" to the radical *Squat* birth journal. She was 23, a midwifery student, and she had a vision: "Though it may be a lifelong undertaking, I dream of the day when I can provide a full scope of reproductive health care to my clients. I am in this profession to better serve women in all their reproductive needs," she wrote.

Dutton-Kenny was an early member of Full Spectrum Doulas in Seattle, which to this day to provides "in-person and telephone support before, during and after an abortion . . . both inside and outside the clinic and at home." *Squat* accepted the essay immediately, and Kenny proposed a workshop on the topic at its upcoming Squatfest conference, to be held in August of that year in San Francisco's historic Women's Building. The "MaestraPeace" mural that covers both facades of the corner Mission Revival building had just been fully cleaned and restored.

Five stories above the entrance is the image by Susan Kelk Cervantes of an enormous nude, pregnant goddess, holding up the sun, its rays shining down the facade. As the mural was being planned in the early 1990s, the San Francisco Landmarks Preservation Advisory Board threatened to pull municipal funds over the image, which they felt was "out of character" with the historic architecture. The artists called the press, and the goddess rose. Cervantes told a reporter, "All women can learn to have control over their own destinies. She holds the sun [symbolizing] that potential."[39]

"It was the first time I'd ever spoken into a microphone," Dutton-Kenny tells me, curled up on her sofa in her new home outside Toronto, where today she is a licensed midwife. Dutton-Kenny is pale and blue-eyed, with long dirty-blond hair and a young face. She blends in easily in her new suburban enclave. Her voice is soft, but opinions and evidence come tumbling out with speed and edge, and she radiates conviction.

In the weeks leading up to the conference, Dutton-Kenny learned that a pre-conference online survey had determined her workshop was among the most popular. "There was a huge demand for this, which was shocking to me," she says.

Speaking before dozens, Dutton-Kenny laid out her vision and the history that informed it. She explained how abortion was used by the newly organized American Medical Association in the mid-1800s to criminalize midwives and displace them as women's primary health care providers. Prior to the spate of laws passed in almost every state by 1880, early abortion was widely practiced and accepted by American society. "Abortion" as we know it wasn't even the terminology; rather, women sought out to "restore the menses," which they did mostly with various herbs and drugs, as they had for millennia.

Historian John Riddle goes back to antiquity and traces the compounds known to "bring on the courses" as they reappear in image and text through to modern times. Herbs like juniper, tansy, and rue are mentioned again and again, though whether they are openly identified as abortifacients depends on the politics of the time, which grow more restrictive. He dismisses the idea that these substances were not effective. For one, controlling knowledge of the "cursed medicines" was the focus of the Church for several centuries. One plant, silphium, was so overharvested for this purpose that it became extinct. Pennyroyal and artemisia appear and reappear on vases and paintings, often next to pregnant women. "We have good reason to believe that contraceptives were effective in reducing family size among ancient peoples," he wrote.[40]

Riddle's scholarship follows the written record of plant knowledge in the West—robust through medieval times, less so into modernity. "The sixteenth and seventeenth centuries seem to have 'deleted from the record' a great deal of knowledge from millennia past," he wrote.[41] As medical training formalized, knowledge of botanical birth control was specifically left out. "The Church regarded it as wrong, and the university was largely an institution of the Church. The physicians' art was for disease and injury, not family planning." Thus, what knowledge remained was in the hands of "old women," that is, midwives, who were the subject of inquisitions and witch burnings. What survived of midwifery and immigrated to the New World was diluted by its persecution, though of course indigenous midwives in the Americas had their plants as well.

In Dutton-Kenny's reading of this history, she makes a connection between illegality and the shift from plants to instruments. While not necessarily cause and effect, these two developments happened contemporaneously in America. In Britain and Ireland, abortion was criminalized by the Ellenborough Act of 1803, which "stated explicitly that the expected means of performing abortions were chemical," Riddle points out. The first American state laws borrowed language from Ellenborough, but when New York passed its law in 1828, it included "any medicine, drug, substance, or thing whatever, or . . . *any instrument or other means*" (my emphasis). That same year, the Ellenborough Act was amended with the American addition verbatim: "any instrument or other means."[42]

What had changed? Riddle observes that by the nineteenth century, male physicians had made a routine of bimanual vaginal examination to diagnose pregnancy. And it was during this time that surgery went from a crude backwater side gig to respectable field of medicine. In 1850, the French surgeon Joseph Récamier introduced the curette to treat cases of abnormal uterine bleeding, but with "disastrous" results, according to one 1895 source.[43] Three deaths from uterine perforation were reported, which led to condemnations by French, German, and English physicians.

The sharp, spoon-like instrument reappeared 15 years later in the hands of J. Marion Sims, at a conference in London—he'd redesigned it and branded it with his name, as he was wont to do, and insisted it is "now recognized as legitimate."[44] Still, it would take another couple decades for others to refine it, and by the end of the century there was a robust medical literature documenting its use for fibroids, endometriosis, cancer, and even "induction of abortion."[45] Dilation and curettage, the D&C, was born, and would became a staple gynecological procedure for the next 100 years.

Riddle reports almost no references to instrumentation of the uterus for this purpose prior to the 1800s. In addition to plants, we also know women used manual massage techniques, and violence to the abdomen, even dehydration. But generally abortion was induced with compounds ingested or applied to the skin or cervix, not through it.

Dutton-Kenny sees the iconic midcentury coat hanger as the logical end of the campaign against not only abortion but also midwifery. As the West became more industrialized, the impulse toward technology (and away from growing medicinal herbs) spilled over. Midwives began inducing abortions with rubber catheters; women resorted to anything long and thin. "Women weren't dying from herbal abortion, they were dying from knitting needles," says Dutton-Kenny. "That concept was introduced by medicine but introduced recklessly, which created the problems which they later solved."

At the very least, illegality staunched innovation, which also put women at more risk. The Scottish physician Sir James Young Simpson is famous for giving chloroform to Queen Victoria in 1853, but that same year he also described making "frequent use" of what he called an "exhausting syringe," which he fashioned out of a thin metal tube, piston, syringe, and glass container to induce menstruation, and possibly also miscarriage. Other physicians followed, and by the turn of the century, medical supply manufacturers "showcased dozens of aspiration units and syringes specifically designed for gynecological purposes," according to Turkish scholar Tanfer Emin Tunc.[46] In other words, the MVA could have been available in North America much earlier.

In 1934, a Hungarian physician claimed the first electric vacuum aspirator, and by the late 1930s this practice would find its way to within walking distance of my current home, at Kings County Hospital in Brooklyn, New York, where a wall-mounted suction unit was installed to manage what must have been a significant number of incomplete abortions (likely induced). According to Tunc, these typically would have been treated with D&C, but at Kings County, "attending physicians often gave interns the task of treating incomplete abortions with electric vacuum aspiration. The patient would usually return home without hospitalization, which was rarely the case with therapeutic D&Cs."

As Leslie Reagan recounted in *When Abortion Was a Crime*, both midwives and physicians continued to perform abortions after they were criminalized in the States. In Chicago, which she uses as a case study by examining media stories and coroner inquests, midwives and physicians performed abortions in equal number and had similar complication rates. In the early years, midwives used herbs and drugs (there were still commercial products, derived from herbs, available in pharmacies), as well as catheters and instruments. Physicians also mixed methods—there was a popular product called Leunbach's paste—but largely favored instruments. Women were mainly dying of infections and internal injuries.

Law enforcement cracked down on the practice after 1900, interrogating women on their deathbeds, arresting lovers, and deputizing physicians, who grew reluctant to get involved in treating women with complications. "As doctors tried to protect themselves from prosecution in abortion cases, women's healthcare suffered," wrote Reagan. "Press coverage of abortion-related deaths warned all women of the dangers of abortion: death and publicity."

Then the Depression hit, making "vivid the relationship between economics and reproduction. Women had abortions on a massive scale." With hardly any midwives left in northern cities, the pressure was on physicians. Reagan reports that most cities had several physician abortion providers and so did many small towns. There was a chain of abortion clinics on the West Coast. In New Jersey, around 1,000 women bought into a "club" that functioned as abortion insurance. Dr. Josephine Gabler ran a clinic in Chicago that performed 18,000 procedures between 1932 and 1941. Even physicians who didn't perform them frequently referred to those who did. They happened in doctor's offices with receptionists just like any other medical procedure. "The proverbial 'back-alley butcher' story of abortion overemphasizes fatalities and limits our understanding of the history of illegal abortion," wrote Reagan.

A handful of physicians wrote books and spoke out about liberalizing abortion law, but by this time the media had turned against the practice. The *New York Times* refused to allow advertisements of one of the books; the New York Public Library carried nothing about abortion on its shelves, and the Academy of Medicine wouldn't let non-physicians see books on the topic. The birth control movement led by Margaret Sanger was also anti-abortion and argued that contraception could eliminate it. "The refusal of American birth controllers to engage in a discussion about liberalizing access to abortion ensured that a public discussion of the idea never developed," wrote Reagan.[47]

The period that we in the twenty-first century associate most with the dark days of illegal abortion began around 1940. Whereas law enforcement had previously worked backward from abortion-related deaths to prosecute incompetent providers, now police were raiding reputable practices, most physician-led. Patients were apprehended by police and forced to undergo exams by colluding gynecologists. Referring physicians were intimidated or arrested. The Red Scare was aligning the country into conformity, and abortion had the stain of communism (it was legal in the Soviet Union). Women were also gaining economic power, wearing pants, and collecting real paychecks while the men were at war. Reagan and others see the crackdown on abortion as a way to keep women's power in check.

"Therapeutic abortion" had long been a workaround for physicians to perform aboveboard procedures. But now hospitals were forming committees to decide which women qualified. Physicians participated as a kind of liability insurance—strength in numbers. As the years wore on, committees approved fewer and fewer cases. As a result, abortions in the 1950s and '60s were "harder to obtain, more expensive, and more dangerous," wrote Reagan.[48] If they could access underground providers, women would often be blindfolded, taken to an unknown location, and subjected to someone with unknown skills or credentials. Tens of thousands of women showed up at hospitals with infections and injuries annually during these years, and as Reagan points out, the rate of abortion-related deaths actually *increased* from previous years, with four times as many black women dying as white women.

But the era of dangerous, illicit abortion was a blip in history, less than 100 years, Dutton-Kenny says. "What I try to remind people is that home abortion is not dangerous, criminalizing traditional providers and taking away their knowledge is dangerous," she says. "The perception of lack of safety of home abortion is the main argument for clinical abortion, it's the main thing *Roe v. Wade* was argued on. But it's a lie. It was always a lie."

At Squatfest, she told her audience, "I truly believe that midwives need to reclaim this aspect of their scope of practice, and in order to reclaim it you need to understand that you were once this provider. It's not that I'm proposing a radical new thing, it's that I'm proposing a return to our traditional scope of practice.

"That was who we were in this society. And we have allowed ourselves to be given the short end of the stick. And the people who are suffering the most are our clients. It is women and people in our communities who need excellent care, who need our model of care to do this, who need us to do this. And we're not doing it. And part of it is outside regulation, and part of it is us rolling over and taking it. And so at what point do we decide, Nope, my scope of practice is wider than this; I will advocate for my community?"

Her audience was "a different kind of midwife" than she'd encountered at larger midwifery conferences. That is, "midwives who were not in it for the sweet babies" but rather who cared about things like racial health disparities, who were looking at pregnancy and childbirth through a social justice lens. "These were my people," she says.

Perhaps it shouldn't have been surprising then, when members of her audience stood up and began sharing stories of inducing their own abortions. "It was clear that this was the first time that anybody had told these stories out loud." They said things like "It never occurred to me that I could have asked for help. I did this scary thing by myself, I didn't know what I was doing, and I like your idea that I could have just called my midwife—she already has all the tools for managing any complication that could have happened, and she could have walked me through the whole thing just like she walked me through my birth." Several of those audience members later reached out to Dutton-Kenny to say, "I want to do this. We should do this."

A SHITTY PLACE TO HAVE A MISCARRIAGE

The D&C, a staple of gynecological practice for a century, is now considered a relic by progressive OB/GYNs. "There should be virtually no use [of the D&C] in my opinion, for either miscarriage or abortion in the first trimester," says Sarah Prager, an OB/GYN and director of the family planning division at the University of Washington who is also advising Ojanen-Goldsmith on her study of community providers. Yet many women leave the ER and even abortion clinics having signed consent forms for a D&C, having been told they had a D&C, though the term is apparently used to describe everything from vacuum suction to use of the curette, to a combination of the two. The code hospitals and physicians use to get reimbursed also does not specify the method of uterine extraction, says Prager; thus there is no reliable data on how prevalent true D&C—with metal instruments—still is.

"This is a really bizarre thing, that the terminology doesn't matter and we don't need to accurately describe the procedure people are getting," says Dutton-Kenny. One of her major points of advocacy is that abortion care and miscarriage management are no different, and midwives are capable of handling both—maybe even more capable than the average emergency room doc. "The ER is a shitty place to have a miscarriage. You're bleeding, you're not a priority, and they offer you a D&C on the spot. Then you're sent home on probably the worst day of your life with no counseling."

The stigma and regulation of abortion have impacted miscarriage treatment, stalling innovation there, too: anything considered an abortion procedure has been ghettoized or even restricted. Catholic hospitals, for instance, often won't evacuate the uterus during a miscarriage if there's a fetal heartbeat—even if the woman's health is at risk. Unless your ER doc was in a progressive residency that taught abortion, they may only know how to do D&C, or may be more comfortable doing a D&C because they didn't get to practice aspiration. It's not clear why everyone isn't offering misoprostol. This means women may get a more crude, traumatic procedure than they need—one that has a higher risk of complications—at a particularly vulnerable moment in their reproductive lives.

According to Philip Darney, a physician at San Francisco General Hospital who went on early missions with USAID to offer MVA, "It's still true in many hospitals around the country and around the world, women who come in suffering from bleeding due to an incomplete abortion, a miscarriage, and wait for hours in the emergency department until they can get into the operating room, and often under general anesthesia have a procedure that's far more dangerous than a simple MVA . . . using electrical equipment that doesn't need to be used at great expense and inconvenience to them."[49]

Prager agrees to a large extent. "There's still much more surgical management of miscarriage than probably needs to happen," and not enough doctors giving the "full complement" of options, from just waiting it out to MVA to misoprostol. Dutton-Kenny suggests avoiding the ER if possible and instead going to an abortion clinic if one needs to conclude a miscarriage. "That's what they're set up for. There's no difference." And that means community providers could also play a role here as well.

The pro-choice establishment has been interestingly silent on the trend of at-home providers, though it is starting to accept the reality of what's known as "self-induced abortion."[50] A group of physicians at University of California, San Francisco, called Advancing New Standards in Reproductive Health have vocally endorsed self-administration of misoprostol and are advocating for both "miso-mifi" and the Pill to go over the counter. "I think a lot of advocates can be totally on board with someone who wants to take medication on their own in their own home," says Ojanen-Goldsmith, "but the idea that we essentially have community-trained health workers who are doing abortions outside of a clinic—people have a very visceral reaction to that."

Prager has no qualms about pills. "Women can read the back of a medication box and figure out if they're safe," she says. "I don't really care if someone gets mifepristone and misoprostol from a physician, from a nurse practitioner, from a midwife, from a lay midwife, from a doula, from a pharmacy, orders it online . . ." she goes on. "We have a lot of data that it works. My only concern around that would be that women are getting appropriate info about what the right way is to take those medicines."

She isn't opposed to herbs either, but "in a perfect world" they'd be studied in a rigorous way. And in terms of midwives and non-clinicians doing manual extractions, there's data that advanced practice clinicians can do it safely, but little data on how those who are trained in the community fare. I ask what her biggest fear would be, what complications might arise. "Number one would be incomplete aspiration of tissue," she says, which would require follow-up care. Number two would be "a perforation that's problematic and not recognized."

She makes no distinction between menstrual extraction (with mason jar and aquatic tubing) and MVA with a professional syringe. "There's no difference" in risk, except perhaps that a non-pregnant uterus is more firm, so less likely to perforate. But there should be no increased risk of infection. The same cannula enters the uterus whether it's ME or MVA or electric suction. "If you are using 'no-touch' technique, I don't care where you are, your risk should be the same." Clinics typically give prophylactic antibiotics, but the baseline risk of infection is low, around 1 in 200—and clinics are institutions with more diverse microbes.

Ten years ago, Prager created a program that trains emergency room doctors and other physicians to offer women miscarrying a range of options, including MVA. "Overall, uterine aspiration is really safe, and it doesn't actually require years and years of medical training to do it," she says. I tell her about my experience with the papaya, and how my teacher encouraged me, and how it echoes the '70s feminist epiphany—*we can do this*. "Anyone can. You don't need to be a physician to do this. I agree with that statement. It's not hard. But you know, just like anyone can build a cabinet, some people can do that a lot more beautifully than others, you know what I mean? And I really do look at it the same way. Some people are more skilled in some areas than others. Not everybody has great hands."

Personally, this network of community providers gives me comfort. That no matter what happens politically, women are taking matters into their own hands, and meanwhile they are redefining quality care and offering what seems to be an informed, affordable, dignified alternative.

Prager agrees, but voices a concern that she's heard spoken by others in the pro-choice community: that by promoting or even condoning at-home abortion, clinic care will be further marginalized—that movement energy will be drawn away from fighting "to make sure safe, legal abortion in medical facilities is accessible and inexpensive," and instead advocates will figure that "people can just go to their local doula and get herbs." But Prager recognizes that fight is being lost, as fewer and fewer clinics can keep their doors open. Clinics "were a great concept in many ways, but what it did was marginalize the procedure outside of normal health care, and we're paying for that now."

While women in the pre-*Roe* era risked their lives to obtain illegal abortions, the greater risk today (and certainly in a post-*Roe* era) is to liberty. The SIA Legal Team has documented 21 arrests of self-inducers since 2000 and is bracing for more. "It is a grave miscalculation to believe that post-*Roe* will look anything like pre-*Roe*. Our nation has spent the intervening 45 years devising a prison-industrial complex that is unparalleled in the world and in which women are the fastest-growing population," wrote Farah Diaz-Tello. "If we want to prevent abortion from being yet another ground for mass imprisonment, the only option is to transform the legal landscape."[51]

"Midwives are an obvious logical abortion provider," says Dutton-Kenny, thinking of how many communities have a known home birth midwife (even in states where the Certified Professional Midwife credential isn't recognized) versus how few have a clinic. "Even if just a fraction of us took this on we could significantly improve access. I also think that midwives work from a model of care that addresses many of the current problems with clinical abortion care. Most women will tell you they left the clinic not pregnant, so that's good, but most don't describe it fondly, for a lot of reasons."

Dutton-Kenny was raised in the Bay Area by artist-activist parents who took her and her siblings to protests. As a teenager, school bored her (she says she sailed through with a 4.0). She tells me she had few friends and was just waiting for it to be over. "They hated me," she says of the school. "I was always in the principal's office saying, 'Hey, we have a problem,' and offering a 10-point solution." She saw problems in the community as well, and one of them was Oakland's dismal abortion clinics (the ones she remembers have since closed). She had friends who had obtained abortions there and vowed to never return, which prompted her to write a research paper on the history of herbal abortion.

Three years later, in 2011, Dutton-Kenny found herself pregnant while studying abroad in Mali, where abortion is very illegal. At the time, she was living with and apprenticing with an elder midwife, a devout Muslim, with whom she dared not share her predicament. Instead, she called a friend in the States, who shipped her herbal tinctures by five-day air—"the most expensive package I've ever shipped." She took them until they ran out, but still didn't begin bleeding.

"I spent my days helping other women bring their babies into the world, and my nights visualizing letting my baby go," Dutton-Kenny wrote in her first essay for *Squat*. "I had brought a handful of midwifery textbooks with me, and flipped through them in desperation, finding nothing helpful. I was confused why there was so little written on abortion by midwives. I felt let down by my community, like I had fallen into a void of fertility that midwives wouldn't touch. I had never before noticed the birthing community's utter silence on abortion; now it was not only noticeable, but palpable and painful."

Now she believes herbs require a lot more patience, but at the time there was too much pressure to resolve the situation before it would require her to leave the country. She finally confided in the program director, who knew of a European-trained doctor who prescribed the mifepristone-misoprostol regimen known as RU-486, which just one pharmacy in the entire city would fill. Within an hour of taking the miso she was throwing up and bleeding, so much so that it began to scare her. "I wanted support, wanted someone else to tell me I was alright. Really what I wanted was a midwife," she wrote.

Squat published her essay on midwives as abortion providers in three parts, in the fall, winter, and spring of 2013 to 2014. In her byline she left her personal email address. Midwives and doulas from across the country flooded her with messages about their own lonely, traumatic abortions and how this made so much sense to them.

When I spoke to several community providers, they told me they look up to Dutton-Kenny as an inspiration, revolutionary, mentor. When midwife Laura Marina Perez, who practices in the Bay Area, heard her message, "to me that was the mandate, that's my job, that's what I really want to do in terms of traditional midwifery," she tells me. To provide services is also the position of the International Confederation of Midwives, she points out.[52]

"I really feel in my heart and in my mind and in my spirit that this is what it means for me to be a midwife, to really have the skills and have the information. And I don't even think it's a midwifery thing. It's a woman thing," says Perez. "Everyone should have a bottle of miso in their house . . . and maybe every woman should have a Del-Em. That does really take a skill set. But I dream of a world where we have that sisterhood and community, where women are like, 'Oh yeah, I can help you.'"

CONCLUSION: THE CASE FOR PHYSIOLOGICAL JUSTICE

ONE MORNING WHEN my son was about nine months old, we headed out to a "babywearing" meet-up. I had been using a long sheet of hand-dyed red cotton to wrap him to my chest since he was born. It was a fail-safe way to calm him down, even when holding him, rocking him, and singing to him didn't do the trick. It was also how I'd negotiate evenings by myself before he could reliably sit up, when he was too restless for the bouncy seat. I'd weave the material over my shoulders, under his legs, around my back and then around his, so that we were belly to belly. Then I'd tie a square knot and go about making dinner. He'd quietly watch my chopping and mixing, then at some point while I was eating, he'd silently nod off.

I didn't consider myself a "babywearer"—I always had a stroller on hand—but wrapping was the closest thing to a superpower I possessed. By nine months, however, my son was getting big enough that my mortal hips couldn't take it for very long, and I purchased a backpack carrier. The hurdle for me was how to get him into it and on my back, without dropping him.

On the way to the meet-up, I met a mom who had used her woven wrap to create a "back-carry" (no buckles required). Not only that, she had created a braid within the front tie and was trying out other flourishes, like a flower tie. She was already part of a tightly knit (pardon the pun) babywearing community, which communicated by a closed Facebook group, shared tips, met for playdates, and even traded wraps (which, like an old pair of jeans, are more valuable when broken in). I didn't have the time (or desire) to make this a hobby. But I marveled at the care and beauty in that braid and couldn't help admiring this sub-subculture of women who had elevated babywearing to an art form.

I also quickly learned of the growing contempt toward this subculture, which is part of a larger phenomenon called attachment parenting. While babywearing (an indigenous tradition around the globe) has gone mainstream in the modern world, for this community it is one expression of a larger philosophy of keeping babies close—very close in the first few weeks and months: in wraps, in bed, at the breast. This is based on instinct as well as research on what's now known as the fourth trimester. The Notre Dame anthropologist James McKenna, who studies how mothers and babies regulate breathing, body temperature, and stress response when they sleep side by side, summarized it this way: "The human infant is the most vulnerable, contact dependent, slowest developing and most dependent primate-mammal of all, largely because humans are born neurologically premature, relative to other primate mammals . . . with only 25 percent of its adult brain volume. This means that its physiological systems are unable to function optimally without contact with the mother's body, which continues to regulate the baby much like it did during gestation."[1]

You'll notice that McKenna referred to "the mother's body" and nobody else's, and the literature generally refers to the "mother-baby dyad." This creates friction with modern egalitarian notions. Thus some feminist scholars and bloggers have denounced the "new maternalism" that has led not only to cosleeping and babywearing, but also to a resurgence in things like knitting and baby food–making and mother-identified organizing (e.g., MomsRising). They've even questioned the science on breastfeeding.

In 2011, sociologist Joan Wolf wrote *Is Breast Best? Taking on the Breastfeeding Experts and the New High Stakes of Motherhood*, in which she calls the science "weak and inconsistent" (and was roundly criticized). "The question I had was how have people who've called themselves feminists dealt with the fact that 'breast is best' and it's a task that cannot be shared?" she told me. Rather than physiology, she traces pro-breastfeeding rationale to deep-seated cultural beliefs about what it means to be a good mother—"the collective fantasy that mothers can and should produce perfect children."

Wolf and others worry this "high-stakes motherhood" creates social pressure, and resulting shame, on those who do things more, shall we say, conventionally. Their bigger concern is that it threatens gender equality, autonomy, and progress, because these women have moved away from the idea of "parenting"—a role that can (theoretically) be divvied up equally between partners—and back to "mothering." As Georgetown legal scholars put it, "it has become increasingly clear that workplace equality for women and household equality for men depend on culturally and legally decoupling family care work from femaleness."[2] In 2016, two medical ethicists argued that "breastfeeding-is-natural" efforts "can inadvertently support biologically deterministic arguments about the roles of men and women in the family (for example, that women should be the primary caretakers of children)." Feminist novelist Erica Jong argued in the *Wall Street Journal* that this "motherphilia" "represents as much of a backlash against women's freedom as the right-to-life movement."[3]

It's true: exclusive breastfeeding requires a mother to be in close proximity to her baby for a period of time—and unless you're Marissa Mayer, who as Yahoo! CEO had a nursery built in her office, this means you are not out there cracking the glass ceiling.

But I do not see this subculture arising out of cultural pressure for female perfection or a reactionary exile to the kitchen, sans shoes. Rather, I see these decisions as active resistance against what I'll call separation ideology, which tells us babies are better off *unattached* from their mothers and is a pervasive force in the United States. It shows up in maternity care and in the delivery room, in the rise of 24-hour daycares, in pro-life legislation that has been used to pit fetus against mother, and, most unconscionably, at our borders, where babies have been quite literally torn from their mothers' arms. Separation ideology denies the physicality of parenting and, specifically, mothering. It denies physiology, period. And it means that resisting separation requires resources, privilege, and, sometimes, attorneys.

Take "fetal rights" legislation, which has succeeded in several states in making the fetus legally separate from the person its life depends on. In Wisconsin, South Carolina, Alabama, and many other states, pregnant women have been charged with "fetal endangerment" or "child abuse" or "child neglect" for drug use. Their fetuses have been granted court-appointed attorneys in utero. And those women have been incarcerated, as if putting a woman in prison won't also punish the fetus living inside her. One pregnant woman in Wisconsin was ordered to solitary confinement (while she was eating for two).

Set aside for the moment that punishing women for the outcomes of their pregnancies (or conversely, compelling medical treatment) treats a person who is pregnant as something other than a fully grown human being with the right to bodily integrity. It also denies the physiology of gestation, as well as the reality of miscarriage. The fetus is being sheltered, nourished, and grown by its mother's body, which has *grown a new organ* (the placenta) to divert blood and nutrients to that baby involuntarily, just as blood and oxygen are circulating without conscious effort. Neglect isn't really possible. Is abuse? (And where do we draw that line? Many prescription medications, including fertility medications, pose a threat.)

Of course, the point of legally separating fetus from mother is to undermine abortion rights, but doing so has much broader implications. And the same thinking that allows us to disconnect the fetus from the person in whom it is growing allows us to disconnect from other physiological realities. It's a fallacy that shows up on the left as well as the right, in the mainstream as well as in the medical community.

In late November 1968, at a chilly YMCA camp outside Chicago, 200 women gathered in the woods for one of the first women's liberation conferences. Shulamith Firestone, a 23-year-old art student, and Ti-Grace Atkinson, philosopher and president of the New York chapter of the National Organization for Women, took to the stage. Twice as many women as expected had shown up at the conference, food was running out, but these speakers had adrenaline to spare. They had come up with a tantalizing antidote to patriarchy: an artificial womb.[4]

Firestone had been studying Marx and had come to this conclusion: if distinctions of class were to be eliminated, so should those of gender. Women were not only oppressed by men, but also by their own bodies, which suffer "barbaric" childbirth and a host of other indignities that limit their equal participation. "Nature produced the fundamental inequality," she would later write in *The Dialectic of Sex*, still widely read as a foundational feminist text. Women needed liberation "from the tyranny of their reproductive biology by every means available."

It wasn't what you'd call pragmatic—and probably wasn't meant to be. In *Dialectic*, Firestone included the caveat that she intended only "to stimulate thinking in fresh areas." But she did believe that, one way or another, sex differences needed eliminating: in her revolution, "genital difference between human beings would no longer matter culturally."[5]

The feminist health movement challenged this framing of biology as oppressive destiny, of difference as an inherent threat to equality. Rather, they saw through "difference" as a social construct, and with speculum in hand set about dismantling it. The poet Adrienne Rich wrote that female biology "has far more radical implications than we have yet come to appreciate. Patriarchal thought has limited female biology to its own narrow specifications. The feminist vision has recoiled from female biology for these reasons; it will, I believe, come to view our physicality as a resource, rather than a destiny."

But after *Roe*, this movement was shunted aside by the dominant "liberal" feminism, which focuses on equality and, like liberal ideology, values mind over body. "Liberal feminism works best to defend women's rights to be like men, to enter into men's worlds, to work at men's jobs for men's pay, to have the rights and privileges of men," wrote sociologist Barbara Katz Rothman. "But what of our rights to be *women*?"

The demands of liberal feminism fit well with capitalism—they fight for equal access to employment and consumption. But those demands are limited in terms of social justice, and they become obvious when women become mothers and hit the "maternal wall." As Katz Rothman explains, arguments of fairness and equality "begin to break down" over women's unique biological needs. "Giving women all the rights of men will not accomplish a whole lot for women facing the demands of pregnancy, birth, and lactation," she wrote, and went further: "For those people (and they may be the most traditional of conservatives or the most radical of feminists) who want to see women—our bodies, our selves, our sexuality, our motherhood—treated with respect, liberal feminism fails."[6]

I remember when my son was about six months old, I was staring at a picture of myself in a white sundress. "Whose boobs are those?" I said to his paternal grandma. "They're his," she said, laughing. It felt so true, and I didn't mind—I was a C-cup for once in my life, and was happy to share. I understand this is not something everyone can or wants to do, nor should anyone be forced or shamed into breastfeeding (or anything else). I was lucky that I had a good birth, that my body and baby obliged, and that I work from home. "Breast is best" campaigns are universally infuriating because they speak to women as if we all have unlimited time off, as if all our bodies are efficient milk machines, as if breastfeeding is simply an individual "choice." Philosopher Fiona Woollard offers a more helpful way to think and talk about it: there are *reasons* to nurse, and *reasons* for policy and culture to support it. Where we get tripped up is mistaking *reason* for *duty*. "I think that if breastfeeding is beneficial, mothers have a reason to breastfeed, but do not have a duty to breastfeed. Once we recognize this, we can see that it is possible to argue for the need to support breastfeeding *without* implying that formula feeders should feel guilty."[7] "Breast is best" sounds like mansplaining. We recognize the condescension as sexist and disrespectful, but it's more difficult to call out the absence of support as equally so.

This book is concerned with much more than pregnancy, birth, and lactation, but the first through fourth trimesters offer an instructive metaphor for how physiology could inform other cultural and policy shifts. Childbirth involves complex, nonlinear chain reactions of various hormones and enzymes that trigger contractions, tweak perception, and make milk flow. The suckling newborn creates more biofeedback, which activates the reward centers in a mother's limbic brain, "imprinting pleasure with infant contact and care," wrote Australian physician Sarah Buckley in a 200-page report on the hormonal physiology of childbirth, in which she surveyed 1,000 studies.[8]

Breast milk has a similar intelligence. It is alive, its composition different depending on the time of day, the age of the baby, and what pathogens mother and baby have been exposed to. Fresh out of the womb the baby gets antibody- and nutrient-rich colostrum, which primes the gut and immune system for life on the outside. Women who give birth prematurely actually produce more colostrum for a longer period of time—the body knows; mother and newborn may be separate but they are still very much in sync.

Our physiology tries mightily to keep mother and baby close in the hours, days, months postpartum. According to Buckley, the mother and fetus/baby "can essentially be seen as one biologic system from pregnancy through the postpartum/newborn period." The umbilical cord, left intact, ensures this proximity in the immediate imprinting moments after birth. Yet we rush to cut the cord, literally and metaphorically.

Freed from its maternal attachment, the baby can be whisked away for measurements, bathing, testing—and away from "bonding." Immediate cord clamping is based on a myth that failing to do so would cause the baby harm, when in fact the opposite is true: the cord blood, rich with stem cells, continues to flow to the baby for several minutes if left intact. Copious research suggests the benefit of not severing the cord so quickly and keeping the baby skin to skin, for sick and preemie babies in particular (in the literature it's called "kangaroo care").[9] But the traditional hospital ritual is for nurses to swaddle the baby in blankets and return it 30 minutes to an hour later, after a pediatrician has examined it—two to three hours later if the birth is surgical.

Separation ideology hits with full force after the baby has been born. So many things come between the dyad: recovery from a C-section or other birth trauma, isolation, exhaustion, formula samples, family leave policy (really, lack thereof), poverty. You have to actually *be* with the baby for breastfeeding to work optimally—and for it to be enjoyable. And companies in the United States don't let most parents be with their babies for more than a few weeks, if they get any paid leave at all. One study found that one-quarter of U.S. mothers go back to work within two weeks of giving birth.[10] If they're lucky, they get time to pump and a "lactation room." (Perhaps this is slowly changing: some 200 companies now allow babies to accompany employees to work, according to the Parenting in the Workplace Institute.)

It's not just a devaluing of human physiology that drives policy; it's a devaluing of human relationships—including our own relationships with ourselves. In separating baby from mother—physiology from society—we are denied optimal maternal health, optimal child development, and another thing we don't tend to associate with women's reproductive capacity: pleasure.

And so the babywearers wrap, resisting the culture that is trying to wrest their babes out of their arms, that wants to deny their biological inheritance. I get it. And I also get the feminist anxiety, the fear that in binding ourselves to our offspring, we're perpetuating a patriarchal bondage.

You can hear echoes of Firestone and Simone de Beauvoir in mainstream contemporary writing. Lindsay Beyerstein has alluded to "a disturbing effort to reduce women to their biological functions in the name of feminism."[11] In an *Atlantic* piece titled "The Case Against Breastfeeding," Hanna Rosin called nursing a "middle class mother's prison."[12] Of younger feminists, Katha Pollitt lamented, "I'm tired of 'body issues' getting so much more emphasis than economic and political ones."[13] Amanda Marcotte, who has lamented "feminist woo" and in this instance was disparaging home birth and fertility awareness, wrote, "As nice as it would be to believe otherwise, nature—which produces mosquitoes and measles and sunburns—is not your friend . . . the human ability to manipulate nature and extract what we want out of it is the defining feature of our species."[14]

But injustice is not rooted in nature. It is rooted in patriarchy. Hostility to breastfeeding, for example, is an understandable reaction to our culture: where breastfeeding is a fight or a career liability or obscene, formula may be liberating. How can we step outside this culture enough to see a path forward where demanding social support for our biology is a feminist act? How can we get to a place "where women can be fully in the world and fully in their bodies," as scholar Fiona Giles eloquently puts it?[15]

Childbearing may be the most dramatic display of how our culture has distanced itself from physiology, but I've illuminated how the pattern repeats throughout the life cycle and remains embedded in the medical standard of care, from "regulating" girls' menstrual cycles to removing menopausal ovaries and uteri. This approach has led us down a path of high-tech fertility intervention and a stunted understanding of basic hormonal physiology that could inform more appropriate and effective treatments for diseases.

In order to truly reclaim our bodies, I think we need to shift the feminist narrative from simply "owning" them and "controlling" them to also knowing them, supporting them—in essence, loving them. Feminist thinker bell hooks writes about how operating from a "love ethic" is difficult in cultures of domination. "Fear is the primary force upholding structures of domination . . . When we are taught that safety lies always with sameness, then difference, of any kind, will appear as a threat. When we choose to love we choose to move against fear—against alienation and separation."[16]

Unlike the radical health feminists, we can't completely take this on ourselves. We need better research so we can better know our bodies. We need health care providers who have a deep understanding of our biology. We need clinicians who focus less on controlling women's fertility and more on enhancing our health. We need skilled pelvic surgeons, and we need maternity care that doesn't leave our bodies and spirits broken as we embark on the epic journey of motherhood.

To do this, we need a new feminist health movement—not isolationist and centered on the self-exam, but rather collaborative, intersectional, and attuned to the broader landscape, the politics and conflicts of interest. That may require people to engage in some ideological self-examination: to acknowledge how ideas about empowerment and oppression have impacted our perspectives of female physiology and on what we deem to be good health care—so that we are making decisions from, as hooks might say, a place of love.

Medical technology offers a tempting workaround for social change, but at a cost. That cost is manifesting in chronic disease, exhaustion, and more pain than pleasure. Engaging with biological reality is one of the best arguments we have for remodeling medical care, reshaping culture, and disrupting the workplace so women don't have to trade power in the public sphere for family.

There's only so much we can ask of our bodies. But the world is what we make it.

NOTES

INTRODUCTION

1. Ashleigh Oxford, Facebook, June 13, 2018; *Switzer v. Rezvina*, Superior Court of New Jersey, Atlantic County, Docket No. 3697–14; Healthy Mothers Matter Too, https://www.healthymothersmattertoo.com; Jennifer Nelson of St. Paul, Minnesota, see chapter 6.
2. Elizabeth and Emily Blackwell, *Medicine as a Profession for Women* (New York: Trustees of the New York Infirmary for Women, 1860), p. 15.
3. William F. Rayburn, *The Obstetrician-Gynecologist Workforce in the United States* (Washington, DC: American Congress of Obstetricians and Gynecologists, 2017), p. 3.
4. National Research Council and Institute of Medicine, *U.S. Health in International Perspective: Shorter Lives, Poorer Health* (Washington, DC: National Academies Press, 2013).
5. Vicki A. Freedman, Douglas A. Wolf, and Brenda C. Spillman, "Disability-free life expectancy over 30 years: A growing female disadvantage in the US population," *American Journal of Public Health* 106, no. 6 (June 1, 2016): 1079–1085.
6. Pamela J. Salsberry, Patricia B. Reagan, and Muriel Z. Fang, "Disparities in women's health across a generation: A mother–daughter comparison," *Journal of Women's Health* 22, no. 7 (2013): 617–624.
7. David A. Kindig and Erika R. Cheng, "Even as mortality fell in most US counties, female mortality nonetheless rose in 42.8 percent of counties from 1992 to 2006," *Health Affairs* 32, no. 3 (2013): 451–458. https://www.healthaffairs.org/doi/full/10.1377/hlthaff.2011.0892.
8. Klea D. Bertakis et al., "Gender differences in the utilization of health care services," *Journal of Family Practice* 49, no. 2 (2000): 147; Kathryn R. Fingar et al., "Most Frequent Operating Room Procedures Performed in U.S. Hospitals, 2003–2012, Statistical Brief #186," Healthcare Cost and Utilization Project (HCUP), Agency for Healthcare Research and Quality, May 2016, www.hcup-us.ahrq.gov/reports/statbriefs/sb186-Operating-Room-Procedures-United-States-2012.jsp; Jennifer LaRue Huget, "Women Prescribed More Drugs Than Men but Don't Always Take Them, Research Shows," *Washington Post*, March 20, 2012.

9. Kelly Mickle, "Why Are So Many Women Being Misdiagnosed?" *Glamour*, August 11, 2017. https://www.glamour.com/story/why-are-so-many-women-being-misdiagnosed.
10. Alix Spiegel, "How a Bone Disease Grew to Fit the Prescription," *All Things Considered*, NPR, December 21, 2009. https://www.npr.org/2009/12/21/121609815/how-a-bone-disease-grew-to-fit-the-prescription.
11. Gina Kolata, "Got a Thyroid Tumor? Most Should Be Left Alone," *New York Times*, August 22, 2016.
12. Thomas J. Moore and Donald R. Mattison, "Adult utilization of psychiatric drugs and differences by sex, age, and race," *JAMA Internal Medicine* 177, no. 2 (2017): 274–275.
13. *The United States for Non-Dependence: An Analysis of the Impact of Opioid Overprescribing in America*, Pacira Pharmaceuticals, Inc., September 26, 2017. https://www.planagainstpain.com/wp-content/uploads/2017/09/PlanAgainstPain_USND.pdf.
14. Sarah J. Buckley, *Hormonal Physiology of Childbearing: Evidence and Implications for Women, Babies, and Maternity Care*, Childbirth Connection Programs, National Partnership for Women & Families (Washington, DC: 2015).
15. Lauren E. Corona et al., "Use of other treatments before hysterectomy for benign conditions in a statewide hospital collaborative," *American Journal of Obstetrics and Gynecology* 212, no. 3 (2015): 304-e1.
16. Susan Perry, "Pap-test frequency guidelines often ignored by doctors, study finds," *MinnPost*, April 10, 2013, https://www.minnpost.com/second-opinion/2013/04/pap-test-frequency-guidelines-often-ignored-doctors-study-finds/; U.S. Preventive Services Task Force, "Cervical Cancer: Screening," January 2003. https://www.uspreventiveservicestaskforce.org/Page/Document/UpdateSummaryFinal/cervical-cancer-screening1.
17. Kirsten Bibbins-Domingo et al., "Screening for gynecologic conditions with pelvic examination: US Preventive Services Task Force recommendation statement," *JAMA* 317, no. 9 (2017): 947–953.
18. American College of Physicians, "American College of Physicians Recommends Against Screening Pelvic Examination in Adult, Asymptomatic, Average Risk, Non-pregnant Women," July 1, 2014. https://www.acponline.org/acp-newsroom/american-college-of-physicians-recommends-against-screening-pelvic-examination-in-adult-asymptomatic.
19. Deepthiman Gowda, "You Don't Need That Annual Pelvic Exam. So Why Is Your Doctor Giving You One?" Reuters, August 5, 2014. https://www.reuters.com/article/idIN335547936520140805.
20. Sandra G. Boodman, "Do You Really Need That Pelvic Exam?" *Washington Post*, October 12, 2015.
21. Naomi Mezey and Cornelia T. L. Pillard, "Against the new maternalism," *Michigan Journal of Gender & Law* 18 (2011): 229.
22. "Global Car & Automobile Manufacturing Industry," IBIS World, December 2017. https://www.ibisworld.com/industry-trends/global-industry-reports/manufacturing/car-automobile-manufacturing.html.
23. Jill B. Becker, Brian J. Prendergast, and Jing W. Liang, "Female rats are not more vari-

able than male rats: A meta-analysis of neuroscience studies," *Biology of Sex Differences* 7, no. 1 (2016): 34.

24. Betty Friedan, *The Feminine Mystique* (New York: W. W. Norton, 2001), p. 462; Judith Thurman's 2010 translation confirms de Beauvoir's attitude toward biology: "Every aspect of the female reproductive system, from puberty to menopause, is approached with the same ferocious disdain," writes Francine du Plessix Gray in her *New York Times* book review. Francine du Plessix Gray, "Dispatches from the Other," *New York Times*, May 27, 2010.
25. Andrea Dworkin, *Right-Wing Women: The Politics of Domesticated Females* (London: Women's Press, 1983), p. 64.
26. Claudia Dreifus, ed., *Seizing Our Bodies: The Politics of Women's Health* (New York: Vintage Books, 1977), pp. xxiv–xxv.

CHAPTER 1

1. Melvin R. Cohen, Irving F. Stein Sr., and Bernard M. Kaye, "Spinnbarkeit: A characteristic of cervical mucus: Significance at ovulation time," *Obstetrical & Gynecological Survey* 7, no. 6 (1952): 892–893.
2. Ibid.
3. Erik Odeblad, "The discovery of different types of cervical mucus and the Billings ovulation method," *Bulletin of the Ovulation Method Research and Reference Centre of Australia* 21, no. 3 (September 1994): 3–35.
4. Ibid.
5. "Family Planning," Rockefeller Foundation: A Digital History. https://rockfound.rockarch.org/family-planning.
6. Peter Rinck, "Europe Celebrates the Forgotten Pioneer of MRI: Dr. Erik Odeblad," AuntMinnieEurope.com, June 19, 2012.
7. Yang Xia and Peter Stilbs, "The first study of cartilage by magnetic resonance: A historical account," *Cartilage* 7, no. 4 (2016): 293–297. https://www.ncbi.nlm.nih.gov/pmc/articles/PMC5029569/.
8. Jan Asplund and Sune Genell, *Proceedings of the Symposium on the Uterine Cervix as a Fertility Factor* (Lund: H. Ohlsson, 1959), preface, p. 1.
9. Erik Odeblad, "The physics of the cervical mucus," *Acta Obstetrica et Gynecologica Scandinavica* 38, suppl. 1 (2009): 44–58.
10. Erik Odeblad et al., "The biophysical properties of the cervical-vaginal secretions," *International Review of Natural Family Planning* 7, no. 1 (1983): 1–56.
11. Robert Jütte, *Contraception: A History* (Cambridge: Polity Press, 2008), p. 31.
12. Case Western Reserve University, "Highlights of the Percy Skuy History of Contraception Gallery." https://www.case.edu/affil/skuyhistcontraception/online-2012/Rhythm-method.html.
13. Birth Control Federation of America, Inc., "Modern Life Is Based on Control and Science," Smith Libraries Exhibits, undated, accessed December 6, 2018, https://libex.smith.edu/omeka/items/show/485.

14. Jonathan Eig, *The Birth of the Pill: How Four Pioneers Reinvented Sex and Launched a Revolution* (New York: Pan Macmillan, 2016).
15. Ibid., p. 3.
16. Ibid., p. 173.
17. Ibid., p. 205.
18. Sheila M. Rothman and David J. Rothman, *The Pursuit of Perfection* (New York: Pantheon, 2003), pp. 13–14.
19. Ibid., pp. 20–29.
20. National Cancer Institute, "Reproductive Cancer History and Risk," updated November 9, 2016. https://www.cancer.gov/about-cancer/causes-prevention/risk/hormones/reproductive-history-fact-sheet.
21. Gaia Pocobelli et al., "Pregnancy history and risk of endometrial cancer," *Epidemiology* 22, no. 5 (2011): 638.
22. Elseline Hoekzema et al., "Pregnancy leads to long-lasting changes in human brain structure," *Nature Neuroscience* 20, no. 2 (2017): 287.
23. For a deep dive into the history of sex hormones, I recommend Bob Ostertag, *Sex Science Self: A Social History of Estrogen, Testosterone, and Identity* (Boston: University of Massachusetts Press, 2016).
24. Jerilynn Prior and Christine Hitchcock, "Manipulating Menstruation with Hormonal Contraception: What Does the Science Say?" Centre for Menstrual Cycle and Ovulation Research, updated April 18, 2014. http://www.cemcor.ubc.ca/resources/manipulating-menstruation-hormonal-contraception-%E2%80%94-what-does-science-say.
25. Daniel R. Mishell et al., "Serum estradiol in women ingesting combination oral contraceptive steroids," *American Journal of Obstetrics and Gynecology* 114, no. 7 (1972): 923–928.
26. Eig, *The Birth of the Pill,* pp. 256–258.
27. Rachel K. Jones, "Beyond birth control: The overlooked benefits of oral contraceptive pills," Alan Guttmacher Institute (2011).
28. Elsimar M. Coutinho and Sheldon J. Segal, *Is Menstruation Obsolete?* (New York: Oxford University Press, 1999).
29. "The Doctor: Learn the History of Dr. Elsimar Coutinho," website of Dr. Elsimar Coutinho. www.elsimarcoutinho.com/o-medico/?lang=en.
30. Malcolm Gladwell, "John Rock's Error," *New Yorker,* March 13, 2000.
31. Lianne Parkin et al., "Risk of venous thromboembolism in users of oral contraceptives containing drospirenone or levonorgestrel: Nested case-control study based on UK General Practice Research Database," *British Medical Journal* 342 (2011): d2139.
32. Cynthia A. Graham et al., "The effects of steroidal contraceptives on the well-being and sexuality of women: A double-blind, placebo-controlled, two-centre study of combined and progestogen-only methods," *Contraception* 52, no. 6 (1995): 363–369.
33. Molly Redden, "The Controversial Doctor Behind the New 'Viagra for Women,'" *Mother Jones,* September 2, 2015. https://www.motherjones.com/politics/2015/09/irwin-goldstein-controversial-doctor-behind-new-viagra-women/.

34. C. W. Skovlund et al., "Association of hormonal contraception with depression," *JAMA Psychiatry* 73, no. 11 (2016): 1154–1162. DOI: 10.1001/jamapsychiatry.2016.2387.
35. Jurate Aleknaviciute et al., "The levonorgestrel-releasing intrauterine device potentiates stress reactivity," *Psychoneuroendocrinology* 80 (2017): 39–45.
36. Melinda Wenner, "Birth Control Pills Affect Women's Taste in Men," *Scientific American*, December 1, 2008. https://www.scientificamerican.com/article/birth-control-pills-affect-womens-taste/.
37. I. F. Godsland et al., "The effects of different formulations of oral contraceptive agents on lipid and carbohydrate metabolism," *New England Journal of Medicine* 323, no. 20 (1990): 1375–1381.
38. Q. Wang et al., "Effects of hormonal contraception on systemic metabolism: Cross-sectional and longitudinal evidence," *International Journal of Epidemiology* 45, no. 5 (October 2016): 1445–1457.
39. Chang Woock Lee, Mark A. Newman, and Steven E. Riechman, "Oral contraceptive use impairs muscle gains in young women," *FASEB Journal* 23, no. 1, suppl. (2009): 955.
40. B. A. Kramer, J. Kintzel, and V. Garikapaty, "Association between contraceptive use and gestational diabetes: Missouri pregnancy risk assessment monitoring system, 2007–2008," *Preventing Chronic Disease* 11 (2014).
41. Sung-Woo Kim et al., "Long-term effects of oral contraceptives on the prevalence of diabetes in post-menopausal women: 2007–2012 KNHANES," *Endocrine* (2016): 1–7.
42. D. Barad et al., "Prior oral contraception and postmenopausal fracture: A Women's Health Initiative observational cohort study," *Fertility and Sterility* 84 (2005): 374–383; Cooper et al., "Oral contraceptive pill use and fractures in women: A prospective study," *Bone* 14 (1993): 41–45; M. Vessey, J. Mant, and R. Painter, "Oral contraception and other factors in relation to hospital referral for fracture: Findings in a large cohort study," *Contraception* 57 (1998): 231–235, cited in Jerilynn C. Prior, "Adolescents' use of combined hormonal contraceptives for menstrual cycle–related problem treatment and contraception: Evidence of potential lifelong negative reproductive and bone effects," *Women's Reproductive Health* 3, no. 2 (2016): 73–92.
43. Jerilynn C. Prior et al., "Oral contraceptive use and bone mineral density in premenopausal women: Cross-sectional, population-based data from the Canadian Multicentre Osteoporosis Study," *Canadian Medical Association Journal* 165, no. 8 (2001): 1023–1029.
44. American College of Obstetricians and Gynecologists, "Depot Medroxyprogesterone Acetate and Bone Effects," Committee Opinion no. 602, June 2014.
45. Cecilie J. Sørensen et al., "Combined oral contraception and obesity are strong predictors of low-grade inflammation in healthy individuals: Results from the Danish Blood Donor Study (DBDS)," *PLOS One* 9, no. 2 (2014): e88196.
46. Jorge Sanchez-Guerrero et al., "Past use of oral contraceptives and the risk of developing systemic lupus erythematosus," *Arthritis & Rheumatism* 40, no. 5 (1997): 804–808.
47. Roni Caryn Rabin, "Birth Control Pills Still Linked to Breast Cancer, Study Finds," *New York Times*, December 6, 2017.

48. Diana Greene Foster, Eleanor Bimla Schwarz, and Daniel Grossman, "Unjustifiable Alarm About Contraceptives," *New York Times*, December 13, 2017.
49. National Cancer Institute, "Oral Contraceptives and Cancer Risk." https://www.cancer.gov/about-cancer/causes-prevention/risk/hormones/oral-contraceptives-fact-sheet.
50. Renee Heffronet et al., "Use of hormonal contraceptives and risk of HIV-1 transmission: A prospective cohort study," *Lancet Infectious Diseases* 12, no. 1 (2012): 19–26.
51. Erik Odeblad, "Some notes on the cervical crypts," *Bulletin of the Ovulation Method Research and Reference Centre of Australia* 24, no. 2 (June 1997): 31.
52. Odeblad, "The discovery of different types of different types of cervical mucus and the Billings ovulation method."
53. Eig, *The Birth of the Pill*, p. 251.
54. Joyce C. Abma and G. M. Martinez, "Sexual Activity and Contraceptive Use Among Teenagers in the United States, 2011–2015," *National Health Statistics Reports* 104 (2017): 1–23.
55. K. Birch Petersen et al., "Ovarian reserve assessment in users of oral contraception seeking fertility advice on their reproductive lifespan," *Human Reproduction* 30, no. 10 (2015): 2364–2375, cited in J. C. Prior, "Adolescents' use of combined hormonal contraceptives for menstrual cycle–related problem treatment and contraception," *Women's Reproductive Health* 3, no. 2 (2016): 73–92.
56. Nayana Talukdar et al., "Effect of long-term combined oral contraceptive pill use on endometrial thickness," *Obstetrics & Gynecology* 120, no. 2 (2012): 348–354.
57. Jill Filipovic, "Critics Can't Decide if Feminists Hate Sex or Are Having Too Much of It," *Guardian*, September 6, 2013. https://www.theguardian.com/commentisfree/2013/sep/06/sweetening-the-pill-book-sets-women-back; Jessica Grose, "Do Not Fear Your Birth Control," Slate, January 22, 2014. https://slate.com/human-interest/2014/01/magazine-stories-about-essure-yaz-and-nuvaring-scaring-you-put-down-the-cosmo-and-talk-to-your-doctor.html.
58. Barbara Seaman, "The Pill and I: 40 Years On, the Relationship Remains Wary," *New York Times*, June 25, 2000.
59. Chandler Marrs, "Real Risk Contraceptive Project: Birth Control and Blood Clots Study," Lucine Health Sciences, Inc., December 1, 2016, citing Dr. John R. McCain speaking at the Nelson Pill Hearings, transcript page 6473. https://www.researchgate.net/publication/329545331_Real_Risk_Contraceptive_Study_Birth_Control_and_Blood_Clots_Phase_1.
60. Ibid., p. 7, citing Dr. Edmond Kassouf speaking at the Nelson Pill Hearings, transcript pages 6108–6133.
61. Eig, *The Birth of the Pill*, p. 158.
62. Susan Jick, "Oral Contraceptives and the Risk of Venous Thromboembolism," in *Medicines for Women*, ed. Mira Harrison-Woolrych (Cham, Switzerland: Adis, 2015), pp. 181–201.
63. C. L. Westhoff et al., "Oral contraceptive discontinuation: Do side effects matter?" *American Journal of Obstetrics and Gynecology* 196, no. 4 (2007): 412-e1; K. Daniels,

W. D. Mosher, and J. Jones, "Contraceptive methods women have ever used: United States, 1982–2010," *National Health Statistics Reports* 62, no. 20 (2013), cited in Marrs, "Real Risk Contraceptive Project," p. 8.

64. Jick, "Oral Contraceptives and the Risk of Venous Thromboembolism."
65. According to the FDA Adverse Event Reporting System (FAERS), as of June 30, 2018, accessed via: https://www.fda.gov/drugs/guidancecomplianceregulatoryinformation/surveillance/adversedrugeffects/ucm070093.htm.
66. Elizabeth Siegel Watkins, "How the Pill became a lifestyle drug: The pharmaceutical industry and birth control in the United States since 1960," *American Journal of Public Health* 102, no. 8 (2012): 1462–1472.
67. Donna Drucker, "The Cervical Cap in the Feminist Women's Health Movement, 1976–1988," NOTCHES, March 24, 2016. http://notchesblog.com/2016/03/24/the-cervical-cap-in-the-feminist-womens-health-movement-1976-1988/.
68. Rebecca Chalker, *The Complete Cervical Cap Guide* (New York: Harper & Row, 1987); A. Chandra et al., "Fertility, family planning, and reproductive health of U.S. Women: Data from the 2002 National Survey of Family Growth," *Vital and Health Statistics*, series 23, Data from the National Survey of Family Growth 25 (2002): 1–160.
69. Vanessa Grigoriadis, "Waking Up from the Pill," *New York* magazine, November 28, 2010.
70. Elaine Tyler May, *America and the Pill: A History of Promise, Peril, and Liberation* (New York: Basic Books, 2010), p. 171.
71. Chelsea B. Polis et al., "An updated systematic review of epidemiological evidence on hormonal contraceptive methods and HIV acquisition in women," *AIDS* 30, no. 17 (2016): 2665.
72. Laura Eldridge, *In Our Control: The Complete Guide to Contraceptive Choices for Women* (New York: Seven Stories Press, 2011), p. 34.
73. Amanda Marcotte, "Pills," RawStory, April 5, 2010. https://www.rawstory.com/2010/04/pandagon-pills/; Amanda Marcotte, "Ricki Lake Starts a Crusade Against Hormonal Birth Control," Slate, June 25, 2015. http://www.slate.com/blogs/xx_factor/2015/06/25/ricki_lake_christian_right_hero_she_s_making_a_documentary_against_hormonal.html; "Sweetening the Pill Kickstarter," YouTube, uploaded June 18, 2018. https://www.youtube.com/watch?v=2bXvR2jpyhY#action=share.
74. Holly Grigg-Spall, *Sweetening the Pill: Or How We Got Hooked on Hormonal Birth Control* (Alresford, UK: John Hunt Publishing, 2013), pp. 9–10.
75. Ibid., p. 19.
76. Lindsay Beyerstein, "The Truth About the Pill," Slate, September 3, 2013. http://www.slate.com/articles/double_x/doublex/2013/09/_sweetening_the_pill_by_holly_grigg_spall_reviewed.html.
77. Jennifer Gunter (@DrJenGunter), "@annejumps do u have a link to your debunking of that atrocious pill book?" Twitter, September 3, 2013, 4:32 p.m.; Jennifer Gunter (@DrJenGunter), "@annejumps @laureneoneal it is sounding increasingly like a pro life

agenda," September 3, 2013, 5:48 p.m. https://twitter.com/DrJenGunter/status/375057828555141120.

78. Janelle Martell, "Tell Zero Books: Birth Control Is Not Sexist and Dangerous," Care2. http://www.thepetitionsite.com/659/006/921/tell-zero-books-birth-control-is-not-sexist-and-dangerous/.
79. Holly Grigg-Spall, "Reproductive Writes: Not Just Another Choice: An Interview with Laura Wershler," Bitchmedia, March 27, 2010, https://www.bitchmedia.org/post/reproductive-writes-not-just-another-choice-an-interview-with-laura-wershler.
80. Rachel K. Jones et al., "Better than nothing or savvy risk-reduction practice? The importance of withdrawal," *Contraception* 79, no. 6 (2009): 407–410. https://www.guttmacher.org/sites/default/files/pdfs/pubs/journals/reprints/Contraception79-407-410.pdf.
81. Hadley Freeman, "Why young women are going off the pill and on to contraception voodoo," *Guardian*, October 29, 2012. https://www.theguardian.com/commentisfree/2013/oct/29/young-women-going-off-pill-contraception-birth-control.
82. ACOG Committee on Adolescent Health Care, "ACOG Committee Opinion No. 349, November 2006: Menstruation in girls and adolescents: Using the menstrual cycle as a vital sign," *Obstetrics and Gynecology* 108, no. 5 (2006): 1323. http://www.acog.org/Resources-And-Publications/Committee-Opinions/Committee-on-Adolescent-Health-Care/Menstruation-in-Girls-and-Adolescents-Using-the-Menstrual-Cycle-as-a-Vital-Sign.
83. These cervix selfies are credited to the Beautiful Cervix Project, beautifulcervix.com.
84. Petra Frank-Herrmann et al., "The effectiveness of a fertility awareness based method to avoid pregnancy in relation to a couples sexual behaviour during the fertile time: A prospective longitudinal study," *Human Reproduction* 22, no. 5 (2007).
85. E. Scherwitzl et al., "Perfect-use and typical use Pearl Index of a contraceptive mobile app," *Contraception* 96, no. 6 (2017): 420–425. https://www.naturalcycles.com/en/hcp/research-and-publications/publications-and-clinical-findings/.
86. Dr. John Billings, "A Story of God's Providence," LifeIssues.net. http://lifeissues.net/writers/bil/bil_02billingshistory.html.
87. R. J. Norman and Adrian Thomas, "James Boyer Brown, 1919–2009," *Human Reproduction Update* 17, no. 2 (March 1, 2011): 139–140. https://doi.org/10.1093/humupd/dmq047; James Boyer Brown's first paper, "A chemical method for the determination of oestriol, oestrone and oestradiol in human urine," *Biochemical Journal* 60, no. 2 (1955), has been cited more than 1,300 times.
88. Margaret Nofziger, *Signs of Fertility: The Personal Science of Natural Birth Control* (Deatsville, Alabama: MND Publishing, Inc., 1998).
89. Lisa Hendrickson-Jack, Fertility Friday, episode 064, "Fertility Awareness, Feminism, and Reproductive Freedoms, Geraldine Matus," posted February 12, 2016. http://fertilityfriday.com/geraldine-matus/.
90. Toni Weschler, *Taking Charge of Your Fertility: The Definitive Guide to Natural Birth Control, Pregnancy Achievement, and Reproductive Health* (New York: Random House, 2003), p. 294.

91. Katie Singer, "Cycles of Hot and Cold," in *Voices of the Women's Health Movement*, vol. 1, ed. Barbara Seaman and Laura Eldridge (New York: Seven Stories Press, 2012), pp. 174–177.

CHAPTER 2

1. Emily L. Que et al., "Quantitative mapping of zinc fluxes in the mammalian egg reveals the origin of fertilization-induced zinc sparks," *Nature Chemistry* 7, no. 2 (2015): 130, in Bec Crew, "Sparks Literally Fly When an Egg Meets Sperm, World-First Images Reveal," Science Alert, December 16, 2014. http://www.sciencealert.com/world-first-images-reveal-sparks-literally-fly-when-an-egg-meets-sperm.
2. Athena Beldecos et al., "The importance of feminist critique for contemporary cell biology," *Feminism and Science* 3, no. 1 (1989): 172.
3. Sheree L. Boulet et al., "Trends in use of and reproductive outcomes associated with intracytoplasmic sperm injection," *JAMA* 313, no. 3 (2015): 255–263.
4. Manon Ceelen et al., "Growth and development of children born after in vitro fertilization," *Fertility and Sterility* 90, no. 5 (2008): 1662–1673.
5. Pamela Schendelaar et al., "The effect of preimplantation genetic screening on neurological, cognitive and behavioural development in 4-year-old children: Follow-up of a RCT," *Human Reproduction* 28, no. 6 (2013): 1508–1518.
6. Michelle Lynne LaBonte, "An analysis of US fertility centre educational materials suggests that informed consent for preimplantation genetic diagnosis may be inadequate," *Journal of Medical Ethics* 38, no. 8 (2012): 479–484.
7. Michèle Hansen et al., "The risk of major birth defects after intracytoplasmic sperm injection and in vitro fertilization," *New England Journal of Medicine* 346 (2002): 725–730.
8. Centers for Disease Control and Prevention, *2015 ART National Summary Report*, pp. 7, 13. https://www.cdc.gov/art/pdf/2015-national-summary-slides/ART_2015_graphs_and_charts.pdf.
9. Jennifer Schneider, Jennifer Lahl, and Wendy Kramer, "Long-term breast cancer risk following ovarian stimulation in young egg donors: A call for follow-up, research and informed consent," *Reproductive Biomedicine Online* 34, no. 5 (2017): 480–485.
10. Elizabeth E. Hatch et al., "Intake of sugar-sweetened beverages and fecundability in a North American preconception cohort," *Epidemiology* 29, no. 3 (2018): 369–378.
11. Gianpiero D. Palermo et al., "Intracytoplasmic sperm injection: State of the art in humans," *Reproduction* 154, no. 6 (2017): f17–f110.
12. Thomas J. Walsh et al., "Increased risk of testicular germ cell cancer among infertile men," *Archives of Internal Medicine* 169, no. 4 (2009): 351–356.
13. CDC, *2015 ART National Summary Report*, p. 7.
14. Charalambos Siristatidis and Siladitya Bhattacharya, "Unexplained infertility: Does it really exist? Does it matter?" *Human Reproduction* 22, no. 8 (2007): 2084–2087.
15. Megan Jula, "4 Lesbians Sue Over New Jersey Rules on Fertility Treatment," *New York Times*, August 8, 2016.
16. Division of Reproductive Health, Centers for Disease Control and Prevention, "Figures

from the 2015 Assisted Reproductive Technology National Summary Report," 2015, p. 17. https://www.cdc.gov/art/pdf/2015-national-summary-slides/ART_2015_graphs_and_charts.pdf.
17. Robin Marantz Henig, "Should You Freeze Your Eggs?" Slate, September 30, 2014. http://www.slate.com/articles/health_and_science/medical_examiner/2014/09/egg_freezing_marketing_campaigns_lie_about_success_rates_of_this_fertility.html.
18. Jessica Bennett, "Company-Paid Egg Freezing Will Be the Great Equalizer," *Time*, October 15, 2014. http://time.com/3509930/company-paid-egg-freezing-will-be-the-great-equalizer/.
19. American Society for Reproductive Medicine, "Can I Freeze My Eggs to Use Later if I'm Not Sick?" Fact sheet, 2014. https://www.reproductivefacts.org/news-and-publications/patient-fact-sheets-and-booklets/documents/fact-sheets-and-info-booklets/can-i-freeze-my-eggs-to-use-later-if-im-not-sick/.
20. Caroline Praderio, "There's a Dark Side to Egg Freezing That No One Is Talking About," *Insider*, March 22, 2017. https://www.thisisinsider.com/egg-freezing-failure-risks-2017-3.
21. Alison Motluk, "Is Egg Donation Dangerous?" *Maisonneuve*, January 21, 2013. https://maisonneuve.org/article/2013/01/21/egg-donation-dangerous/.
22. Lisa Miller, "Parents of a Certain Age," *New York*, September 25, 2011.

CHAPTER 3

1. Linda Gordon, *The Moral Property of Women: A History of Birth Control Politics in America* (Chicago: University of Illinois Press, 2002), p. 21.
2. Barbara Diane Reed et al., "Prevalence and demographic characteristics of vulvodynia in a population-based sample," *American Journal of Obstetrics and Gynecology* 206, no. 2 (2012): 170-e1.
3. Veronica Manchester, "Let Who Put What Where? Finding a Cure for Pelvic Pain," *Elle*, August 27, 2013. https://www.elle.com/beauty/health-fitness/advice/a26316/cure-pelvic-pain/.
4. Chloe Angyal, "When Sex Wouldn't Stop Hurting," Salon, December 10, 2010. https://www.salon.com/2010/12/10/sex_chronic_pain/.
5. Jeffrey R. Harris and Robert B. Wallace, "The Institute of Medicine's new report on living well with chronic illness," *Preventing Chronic Disease* 9 (2012).
6. C. Veasley et al., "Impact of Chronic Overlapping Pain Conditions on Public Health and the Urgent Need for Safe and Effective Treatment: 2015 Analysis and Policy Recommendations," Chronic Pain Research Alliance (2015), p. 5.
7. Jacob Bornstein et al., "2015 ISSVD, ISSWSH, and IPPS consensus terminology and classification of persistent vulvar pain and vulvodynia," *Journal of Sexual Medicine* 13, no. 4 (2016): 607–612.
8. Denniz A. Zolnoun et al., "Overlap between orofacial pain and vulvar vestibulitis syndrome," *Clinical Journal of Pain* 24, no. 3 (2008): 187.
9. Andrew Goldstein et al., "Polymorphisms of the androgen receptor gene and hormonal

contraceptive induced provoked vestibulodynia," *Journal of Sexual Medicine* 11, no. 11 (2014): 2764–2771.

10. Camran Nezhat, Farr Nezhat, and Ceana Nezhat, "Endometriosis: Ancient disease, ancient treatments," *Fertility and Sterility* 98, no. 6 (2012): S1–S62.
11. David Redwine, "Redefining Endometriosis in the Modern Era: An Overview of the Origin, History, Diagnosis, and Treatment of Endometriosis," *Endopaedia.* http://endopaedia.info/origin1.html.
12. Sherry E. Rier et al., "Endometriosis in rhesus monkeys (*Macaca mulatta*) following chronic exposure to 2, 3, 7, 8-tetrachlorodibenzo-p-dioxin," *Toxicological Sciences* 21, no. 4 (1993): 433–441.
13. Hifsa Mobeen, Nadeem Afzal, and Muhammad Kashif, "Polycystic Ovary Syndrome May Be an Autoimmune Disorder," *Scientifica* (2016).
14. Lena Dunham, "In Her Own Words: Lena Dunham on Her Decision to Have a Hysterectomy at 31," *Vogue*, February 14, 2018. https://www.vogue.com/article/lena-dunham-hysterectomy-vogue-march-2018-issue.
15. Julie K. Bower et al., "Black–white differences in hysterectomy prevalence: The CARDIA study," *American Journal of Public Health* 99, no. 2 (2009): 300–307.
16. Lynne T. Shuster et al., "Prophylactic oophorectomy in premenopausal women and long-term health," *Menopause International* 14, no. 3 (2008): 111–116; B. Rizk et al., "Recurrence of endometriosis after hysterectomy," *Facts, Views & Vision in ObGyn* 6, no. 4 (2014): 219.
17. Jennifer Block and Fernanda Camarena, "Her Own Devices: Is a Contraceptive Implant Making Us Sick?" *Reveal*, Center for Investigative Reporting, July 29, 2017. https://www.revealnews.org/episodes/her-own-devices-is-a-contraceptive-implant-making-us-sick/.
18. AAGL Advancing Minimally Invasive Gynecology Worldwide, "AAGL practice report: Practice guidelines on the prevention of apical prolapse at the time of benign hysterectomy," *Journal of Minimally Invasive Gynecology* 21, no. 5 (2014): 715–722. http://www.aagl.org/wp-content/uploads/2013/03/Aprical-Prolapse-in-JMIG.pdf.
19. Abraham Shahoua, "Da Vinci Robotic Surgery for Hysterectomy," YouTube, November 23, 2009. https://www.youtube.com/watch?v=UFb-1XDpYkU.
20. Stefano Uccella et al., "Vaginal cuff closure after minimally invasive hysterectomy: Our experience and systematic review of the literature," *American Journal of Obstetrics and Gynecology* 205, no. 2 (2011): 119–e1.
21. Sarah L. Cohen et al., "Outpatient hysterectomy volume in the United States," *Journal of Minimally Invasive Gynecology* 24, no. 7 (2017): S181; Marisa R. Adelman and Howard T. Sharp, "Ovarian conservation vs. removal at the time of benign hysterectomy," *American Journal of Obstetrics and Gynecology* 218, no. 3 (2018): 269–279.
22. Risa Lonnée-Hoffmann and Ingrid Pinas, "Effects of hysterectomy on sexual function," *Current Sexual Health Reports* 6, no. 4 (2014): 244–251.
23. Federation of Feminist Women's Health Centers, *A New View of a Woman's Body: A Fully Illustrated Guide* (New York: Simon & Schuster, 1981), p. 50.

24. Brian E. Schirf et al., "Complications of uterine fibroid embolization," *Seminars in Interventional Radiology* 23, no. 2 (2006): 143. https://www.ncbi.nlm.nih.gov/pmc/articles/PMC3036365.
25. Mindy K. Longinotti et al., "Probability of hysterectomy after endometrial ablation," *Obstetrics & Gynecology* 112, no. 6 (2008): 1214–1220. https://www.ncbi.nlm.nih.gov/pubmed/19037028.
26. Walter A. Rocca et al., "Long-term effects of bilateral oophorectomy on brain aging: Unanswered questions from the Mayo Clinic cohort study of oophorectomy and aging," *Women's Health* 5, no. 1 (2009): 39–48.
27. Shuster et al., "Prophylactic oophorectomy in premenopausal women and long-term health."
28. Eve Agee, *The Uterine Health Companion: A Holistic Guide to Lifelong Wellness* (New York: Celestial Arts, 2010), pp. 32–34.
29. Whitney R. Robinson et al., "For us black women, shift of hysterectomy to outpatient settings may have lagged behind white women: A claims-based analysis, 2011–2013," *BMC Health Services Research* 17, no. 1 (2017): 526.
30. Harriet A. Washington, *Medical Apartheid: The Dark History of Medical Experimentation on Black Americans from Colonial Times to the Present* (New York: Doubleday, 2006), pp. 202–203.
31. Mary Daly, *Gyn/ecology: The Metaethics of Radical Feminism* (Boston: Beacon Press, 1990), pp. 227–228.
32. Harvey Graham, *Eternal Eve* (New York: Doubleday, 1951), p. 519.
33. Ibid., pp. 421–453.
34. Ibid., p. 623.
35. Deborah Larned, "The Epidemic in Unnecessary Hysterectomy," in *Seizing Our Bodies: The Politics of Women's Health*, ed. Claudia Dreifus (New York: Vintage Books, 1978), p. 198.
36. R. C. Wright, "Hysterectomy: Past, present, and future," *Obstetrics and Gynecology* 33, no. 4 (1969): 560–563, quoted in Larned, "The Epidemic in Unnecessary Hysterectomy."
37. Daly, *Gyn/ecology*, p. 239.
38. Lee Rothberg, "Hysterectomy: The Shocking Truth," *Woman's Newspaper*, Princeton, NJ, 1986. http://www.whale.to/a/coffey.html.
39. Jennifer Gunter, "Surprise! When it comes to a vaginal hysterectomy, this insurance company gets it right," KevinMD.com, March 16, 2015. http://www.kevinmd.com/blog/2015/03/surprise-comes-vaginal-hysterectomy-insurance-company-gets-right.html.
40. International Society of Cosmetogynecology Faculty, Marco A. Pelosi II, MD. http://www.iscgyn.com/en/marco_pelosi1.
41. Klim McPherson, Giorgia Gon, and Maggie Scott, "International Variations in a Selected Number of Surgical Procedures," OECD Health Working Paper 61 (2013), p. 23.
42. Vicki Hufnagel with Susan Golant, *No More Hysterectomies* (New York: Dutton Adult, 1988), p. 4.
43. Lauren A. Wise et al., "Perceived racial discrimination and risk of uterine leiomyomata," *Epidemiology* 18, no. 6 (2007): 747–757.

CHAPTER 4

1. Hanna E. Bloomfield et al., *Screening Pelvic Examinations in Asymptomatic Average Risk Adult Women*, Department of Veterans Affairs, Health Services Research & Development Service, 2013. https://www.hsrd.research.va.gov/publications/esp/pelvic-exam.pdf.
2. "ACOG Statement on USPSTF Draft Recommendations on Pelvic Exams," American College of Obstetricians and Gynecologists, June 28, 2016. https://www.acog.org/About-ACOG/News-Room/Statements/2016/ACOG-Statement-on-USPSTF-Draft-Recommendations-on-Pelvic-Exams.
3. Jillian T. Henderson et al., "Routine bimanual pelvic examinations: Practices and beliefs of US obstetrician-gynecologists," *American Journal of Obstetrics and Gynecology* 208, no. 2 (2013): 109-e1. https://www.ajog.org/article/S0002-9378(12)02070-4/fulltext.
4. Terri Kapsalis, *Public Privates: Performing Gynecology from Both Ends of the Speculum* (Durham, NC: Duke University Press, 1997), p. 70.
5. American College of Obstetricians and Gynecologists, Committee on Ethics, "Professional Responsibilities in Obstetric-Gynecologic Medical Education and Training," No. 500, August 2011. https://www.acog.org/Clinical-Guidance-and-Publications/Committee-Opinions/Committee-on-Ethics/Professional-Responsibilities-in-Obstetric-Gynecologic-Medical-Education-and-Training; Phoebe Friesen, "Educational pelvic exams on anesthetized women: Why consent matters," *Bioethics* 32, no. 5 (2018): 298–307. https://onlinelibrary.wiley.com/doi/full/10.1111/bioe.12441.
6. U.S. Preventive Services Task Force, "Final Recommendation Statement: Breast Cancer: Screening," November 2016. https://www.uspreventiveservicestaskforce.org/Page/Document/RecommendationStatementFinal/breast-cancer-screening1.
7. Calonge's analogy is borne out by a 2014 study in *JAMA*, which estimated that under the old yearly mammogram guidelines, for every five lives saved by "early detection," some 6,000 patients dealt with false-positive results: L. E. Pace and N. L. Keating, "A systematic assessment of benefits and risks to guide breast cancer screening decisions," *JAMA* 311, no. 13 (2014): 1327–1335; Carey Goldberg, "Mammogram? 50 Years of Data and Decision Aids to Help You Think Through," WBUR CommonHealth, April 1, 2014. http://www.wbur.org/commonhealth/2014/04/01/mammogram-decision-jama.
8. C. Harding et al., "Breast cancer screening, incidence, and mortality across US counties," *JAMA Internal Medicine* 175, no. 9 (2015): 1483–1489, DOI: 10.1001/jamainternmed.2015.3043.
9. U.S. Preventive Services Task Force, "Final Recommendation Statement: Cervical Cancer: Screening," August 2018. https://www.uspreventiveservicestaskforce.org/Page/Document/UpdateSummaryFinal/cervical-cancer-screening2.
10. Carolyn L. Westhoff, Heidi E. Jones, and Maryam Guiahi, "Do new guidelines and technology make the routine pelvic examination obsolete?" *Journal of Women's Health* 20, no. 1 (January 2011): 5–10. https://doi.org/10.1089/jwh.2010.2349.
11. Sandra G. Boodman, "Do You Really Need That Pelvic Exam?" *Washington Post*, October 12, 2015. https://www.washingtonpost.com/national/health-science/do-you

-really-need-that-pelvic-exam/2015/10/12/8c79942e-3b7e-11e5-8e98-115a3cf7d7ae_story.html?utm_term=.cd2c4f2f8f10.
12. Howard Kelly, *Medical Gynecology* (New York: D. Appleton & Company, 1908), p. 1.
13. Ibid., p. 3.
14. Ronald M. Cyr, "History of Obstetrics and Gynecology." http://history-of-obgyn.com/.
15. U.S. Preventive Services Task Force, "Final Recommendation Statement: Screening for Gynecologic Conditions with Pelvic Examination," March 2017. https://www.uspreventiveservicestaskforce.org/Announcements/News/Item/final-recommendation-statement-screening-for-gynecologic-conditions-with-pelvic-examination.
16. Westhoff, Jones, and Guiahi, "Do new guidelines and technology make the routine pelvic examination obsolete?"
17. George F. Sawaya et al., "Effect of professional society recommendations on women's desire for a routine pelvic examination," *American Journal of Obstetrics and Gynecology* 217, no. 3 (2017): 338-e1.
18. P. A. Ubel, C. Jepson, and A. Silver-Isenstadt, "Don't ask, don't tell: A change in medical student attitudes after obstetrics/gynecology clerkships toward seeking consent for pelvic examinations on an anesthetized patient," *American Journal of Obstetrics and Gynecology* 188, no. 2 (2003): 575.
19. Gina Kolata, "Why 'Useless' Surgery Is Still Popular," *New York Times*, August 3, 2016. https://www.nytimes.com/2016/08/04/upshot/the-right-to-know-that-an-operation-is-next-to-useless.html?_r=0.
20. Katie Hafner and Griffin Palmer, "Skin Cancers Rise, Along with Questionable Treatments," *New York Times*, November 20, 2017.
21. National Academies, "What's Possible for Health Care?" Infographic, revised March 2013. http://www.nationalacademies.org/hmd/Reports/2012/Best-Care-at-Lower-Cost-The-Path-to-Continuously-Learning-Health-Care-in-America/Infographic.aspx.
22. R. Nash et al., "State variation in the receipt of a contralateral prophylactic mastectomy among women who received a diagnosis of invasive unilateral early-stage breast cancer in the United States," *JAMA Surgery* 152, no. 7 (2017): 648–657. DOI: 10.1001/jamasurg.2017.0115.
23. Amanda Carson Banks, *Birth Chairs, Midwives, and Medicine* (Jackson: University Press of Mississippi, 2012), p. 68.
24. Richard W. Wertz and Dorothy C. Wertz, *Lying-In: A History of Childbirth in America* (New Haven, CT: Yale University Press, 1989), p. 66.
25. Barbara Ehrenreich and Deirdre English, *For Her Own Good* (New York: Anchor, 1978), p. 97.
26. Banks, *Birth Chairs, Midwives, and Medicine*, p. 39.
27. Harvey Graham, *Eternal Eve* (New York: Doubleday, 1951), p. 617.
28. Laura Helmuth, "The Disturbing, Shameful History of Childbirth Deaths," Slate, September 10, 2013. http://www.slate.com/articles/health_and_science/science_of_longevity/2013/09/death_in_childbirth_doctors_increased_maternal_mortality_in_the_20th_century.html.

29. Jennifer Block, *Pushed: The Painful Truth About Childbirth and Modern Maternity Care* (Cambridge, MA: Da Capo Press, 2007), pp. 214–215.
30. Ehrenreich and English, *For Her Own Good*, p. 98.
31. Deirdre Cooper Owens, *Medical Bondage: Race, Gender, and the Origins of American Gynecology* (Athens: University of Georgia Press, 2018), p. 4.
32. Ibid., pp. 18, 31–32.
33. Ibid., p. 20.
34. Ibid., p. 31.
35. Ibid., p. 28.
36. Leyland A. Robinson, "The evolution of the gynecologist," *BJOG* 58, no. 1 (1951): 50–72.
37. Sam Gordon Berkow, "After office hours: Obstetrics, Cinderella of medicine," *Obstetrics and Gynecology* (1954): 222–224. http://history-of-obgyn.com/uploads/3/5/3/8/3538227/1954-berkow-obs_cinderella-rev-feb2015.pdf.
38. Paul Titus, "American Association of Obstetricians, Gynecologists and Abdominal Surgeons: Presidential address: Obstetrics and gynecology as a united specialty," *American Journal of Obstetrics and Gynecology* 37, no. 4 (1939): 545–558.
39. Ibid.
40. Ralph W. Hale, "The obstetrician and gynecologist: Primary care physician or specialist?" *American Journal of Obstetrics and Gynecology* 172, no. 4 (1995): 1181–1183; William Hurd, Sheela M. Barhan, and Robert E. Rogers, "Obstetrician-gynecologist as primary care provider," *American Journal of Managed Care* 7 (2001): SP19–24.
41. Sarah L. Cohen and Emily Hinchcliff, "Is surgical training in ob/gyn residency adequate?" *Contemporary OB/GYN* 61, no. 8 (2016): 24.
42. Sandy Hingston, "What Are the Chances?" *Boston Magazine*, March 20, 2016.
43. Cook Urological Inc., Cook Tissue Morcellator, FDA 510K Premarket Notification K925851, filed November 17, 1992, approved May 21, 1993. https://www.accessdata.fda.gov/scripts/cdrh/cfdocs/cfPMN/pmn.cfm?ID=K925851.
44. Matthew Bin Han Ong, "Amy Reed, Physician and Patient Who 'Moved Mountains' to End Widespread Use of Power Morcellation, Dies at 44," *Cancer Letter*, May 26, 2017. https://cancerletter.com/articles/20170526_1/.
45. Michael A. Seidman et al., "Peritoneal dissemination complicating morcellation of uterine mesenchymal neoplasms," *PLOS One* 7, no. 11 (2012): e50058. http://journals.plos.org/plosone/article?id=10.1371/journal.pone.0050058.
46. Vrunda B. Desai et al., "Occult gynecologic cancer in women undergoing hysterectomy or myomectomy for benign indications," *Obstetrics & Gynecology* 131, no. 4 (2018): 642–651. https://journals.lww.com/greenjournal/Abstract/publishahead/Occult_Gynecologic_Cancer_in_Women_Undergoing.98119.aspx.
47. FDA Center for Devices and Radiological Health Medical Devices Advisory Committee, Obstetrics and Gynecology Devices Panel, July 11, 2014.
48. "FDA in Brief: FDA Releases New Findings on the Risks of Spreading Hidden Uterine Cancer Through the Use of Laparoscopic Power Morcellators," December 14, 2017. https://www.fda.gov/newsevents/newsroom/fdainbrief/ucm589137.htm.

49. Jennifer Block, "The Battle over Essure," *Washington Post Magazine*, July 26, 2017.
50. Vikki Ortiz Healy, "'We Want to Make Our Voices Heard': Women Battle FDA over Contraceptive Device They Say Made Them Sick," *Chicago Tribune*, May 8, 2018. http://www.chicagotribune.com/lifestyles/health/98365218-132.html.
51. *The Bleeding Edge*, dir. Kirby Dick, Netflix Original Documentary, 2018, 18:45 minutes.
52. FDA, "Enforcement Report," March 17, 1999, quoted in Jane Akre, "ProteGen—The First Mesh, a 20 Year History," Mesh News Desk, July 25, 2016. https://www.meshmedicaldevicenewsdesk.com/protegen-first-mesh-20-year-history/.
53. Husam Abed et al., "Incidence and management of graft erosion, wound granulation, and dyspareunia following vaginal prolapse repair with graft materials: A systematic review," *International Urogynecology Journal* 22, no. 7 (2011): 789–798.
54. Cheryl B. Iglesia et al., "Vaginal mesh for prolapse: A randomized controlled trial," *Obstetrics & Gynecology* 116, no. 2 (2010): 293–303.
55. Lindsay Beyerstein, "A Female Surgical Nightmare," *In These Times*, June 13, 2012. http://inthesetimes.com/article/13353/a_female_surgical_nightmare/.
56. Elaine Silvestrini, "Transvaginal Mesh Lawsuits," DrugWatch. https://www.drugwatch.com/transvaginal-mesh/lawsuits/.
57. Hannah Devlin, "Revealed: Johnson & Johnson's 'Irresponsible' Actions over Vaginal Mesh Implant," *Guardian*, September 29, 2017. https://www.theguardian.com/society/2017/sep/29/revealed-johnson-johnsons-irresponsible-actions-over-vaginal-mesh-implant.
58. Hooman Noorchashm, "An Open Letter to the American College of Surgeons: Residency Training in Gynecology Is Dangerously Deficient," Medium, October 1, 2017. https://medium.com/@noorchashm/an-open-letter-to-the-american-college-of-surgeons-residency-training-in-gynecology-is-dangerously-e1c4524ad638.
59. Tanya Basu, "The Million-Dollar Deal Behind the Vaginal Mesh Implant Mess," Daily Beast, October 13, 2018. https://www.thedailybeast.com/the-million-dollar-deal-behind-the-vaginal-mesh-implant-mess.
60. "Prolift Mesh: What Did Johnson & Johnson Know?" YouTube, February 16, 2017. https://www.youtube.com/watch?v=lBxj4h8C36M.
61. Jonathan Gornall, "Vaginal mesh implants: Putting the relations between UK doctors and industry in plain sight," *British Medical Journal* 363 (2018): k4164.
62. "Prolift Mesh: What Did Johnson & Johnson Know?" YouTube.
63. Nicholas Fogelson, "On Hysterectomies and Hysterectomy Alternatives," *Academic OB/GYN*, June 18, 2017. https://academicobgyn.com/2017/06/18/on-hysterectomies-and-hysterectomy-alternatives/#more-1865.
64. Jennifer Levitz and Betsy McKay, "CDC Eyes Review of Gynecological Cancer Screens," *Wall Street Journal*, May 2, 2018. https://www.wsj.com/articles/cdc-eyes-review-of-gynecological-cancer-screens-1525318834.
65. Rebecca Chalker, *The Clitoral Truth* (New York: Seven Stories Press, 2000), p. 77.
66. Bonnie Fortune, "Temporary Conversations: Suzann Gage" (Temporary Services at

Half Letter Press, 2009), p. 15. http://www.bonniefortune.info/overview/temporary-conversations-suzann-gage/.

67. Chalker, *The Clitoral Truth*, p. 84.
68. "Cliteracy," Huffington Post. http://projects.huffingtonpost.com/cliteracy.
69. Federation of Feminist Women's Health Centers, *A New View of a Woman's Body: A Fully Illustrated Guide* (New York: Simon & Schuster, 1981), pp. 39–41.
70. Ibid., p. 47.
71. "Cliteracy."
72. Tomasz Frymorgen, "This Woman Is Creating Clitoris Street Art to Get People Talking About Female Pleasure," BBC News, March 27, 2018. http://www.bbc.co.uk/bbcthree/item/08917f1e-e93c-4d3a-aa10-bbb29f0eaaf4.
73. Helen E. O'Connell et al., "Anatomical relationship between urethra and clitoris," *Journal of Urology* 159, no. 6 (1998): 1892–1897.
74. Emmanuele A. Jannini, Odile Buisson, and Alberto Rubio-Casillas, "Beyond the G-spot: Clitourethrovaginal complex anatomy in female orgasm," *Nature Reviews Urology* 11, no. 9 (2014): 531.
75. Sharon Mascall, "Time for Rethink on the Clitoris," BBC News, June 11, 2006. http://news.bbc.co.uk/go/pr/fr/-/2/hi/health/5013866.stm.
76. "History: The Clitoris' Vanishing Act," Huffington Post. http://projects.huffingtonpost.com/cliteracy.
77. Robbie Gonzalez, "Until 2009, the Human Clitoris Was an Absolute Mystery," io9, January 16, 2012. https://io9.gizmodo.com/5876335/until-2009-the-human-clitoris-was-an-absolute-mystery.
78. David A. Frederick et al., "Differences in orgasm frequency among gay, lesbian, bisexual, and heterosexual men and women in a US national sample," *Archives of Sexual Behavior* 47, no. 1 (2018): 273–288.
79. Helen E. O'Connell, Kalavampara V. Sanjeevan, and John M. Hutson, "Anatomy of the clitoris," *Journal of Urology* 174, no. 4 (2005): 1189–1195. https://www.skepticink.com/incredulous/2013/08/12/the-clitoris-revealed-and-how-io9-got-it-wrong/.
80. "Anatomy of a Revolution," *Sydney Morning Herald,* September 8, 2005. http://www.smh.com.au/news/health/anatomy-of-a-revolution/2005/09/08/1125772617200.html.

CHAPTER 5

1. Consumer Reports, "Consumer Reports Analysis: Most U.S. Hospitals' C-Section Rates Exceeding National Targets," May 16, 2017; "Compare: Tri-County Hospitals and Birthing Centers," *Sun Sentinel*, April 5, 2018. http://www.sun-sentinel.com/features/south-florida-parenting/sfp-tri-county-hospitals-and-birthing-centers-story.html.
2. Diana R. Jolles et al., "Outcomes of childbearing Medicaid beneficiaries engaged in care at Strong Start birth center sites between 2012 and 2014," *Birth* 44, no. 4 (2017): 298–305.
3. Susan Morse, "Half of states report 50 percent or more of births financed by Medicaid," *Healthcare Finance*, March 30, 2017. https://www.healthcarefinancenews.com/news/half-states-report-50-or-more-births-financed-medicaid.

4. Florida Department of Health, Bureau of Vital Statistics, "Cesarean Section Deliveries," 2017. http://www.flhealthcharts.com/charts/DataViewer/BirthViewer/BirthViewer.aspx?cid=443.
5. Michelle J. K. Osterman and Joyce A. Martin, "Trends in low-risk cesarean delivery in the United States, 1990–2013," National Vital Statistics Reports, November 5, 2014. https://www.cdc.gov/nchs/data/nvsr/nvsr63/nvsr63_06.pdf.
6. Tara Haelle, "Childbirth: What to Reject When You're Expecting: 9 Procedures to Think Twice About During Your Pregnancy," Consumer Reports, May 16, 2017. https://www.consumerreports.org/pregnancy-childbirth/childbirth-what-to-reject-when-youre-expecting/.
7. Florida Agency for Health Care Administration, "Newborns and Cesarean Rates 2000–2016," FloridaHealthFinder.gov. http://www.floridahealthfinder.gov/researchers/QuickStat/cesarean-buffer.aspx.
8. "11 Hospitals to Avoid if You Don't Want a C-Section Birth," Consumer Reports, June 9, 2016. https://finance.yahoo.com/news/11-hospitals-avoid-dont-want-100007513.html.
9. "Consumer Reports Analysis: Most U.S. Hospitals' C-Section Rates Exceeding National Targets."
10. American College of Obstetricians and Gynecologists and the Council on Patient Safety in Women's Health Care, Patient Safety Bundles, "Safe Reduction of Primary Cesarean Birth (+AIM)." https://safehealthcareforeverywoman.org/patient-safety-bundles/safe-reduction-of-primary-cesarean-birth/.
11. Eugene R. Declercq et al., *Listening to Mothers III: Pregnancy and Birth* (New York: Childbirth Connection, 2013).
12. Aaron B. Caughey et al. and the American College of Obstetricians and Gynecologists, "Safe prevention of the primary cesarean delivery," *American Journal of Obstetrics and Gynecology* 210, no. 3 (2014): 179–193.
13. Carol Sakala et al., *Listening to Mothers in California: A Population-Based Survey of Women's Childbearing Experiences* (Washington, DC: National Partnership for Women & Families, 2018), p. 50.
14. Carol Sakala, Eugene R. Declercq, and Maureen P. Corry, "Listening to mothers: The first national US survey of women's childbearing experiences," *Journal of Obstetric, Gynecologic, & Neonatal Nursing* 31, no. 6 (2002): 633–634.
15. National Institutes of Health, "State-of-the-Science Conference Statement: Cesarean Delivery on Maternal Request," *Obstetrics & Gynecology* 107 (2006): 1386–1397.
16. Jennifer Block, *Pushed: The Painful Truth About Childbirth and Modern Maternity Care* (Cambridge, MA: Da Capo Press, 2007), p. 72.
17. Ricki Lake, Jennifer Block, and Abby Epstein, "Docs to Women: Pay No Attention to Ricki Lake's Home Birth," Huffington Post, June 26, 2008. https://www.huffingtonpost.com/ricki-lake-jennifer-block-and-abby-epstein/docs-to-women-pay-no-atte_b_107845.html.
18. Committee on Obstetric Practice, "Committee opinion no. 697: Planned home birth," *Obstetrics and Gynecology* 129, no. 4 (2017): e117. https://www.acog.org/-/media

/Committee-Opinions/Committee-on-Obstetric-Practice/co697.pdf?dmc=1&ts=20170506T1034060833.

19. The technical term is "NTSV"—nulliparous term singleton vertex.
20. Mary E. D'Alton et al., "Putting the 'M' back in maternal–fetal medicine," *American Journal of Obstetrics and Gynecology* 208, no. 6 (2013): 442–448.
21. Block, *Pushed*, pp. 109–111.
22. Robin Fields and Joe Sexton, "How Many American Women Die from Causes Related to Pregnancy or Childbirth? No One Knows," ProPublica, October 23, 2017. https://www.propublica.org/article/how-many-american-women-die-from-causes-related-to-pregnancy-or-childbirth.
23. Marian F. MacDorman et al., "Is the United States maternal mortality rate increasing? Disentangling trends from measurement issues," *Obstetrics and Gynecology* 128, no. 3 (2016): 447.
24. Nina Martin and Renée Montagne, "The Last Person You'd Expect to Die in Childbirth," *ProPublica* and NPR, May 12, 2017. https://www.propublica.org/article/die-in-childbirth-maternal-death-rate-health-care-system.
25. Alison Young, Laura Ungar, and Christopher Schnaars, "Deadly Deliveries," *USA Today*, July 26, 2018. https://www.usatoday.com/in-depth/news/investigations/deadly-deliveries/2018/07/26/maternal-mortality-rates-preeclampsia-postpartum-hemorrhage-safety/546889002/.
26. "Reproductive Injustice: Racial and Gender Discrimination in U.S. Health Care," Center for Reproductive Rights, SisterSong, National Latina Institute for Reproductive Health, 2014, p. 13. https://www.reproductiverights.org/sites/crr.civicactions.net/files/documents/CERD_Shadow_US_6.30.14_Web.pdf.
27. Robin Fields, "New York City Launches Committee to Review Maternal Deaths," ProPublica, November 15, 2017. https://www.propublica.org/article/new-york-city-launches-committee-to-review-maternal-deaths.
28. Annalisa Merelli, "What's Killing America's New Mothers?" Quartz, October 29, 2017. https://qz.com/1108193/whats-killing-americas-new-mothers/.
29. Myra J. Tucker et al., "The black–white disparity in pregnancy-related mortality from 5 conditions: Differences in prevalence and case-fatality rates," *American Journal of Public Health* 97, no. 2 (2007): 247–251.
30. Linda Villarosa, "Why America's Black Mothers and Babies Are in a Life-or-Death Crisis," *New York Times Magazine*, April 11, 2018.
31. Ellen D. Hodnett et al., "Continuous support for women during childbirth," *Cochrane Database of Systematic Reviews* 10 (2012).
32. Saraswathi Vedam et al., "Mapping integration of midwives across the United States: Impact on access, equity, and outcomes," *PLOS One* 13, no. 2 (2018): e0192523.
33. American College of Obstetricians and Gynecologists, "New Guidelines to Prevent Blood Clots in Pregnant Women," August 26, 2011.
34. Committee on Obstetric Practice, "Committee opinion no. 529: placenta accreta," *Obstetrics and Gynecology* 120, no. 1 (2012): 207. https://www.acog.org/Clinical-Guidance

-and-Publications/Committee-Opinions/Committee-on-Obstetric-Practice/Placenta-Accreta.

35. American College of Obstetricians and Gynecologists, "New VBAC guidelines: What they mean to you and your patients," *ACOG Today*, August 2010. https://www.acog.org/-/media/ACOG-Today/acogToday0810.pdf?dmc=1&ts=20180802T1503091858.
36. Lindsay Switzer to Somers Manor OB/GYN, letter, June 4, 2013. https://www.healthymothersmattertoo.com/uploads/6/5/3/3/65336197/letter_to_somers_manor.pdf; Letters, complaint, doula notes, et cetera, posted here: Lindsay Switzer, "Healthy Mothers Matter Too." https://www.healthymothersmattertoo.com.
37. Beth Greenfield, "Mom Sues Doctor over C-Section Fight: 'I Was Treated Like a Child,'" Yahoo! News, October 6, 2015. https://www.yahoo.com/news/mom-sues-doctor-over-c-section-fight-i-was-090037592.html.
38. Beth Greenfield, "Woman Sues Hospital over Traumatic Birth That 'Turned Our Family Life Upside Down,'" Yahoo! News, November 19, 2015. https://www.yahoo.com/news/woman-sues-hospital-for-traumatic-birth-that-201605478.html?ref=gs.
39. Anna Claire Vollers, "Caroline Malatesta Opens Up About Birth Trauma, Bait-and-Switch Advertising of Alabama Hospital," Alabama Media Group, August 9, 2016. https://www.al.com/living/index.ssf/2016/08/malatesta_opens_up_about_birth.html.
40. "Birth Video Epidural and Episiotomy," YouTube, August 27, 2014. https://www.youtube.com/watch?v=lCfXxtoAN-I.
41. Beth Greenfield, "Woman Forced into Violent Episiotomy Settles with Doctor," Yahoo! News, March 15, 2017. https://www.yahoo.com/news/woman-forced-into-violent-episiotomy-settles-with-doctor-182947205.html.
42. Sarah Yahr Tucker, "There Is a Hidden Epidemic of Doctors Abusing Women in Labor, Doulas Say," Broadly, May 8, 2018. https://broadly.vice.com/en_us/article/evqew7/obstetric-violence-doulas-abuse-giving-birth.
43. American College of Obstetricians and Gynecologists, "Refusal of Medically Recommended Treatment During Pregnancy," *American College of Obstetricians and Gynecologists* 664 (2016). https://www.acog.org/-/media/Committee-Opinions/Committee-on-Ethics/co664.pdf?dmc=1&ts=20170812T0253370666.
44. Greenfield, "Mom Sues Doctor over C-Section Fight."
45. Cristen Pascucci, "ACOG to Docs: Women's Right to Say 'No' Comes First," *Birth Monopoly*, May 31, 2016. http://birthmonopoly.com/no/.
46. Elisa Albert, "Confessions of a Radical Doula," The Cut, March 2016. https://www.thecut.com/2016/03/confessions-of-a-radical-doula-c-v-r.html.
47. Declercq et al., *Listening to Mothers III*.

CHAPTER 6

1. James E. Causey and Mary Spicuzza, "HIV, Syphilis Cluster in Teens, Adults Found in Milwaukee," *USA Today*, March 8, 2018. https://www.usatoday.com/story/news/nation-now/2018/03/08/hiv-syphilis-cluster-milwaukee/405648002/.

2. Sandra Morgen, *Into Our Own Hands: The Women's Health Movement in the United States, 1969–1990* (New Brunswick, NJ: Rutgers University Press, 2002), p. 72.
3. Marion Banzhaf, ACT-UP Oral History Project, April 18, 2007, p. 17. www.actuporalhistory.org/interviews/images/banzhaf.pdf.
4. Cassie Frank et al., "Era of faster FDA drug approval has also seen increased black-box warnings and market withdrawals," *Health Affairs* 33, no. 8 (2014): 1453–1459. https://www.healthaffairs.org/doi/full/10.1377/hlthaff.2014.0122.
5. Center for Drug Evaluation and Research, U.S. Food and Drug Administration, "The Voice of the Patient: A Series of Reports from the U.S. Food and Drug Administration's Patient-Focused Drug Development Initiative," Female Sexual Dysfunction, Public Meeting, October 27, 2014. https://www.fda.gov/downloads/drugs/newsevents/ucm453718.pdf.
6. Female Sexual Dysfunction Patient-Focused Drug Development Public Meeting, October 27, 2014, Capital Reporting Company.
7. Jennifer Block and Liz Canner, "The 'Grassroots Campaign' for 'Female Viagra' Was Actually Funded by Its Manufacturer," The Cut, September 8, 2016. https://www.thecut.com/2016/09/how-addyi-the-female-viagra-won-fda-approval.html
8. Alycia Hogenmiller, Alessandra Hirsch, and Adriane Fugh-Berman, "The Score Is Even," Hastings Bioethics Forum, June 14, 2017. https://www.thehastingscenter.org/the-score-is-even/.
9. Sabrina Tavernise and Andrew Pollack, "Aid to Women, or Bottom Line? Advocates Split on Libido Pill," *New York Times*, June 13, 2015. http://www.nytimes.com/2015/06/14/us/aid-to-women-or-bottom-line-advocates-split-on-libido-pill.html?_r=0.
10. Azeen Ghorayshi, "How Big Pharma Used Feminism to Get the 'Female Viagra' Approved," BuzzFeed, August 18, 2015. https://www.buzzfeednews.com/article/azeenghorayshi/fda-approves-flibanserin.
11. Weronika Chańska and Katarzyna Grunt-Mejer, "The unethical use of ethical rhetoric: The case of flibanserin and pharmacologisation of female sexual desire," *Journal of Medical Ethics* 42 (2016): 701–704.
12. Derek Bagley, "Hormone Health Network Partners with Red Hot Mamas," *Endocrine News*, June 2015. https://endocrinenews.endocrine.org/hhn-partners-with-red-hot-mamas/; Endocrine Society, "The Corporate Liaison Board." https://www.endocrine.org/corporate-relations/corporate-liaison-board.
13. "Impotence," *His and Her Health*. http://www.hisandherhealth.com/impotence.html.
14. Andrew Pollack, "FDA Approves Addyi, a Libido Pill for Women," *New York Times*, August 18, 2015.
15. Matthew Herper, "Novartis Calls Wonder Woman," *Forbes*, December 5, 2002. https://www.forbes.com/2002/12/05/cx_mh_1205nvs.html#5778e6dd339f.
16. Alicia Mundy, "Hot Flash, Cold Cash," *Washington Monthly*, January 1, 2001. https://washingtonmonthly.com/2001/01/01/hot-flash-cold-cash/.
17. Rebecca Mayer Knutsen, "Therapeutic Focus: Women's Health," MM&M, August 19,

2015. https://www.mmm-online.com/home/resources/therapeutic-focus/therapeutic-focus-womens-health/.

18. L. Jaspers et al., "Efficacy and safety of flibanserin for the treatment of hypoactive sexual desire disorder in women: A systematic review and meta-analysis," *JAMA Internal Medicine* 176, no. 4 (2016): 453–462. https://jamanetwork.com/journals/jamainternalmedicine/fullarticle/2497781#120766726.
19. HealthyWomen, "New National Survey Reveals 82 Percent of Postmenopausal Women Miss Critical Connection Between Osteoporosis and Bone Fractures," August 10, 2017. http://www.healthywomen.org/content/press-release/new-national-survey-reveals-82-percent-postmenopausal-women-miss-critical.
20. Susan Kelleher, "Osteoporosis Screenings a Marketing Juggernaut," *Seattle Times*, July 27, 2005.
21. Ray Moynihan and Alan Cassels, *Selling Sickness: How the World's Biggest Pharmaceutical Companies Are Turning Us All into Patients* (New York: Nation Books, 2005), p. 140.
22. HealthyWomen, "Corporate Advisory Board," web archive. https://web.archive.org/web/20111102082323/http://www.healthywomen.org/about-us/corporate-advisory-board.
23. HealthyWomen, "Our Founder." http://www.healthywomen.org/about-us/our-founder.
24. Palatin Technologies, Inc., "New Survey Reveals That Low Sexual Desire Disrupts Relationships," PR Newswire, May 20, 2014. https://www.prnewswire.com/news-releases/new-survey-reveals-that-low-sexual-desire-disrupts-relationships-259933261.html.
25. Jason D. Wright et al., "Robotically assisted vs. laparoscopic hysterectomy among women with benign gynecologic disease," *JAMA* 309, no. 7 (2013): 689–698.
26. Gary Schwitzer, "Local news hype of robotic surgery doesn't match many hysterectomy patients' experiences," Health News Review, July 17, 2018. https://www.healthnewsreview.org/2018/07/local-news-hype-of-robotic-surgery-doesnt-match-many-hysterectomy-patients-experiences/.
27. Marie N. Stagnitti and Doris Lefkowitz, "Trends in Hormone Replacement Therapy Drugs Utilization and Expenditures for Adult Women in the US Civilian Noninstitutionalized Population, 2001–2008" (Agency for Healthcare Research and Quality, 2011).
28. Women's Health Initiative, "Executive Summary and Questions and Answers." https://www.whi.org/SitePages/WHI Hormone Trial Findings Questions and Answers.aspx.
29. Jennifer Block, "Will This Pill Fix Your Sex Life?" *Newsweek*, April 30, 2013.
30. Mundy, "Hot Flash, Cold Cash."
31. Alan Altman, "Postmenopausal dyspareunia—A problem for the 21st century." *OBG Management* 21, no. 3 (2009): 37. https://www.scribd.com/document/201198976/2103OBGM-Article3. Author disclosure accessed September 4, 2018.
32. Faculty disclosures in "Talking to Female Patients About Sexual Health: Overcoming Common Communication Challenges," Medscape Education Ob/Gyn & Women's Health, May 25, 2010. http://www.medscape.org/viewarticle/721398; PBS *Need to Know* transcript, July 2, 2010. http://www.pbs.org/wnet/need-to-know/uncategorized/need-to-know-transcript-july-2-2010/2085/.

33. Jaime Holguin, "The Hormone Hype," CBS, November 20, 2002. https://www.cbsnews.com/news/the-hormone-hype/.
34. Anita H. Clayton, MD, bio, Huffington Post. https://www.huffingtonpost.com/author/anita-h-clayton-md.
35. Michael L. Power, Britta L. Anderson, and Jay Schulkin, "Attitudes of obstetrician-gynecologists towards the evidence from the WHI HT trials remain generally skeptical," *Menopause* 16, no. 3 (2009): 500.
36. "Perimenopause: Rocky Road to Menopause," Harvard Women's Health Watch, updated August 24, 2018. https://www.health.harvard.edu/womens-health/perimenopause-rocky-road-to-menopause.
37. John Carreyrou, "Questions on Efficacy Cloud a Cancer Vaccine: Merck Predicts Big Fall in Cervical Lesions, But Data Are Complex," *Wall Street Journal*, April 16, 2007. https://www.wsj.com/articles/SB117668541991270825.
38. Jeanne Lenzer, "How Effective Is the HPV Vaccine at Preventing Cancer? A Closer Look," *Discover*, November 23, 2011. http://blogs.discovermagazine.com/crux/2011/11/23/how-effective-is-the-hpv-vaccine-at-preventing-cancer-a-closer-look/.
39. National Cancer Institute, Surveillance, Epidemiology, and End Results Program, "Cancer Stat Facts: Cervical Cancer." https://seer.cancer.gov/statfacts/html/cervix.html.
40. Judith Siers-Poisson, "The Politics and PR of Cervical Cancer," PR Watch, July 15, 2007. https://www.alternet.org/story/55821/the_politics_and_pr_of_cervical_cancer.
41. Judith Siers-Poisson, "Women in Government, Merck's Trojan Horse: Part Three in a Series on the Politics and PR of Cervical Cancer," PR Watch, July 17, 2007. https://www.alternet.org/story/56679/women_in_government percent2C_merck percent27s_trojan_horse_percent3A_part_three_in_a_series_on_the_politics_and_pr_of_cervical_cancer.
42. Ibid.
43. Terry J. Allen, "Merck's Murky Dealings: HPV Vaccine Lobby Backfires," Corpwatch, March 7, 2007. https://corpwatch.org/article/mercks-murky-dealings-hpv-vaccine-lobby-backfires.
44. Sheila M. Rothman and David J. Rothman, "Marketing HPV vaccine: Implications for adolescent health and medical professionalism," *JAMA* 302, no. 7 (2009): 781–786, DOI: 10.1001/jama.2009.1179.
45. Tasha N. Dubriwny, *The Vulnerable Empowered Woman: Feminism, Postfeminism, and Women's Health* (New Brunswick, NJ: Rutgers University Press, 2012), p. 117.
46. Judith Siers-Poisson, "Research, Develop, and Sell, Sell, Sell: Part Two in a Series on the Politics and PR of Cervical Cancer," PR Watch, July 16, 2007. https://www.alternet.org/story/56677/research percent2C_develop percent2C_and_sell percent2C_sell_percent2C_sell_percent3A_part_two_in_a_series_on_the_politics_and_pr_of_cervical_cancer.
47. Jeanne Lenzer, "Should Boys Be Given the HPV Vaccine? The Science Is Weaker Than the Marketing," *Discover*, November 14, 2011. http://blogs.discovermagazine.com/crux/2011/11/14/should-boys-be-given-the-hpv-vaccine-the-science-is-weaker-than-the-marketing/.

48. Lars Jørgensen, Peter C. Gøtzsche, and Tom Jefferson, "The Cochrane HPV vaccine review was incomplete and ignored important evidence of bias," *BMJ Evidence-Based Medicine* 23, no. 5 (2018): 165–168; Lars Jørgensen, Peter Doshi, Peter Gøtzsche, and Tom Jefferson, "Challenges of independent assessment of potential harms of HPV vaccines," *British Medical Journal* 362 (2018): k3694; Tom Jefferson and Lars Jørgensen, "Human papillomavirus vaccines, complex regional pain syndrome, postural orthostatic tachycardia syndrome, and autonomic dysfunction—A review of the regulatory evidence from the European Medicines Agency," *Indian Journal of Medical Ethics* 2, no. 1 (2017): 30–37.

49. Catherine Riva, Serena Tinari, and Jean-Pierre Spinosa, "Lessons learnt on transparency, scientific process and publication ethics. The short story of a long journey to get into the public domain unpublished data, methodological flaws and bias of the Cochrane HPV vaccines review," *BMJ Evidence-Based Medicine*, published online: December 16, 2018.

50. Frederik Joelving, "What the Gardasil Testing May Have Missed," Slate, December 17, 2017. https://slate.com/health-and-science/2017/12/flaws-in-the-clinical-trials-for-gardasil-made-it-harder-to-properly-assess-safety.html.

51. "National Organization for Women Foundation," SourceWatch. https://www.sourcewatch.org/index.php/National_Organization_for_Women_Foundation; Sylvia Law, "Human Papillomavirus Vaccination, Private Choice, and Public Health," *UC Davis Law Review* 41 (2007): 1740.

52. Quoted in Siers-Poisson, "Women in Government, Merck's Trojan Horse," 2007.

53. Ellen Goodman, "A Dose of Reality on HPV Vaccine," *Boston Globe*, March 2, 2007.

54. Daron G. Ferris et al., "4-valent human papillomavirus (4vHPV) vaccine in preadolescents and adolescents after 10 years," *Pediatrics* (2017): e20163947.

55. Medical College of Georgia at Augusta University, "HPV Vaccine Is Effective, Safe 10 Years After It's Given, Study Shows," *Science Daily*, November 29, 2017. https://www.sciencedaily.com/releases/2017/11/171129131400.htm.

56. Warner K. Huh et al., "Final efficacy, immunogenicity, and safety analyses of a nine-valent human papillomavirus vaccine in women aged 16–26 years: A randomised, double-blind trial," *Lancet* 390, no. 10108 (2017): 2143–2159.

57. University of Alabama at Birmingham, "Vaccine to prevent most cervical cancers shows long-term effectiveness," Public release, September 5, 2017. https://www.eurekalert.org/pub_releases/2017-09/uoaa-vtp090517.php.

58. Stephanie Soucheray, "HPV vaccine may protect against 90 percent of cervical cancers," Center for Infectious Disease Research and Policy, September 6, 2017. http://www.cidrap.umn.edu/news-perspective/2017/09/hpv-vaccine-may-protect-against-90-cervical-cancers.

59. Thea Tympanick, "Why Your Daughters (and Sons) Need the HPV Vaccine," Consumer Reports, August 9, 2017. https://www.consumerreports.org/hpv-vaccine/why-your-daughters-and-sons-need-the-hpv-vaccine/.

60. Joint Meeting on the Reproductive Health Drugs Advisory Committee and the Drug Safety and Risk Management Advisory Committee Meeting Announcement, transcript, December 8, 2011, pp. 237–238. https://wayback.archive-it.org/7993/20170404150052/https://www.fda.gov/AdvisoryCommittees/Calendar/ucm273236.htm.
61. John Pickett, "Former FDA Commish: Bayer Hid Yasmin Data," Expert Briefings, December 6, 2011. http://www.expertbriefings.com/news/former-fda-commish-bayer-hid-yasmin-data/.
62. Richard Knox, "With Doubts, FDA Panel Votes for Yaz and Related Contraceptives," NPR, December 9, 2011. https://www.npr.org/sections/health-shots/2011/12/09/143434891/with-doubts-fda-panel-votes-for-yaz-and-related-contaceptives.
63. Jeanne Lenzer and Keith Epstein, "The Yaz Men: Members of FDA Panel Reviewing the Risks of Popular Bayer Contraceptive Had Industry Ties," *Washington Monthly*, January 9, 2012.
64. Joint Meeting on the Reproductive Health Drugs Advisory Committee and the Drug Safety and Risk Management Advisory Committee Meeting Announcement, transcript, December 8, 2011, pp. 255–256.
65. Natasha Singer, "A Birth Control Pill That Promised Too Much," *New York Times*, February 10, 2009.
66. Ibid.
67. Roni Caryn Rabin, "Bayer's Essure Contraceptive Implant, Now with a Warning," *New York Times*, November 21, 2016.
68. Lenzer and Epstein, "The Yaz Men."
69. Larry Husten, "Oops, She Did It Again! FDA Disinvites Another Advisor," *Forbes*, December 8, 2011. https://www.forbes.com/sites/larryhusten/2011/12/08/oops-she-did-it-again-fda-disinvites-another-advisor/#36e8bfb87fb5.
70. Judith Bruce and S. Bruce Shearer, "Contraceptives and Common Sense: Conventional Methods Reconsidered" (1979), quoted in Betsy Hartmann, *Reproductive Rights and Wrongs: The Global Politics of Population Control* (Boston: South End Press, 1995), p. 177.
71. Kathryn Joyce, "The New War on Birth Control," Pacific Standard, August 17, 2017. https://psmag.com/magazine/new-war-on-birth-control.
72. Karen Weise, "Warren Buffett's Family Secretly Funded a Birth Control Revolution," Bloomberg Businessweek, July 30, 2015.
73. ACOG Committee Opinion no. 539, October 2012, since replaced by ACOG Committee Opinion no. 735, American College of Obstetricians and Gynecologists, May 2018. https://www.acog.org/Clinical-Guidance-and-Publications/Committee-Opinions/Committee-on-Adolescent-Health-Care/Adolescents-and-Long-Acting-Reversible-Contraception.
74. Sabrina Tavernise, "Colorado's Effort Against Teenage Pregnancies Is a Startling Success," *New York Times*, July 5, 2015, https://www.nytimes.com/2015/07/06/science/colorados-push-against-teenage-pregnancies-is-a-startling-success.html; Jason Salzman, "Teen Pregnancy, Abortion Rates Plummet in Colorado Thanks to Contraception

Program," Rewire News, December 4, 2017. https://rewire.news/article/2017/12/04/colorado-program-continues-reduce-teen-abortion-pregnancy-rates/.

75. Anu Manchikanti Gomez, Liza Fuentes, and Amy Allina, "Women or LARC first? Reproductive autonomy and the promotion of long-acting reversible contraceptive methods," *Perspectives on Sexual and Reproductive Health* 46, no. 3 (2014): 171–175.

76. Ashleigh Oxford, Facebook post, June 13, 2018. https://www.facebook.com/ashleigh.oxford/posts/10216688088344817.

77. Julia Strasser et al., "Access to removal of long-acting reversible contraceptive methods is an essential component of high-quality contraceptive care," *Women's Health Issues* 27, no. 3 (2017): 253–255. https://www.whijournal.com/article/S1049-3867(17)30072-5/fulltext.

78. South Dakota Department of Social Services, "South Dakota Medicaid Professional Services Billing Manual October 2018." https://dss.sd.gov/formsandpubs/docs/medsrvcs/professional.pdf.

79. Adele Oliveira, "What Happens When You Give Teenage Girls Free IUDs?" Jezebel, March 24, 2015. https://jezebel.com/what-happens-when-you-give-teenage-girls-free-iuds-1691995183.

80. Elizabeth Dawes Gay, "DIY Birth Control Shot Can Help Advance Reproductive Justice," Rewire News, January 24, 2018. https://rewire.news/article/2018/01/24/diy-birth-control-shot-can-help-advance-reproductive-justice/.

81. Justine P. Wu, Michelle H. Moniz, and Allison N. Ursu, "Long-acting reversible contraception—highly efficacious, safe, and underutilized," *JAMA* 320, no. 4 (2018): 397–398. https://jamanetwork.com/journals/jama/fullarticle/2687700?utm_source=silverchair.

82. Linda Gordon, *The Moral Property of Women: A History of Birth Control Politics in America* (Chicago: University of Illinois Press, 2002), p. 189.

83. Hartmann, *Reproductive Rights and Wrongs*, p. 99.

84. Gordon, *The Moral Property of Women*, pp. 171–189.

85. Hartmann, *Reproductive Rights and Wrongs*, pp. 110–113.

86. "Norplant and Contraceptive Pricing: Conflict of Interest, Protection of Public Ownership in Drug Development Deals Between Tax-Exempt, Federally Supported Labs and the Pharmaceutical Industry," Hearing Before the Subcommittee on Regulation, Business Opportunities, and Technology of the Committee on Small Business, House of Representatives, 103rd Cong., 1st Sess., Part 3. U.S. Government Printing Office, January 1, 1994, p. 7; "FDA board investigates Depo-Provera safety," *Contraceptive Technology Update* 4, no. 3 (1983): 25–27.

87. Joyce, "The New War on Birth Control."

88. Hartmann, *Reproductive Rights and Wrongs*, p. 165.

89. Joyce, "The New War on Birth Control": "One 2005 study found that 84 percent of Depo users were black, 74 percent low-income, and 33 percent under 19 years of age."

90. Ibid.

CHAPTER 7

1. Maureen Paul and Kristin Nobel, "Papaya: A Simulation Model for Training in Uterine Aspiration," *Family Medicine* (April 2005); "Training in MVA Using Papayas," Reproductive Health Access Project. http://www.reproductiveaccess.org/wp-content/uploads/2014/12/mva_training_using_papayas.pdf.
2. Jane E. Brody, "Lunch Hour Abortion Devised," *New York Times*, December 20, 1973.
3. Ipas, "Ipas Official Update," Family Planning 2020, October 16, 2015. https://www.familyplanning2020.org/news/ipas-official-update.
4. Patty Skuster, *Who Can Provide Abortion Care? Considerations for Law and Policy Makers* (Chapel Hill, NC: Ipas, 2015).
5. World Health Organization, *Safe Abortion: Technical and Policy Guidance for Health Systems*, 2nd ed. (Geneva: World Health Organization, 2012).
6. Lizzie Presser, "Whatever's Your Darkest Question, You Can Ask Me: A Secret Network of Women Is Working Outside the Law and the Medical Establishment to Provide Safe, Cheap Home Abortions," *California Sunday Magazine*, March 28, 2018.
7. Francine Coeytaux and Elisa Wells, "Misoprostol Is a Game-Changer for Safe Abortion and Maternal Health Care. Why Isn't It More Widely Available?" Rewire News, May 28, 2013. https://rewire.news/article/2013/05/28/why-arent-we-taking-advantage-of-the-potentially-game-changing-drug-misoprostol/.
8. Presser, "Whatever's Your Darkest Question, You Can Ask Me."
9. Marisa Crawford, "The Back-Alley Abortion That Almost Didn't Make It into 'Dirty Dancing,'" Broadly, August 21, 2017. https://broadly.vice.com/en_us/article/433a99/the-back-alley-abortion-that-almost-didnt-make-it-into-dirty-dancing.
10. Leslie J. Reagan, *When Abortion Was a Crime: Women, Medicine, and Law in the United States, 1867–1973* (Berkeley: University of California Press, 1997), pp. 249–250.
11. Jessica Ravitz, "Abortion Pills Now Available by Mail in US—but FDA Is Investigating," CNN, October 23, 2018.
12. Ninia Baehr, *Abortion Without Apology: A Radical History for the 1990s* (Boston: South End Press, 1990), p. 47.
13. Dennis Hevesi, "Constance E. Cook, 89, Who Wrote Abortion Law, Is Dead," *New York Times*, January 24, 2009.
14. Carole Joffe, *Doctors of Conscience: The Struggle to Provide Abortion Before and After* Roe v. Wade (Boston: Beacon Press, 1996), p. 132.
15. Baehr, *Abortion Without Apology*, p. 33.
16. Ibid., p. 42.
17. Lucinda Cisler, "Abortion Law Repeal (Sort Of): A Warning to Women," Women's Liberation, 1974. http://www.womensliberation.org/images/stories/abortion/abortion.law.repeal.pdf.
18. Ruth Rosen, *The World Split Open: How the Modern Women's Movement Changed America* (New York: Viking, 2013), p. 158.
19. Baehr, *Abortion Without Apology*, p. 44.

20. Lucinda Cisler, "A Room of One's Own: The Architecture of Choice," *Vassar Quarterly* L, no. 4 (April 1, 1965). http://newspaperarchives.vassar.edu/cgi-bin/vassar?a=d&d=vq19650401-01.2.10.
21. Lucinda Cisler and James Clapp, "Abortion Ruling: Some Good News . . . and Some Bad News," ALF discussion paper, Association of Libertarian Feminists, New York, 1976.
22. Lucinda Cisler and James Clapp, "Abortion: Inside and Outside the Hospital," Pacifica Radio Archives, episode 2, January 8, 1969. https://archive.org/details/pacifica_radio_archives-BB2031.
23. Baehr, *Abortion Without Apology*, p. 22.
24. Elizabeth Fishel, "Women's Self-Help Movement," *Ramparts Magazine*, November 1973.
25. Interview by Rebecca Sharpless, transcript of audio recording, October 8–9, 2002. Population and Reproductive Health Oral History Project, Sophia Smith Collection, Smith College, Northampton, Massachusetts, p. 74, quoted in Michelle Goldberg, *The Means of Reproduction: Sex, Power, and the Future of the World* (New York: Penguin, 2009), p. 38.
26. Harvey Karman and Malcolm Potts, "Very early abortion using syringe as vacuum source," *Lancet* 299, no. 7759 (1972): 1051–1052.
27. Tanfer Emin Tunc, "Designs of devices: The vacuum aspirator and American abortion technology," *Dynamis* 28 (2008): 353–376.
28. Goldberg, *The Means of Reproduction*, p. 39.
29. Ann Furedi and Mick Hume, eds., *Abortion Law Reformers: Pioneers of Change* (Birth Control Trust, 1997). http://www.abortionreview.org/images/uploads/Abortion_Pioneers_(1).pdf.
30. "A statement on abortion by one hundred professors of obstetrics," *American Journal of Obstetrics and Gynecology* 112 (1972): 992–998.
31. Heather Rogers, "Pro-choice timidity in fighting shortage of abortion providers," Reproductive Health Services, March 13, 2013. http://www.remappingdebate.org/article/pro-choice-timidity-fighting-shortage-abortion-providers.
32. Carole E. Joffe, Tracy A. Weitz, and Chris L. Stacey, "Uneasy allies: Pro-choice physicians, feminist health activists and the struggle for abortion rights," *Sociology of Health & Illness* 26, no. 6 (2004): 775–796.
33. Katrina Kimport, Kate Cockrill, and Tracy A. Weitz, "Analyzing the impacts of abortion clinic structures and processes: A qualitative analysis of women's negative experience of abortion clinics," *Contraception* 85, no. 2 (2012): 204–210.
34. Alison Ojanen-Goldsmith and Sarah Prager, "Beyond the clinic: Preferences, motivations, and experiences with alternative abortion care in North America," *Contraception* 94, no. 4 (2016): 398–399.
35. K. White et al., "First-trimester surgical abortion practices in the United States," *Contraception* 92, no. 4 (2015): 368.
36. Brody, "Lunch Hour Abortion Devised."

37. Early Options, "Softouch FAQ." https://www.earlyabortionoptions.com/early-abortion-options/softouch-natural-abortion/.
38. Rachel K. Jones and Jenna Jerman, "Abortion incidence and service availability in the United States, 2014," *Perspectives on Sexual and Reproductive Health* 49, no. 1 (2017): 17–27.
39. Diana Scott, "Unfurling a Maestrapeace: Mythic and Mortal Female Ancestors Grace This San Francisco Landmark," *On the Issues* (Winter 1995). http://www.ontheissuesmagazine.com/1995winter/win95_scott.php.
40. John M. Riddle, *Eve's Herbs: A History of Contraception and Abortion in the West* (Cambridge, MA: Harvard University Press, 1999), pp. 156, 158.
41. Ibid., p. 166.
42. Ibid., pp. 207–210.
43. J. W. Ballantyne, "Curettage of the uterus: History, indications, and technique," *Edinburgh Medical Journal* 41, no. 10 (1896): 908.
44. Ibid., p. 70.
45. Joffe, *Doctors of Conscience*; Reagan, *When Abortion Was a Crime*, pp. 123–149.
46. Tunc, "Designs of Devices," pp. 356–357.
47. Reagan, *When Abortion Was a Crime*, p. 193.
48. Ibid.
49. "History of MVA," Papaya Workshop. https://papayaworkshop.org/workshop-teaching-resources/history-of-mva/.
50. Presser, "Whatever's Your Darkest Question, You Can Ask Me." Planned Parenthood and NARAL offered no comment.
51. Farah Diaz-Tello, "How to Prepare for a Post-Roe America," *In These Times*, August 27, 2018.
52. International Confederation of Midwives, "Position Statement: Midwives' Provision of Abortion-Related Services," Reviewed and adopted at Prague Council meeting, 2014. https://www.internationalmidwives.org/assets/files/statement-files/2018/04/midwives-provision-of-abortion-related-services-eng.pdf.

CONCLUSION

1. Arianna Huffington, "My Conversation with Co-Sleeping Expert James McKenna," Huffington Post, April 22, 2015.
2. Naomi Mezey and Cornelia T. L. Pillard, "Against the New Maternalism," *Michigan Journal of Gender & Law* 18 (2011): 229.
3. Erica Jong, "Mother Madness," *Wall Street Journal*, November 6, 2010.
4. Wendy Kline, *Bodies of Knowledge: Sexuality, Reproduction, and Women's Health in the Second Wave* (Chicago: University of Chicago Press, 2010), p. 66.
5. Susan Faludi, "Death of a Revolutionary," *New Yorker*, April 15, 2013.
6. Barbara Katz Rothman, *Recreating Motherhood* (New Brunswick, NJ: Rutgers University Press, 2000), pp. 194–196.

7. Lisa Bortolotti, "The Philosophy of Early Motherhood: Interview with Fiona Woollard," Imperfect Cognitions, March 30, 2017. http://imperfectcognitions.blogspot.com/2017/03/the-philosophy-of-early-motherhood.html.
8. Sarah J. Buckley, *Hormonal Physiology of Childbearing: Evidence and Implications for Women, Babies, and Maternity Care,* Childbirth Connection Programs, National Partnership for Women & Families (Washington, DC: 2015).
9. Eileen K. Hutton and Eman S. Hassan, "Late vs early clamping of the umbilical cord in full-term neonates: Systematic review and meta-analysis of controlled trials," *JAMA* 297, no. 11 (2007): 1241–1252; Judith S. Mercer et al., "Delayed cord clamping in very preterm infants reduces the incidence of intraventricular hemorrhage and late-onset sepsis: A randomized, controlled trial," *Pediatrics* 117, no. 4 (2006): 1235–1242.
10. Sharon Lerner, "The Real War on Families: Why the U.S. Needs Paid Leave Now," *In These Times*, August 18, 2015. http://inthesetimes.com/article/18151/the-real-war-on-families.
11. Lindsay Beyerstein, "The Truth About the Pill," Slate, September 3, 2013. http://www.slate.com/articles/double_x/doublex/2013/09/_sweetening_the_pill_by_holly_grigg_spall_reviewed.html.
12. Hanna Rosin, "The Case Against Breast-Feeding," *The Atlantic*, April 2009.
13. Katha Pollitt, "Feminist Mothers, Flapper Daughters?" *The Nation*, September 30, 2010.
14. Amanda Marcotte, "Ricki Lake Starts a Crusade Against Hormonal Birth Control," Slate, June 25, 2015. https://slate.com/human-interest/2015/06/ricki-lake-christian-right-hero-she-s-making-a-documentary-against-hormonal-birth-control.html.
15. In *Breastmilk*, directed by Dana Ben-Ari, 2014.
16. bell hooks, *All About Love: New Visions* (New York: William Morrow, 2000), p. 93.

INDEX